PLAYBOY'S BOOK OF FITNESS FOR MEN

Bob --

Now that you are a tennis maven, you really don't need this!!

Marty

PLAYBOY'S BOOK OF FITNESS FOR MEN

•••••••••••••

Ralph and Valerie Carnes

PBP

A PLAYBOY PRESS BOOK

To Comrade in Arms, Curt Clemmer (aka "Red Beard"), veteran of Frankencon,
to all the members of the Dorsai Irregulars,
and to the Hole in the Deck Gang.

Copyright © 1980 by Ralph Carnes and Valerie Carnes

All rights reserved. No part of this book may be reproduced, stored in a retrieval system or transmitted in any form by an electronic, mechanical, photocopying, recording means or otherwise, without prior written permission of the author. Published simultaneously in the United States and Canada by Playboy Press, Chicago, Illinois. Printed in the United States of America.

FIRST EDITION

Playboy and Rabbit Head are trademarks of Playboy, 919 North Michigan Avenue, Chicago, Illinois 60611 (U.S.A.) reg. U.S. Pat., marca registrada, marque dépośee.

Designed by Tere LoPrete

Library of Congress Cataloging in Publication Data

Carnes, Ralph L.
Playboy's book of fitness for men.

"A Playboy Press book."
1. Physical fitness. 2. Exercise. I. Carnes, Valerie, joint author. II. Title. III. Title: Book of fitness for men.
GV481.C3 613.7′044 79-90918
ISBN 0-87223-596-3
ISBN 0-87223-599-8 (pbk.)

ACKNOWLEDGMENTS

We would like to express our appreciation to the following people who provided services, encouragement, and good advice as we put our book together:

PHILLIP C. ZERRILLO: weight trainer, budding economist, physical training instructor, dynamic, all-around terrific guy. Phil was the principal model for the exercise photos. That's him doing the concentrated curls with the dumbbell.

DANNY TOBOL: Teenage Mr. America, 1974, manager of the Houston flagship of the Presidents/First Lady Spa chain, shrewd businessman and strong, silent type. That's Danny doing the squats.

CARLOS BLACKWELL: Mr. Southwest, 1978, Junior Mr. Texas, 1978, physical training instructor, topnotch bodybuilder, sharp and solid in mind and body. That's Carlos doing the shoulder shrugs.

CARL SILVANI, owner of the Presidents/First Lady Spa and health club chain in Houston: a hard-driving former pro football player who runs one of the finest health club operations in the country. Carl provided space and equipment for the photos.

BUD and BILL HALBERT, whose superclean, cordial and beautiful Omega Health Club provided the backdrop for photos of the crossover pulley machine and the dance and yoga stretches.

PATRICIA MOSS, who heads Creative Illustrations, and whose sure hand and expertise was responsible for Valerie's makeup in the dance and yoga photos.

GAYNELL CAMPISI, owner of Just Hair and the best stylist in Houston, who created Valerie's coiffure.

JOSEPH COCO: district manager of the Presidents/First Lady Health Spa chain in Houston, sharp salesman, cool manager, ace troubleshooter. That's him on the cover doing seated concentrated curls with the dumbbell.

And especially to Dominick Abel, just for being Dominick Abel.

CONTENTS

PREFACE

•

Shape up! You've all heard the words, and most of you want to put them into action. Shaping up means being more active, being in better physical condition, and being able to do all the things you want to do.

Shaping up means something else, too: it means, literally, changing your shape. Besides being in better physical condition, one of the chief benefits of shaping up is that you really have a younger, more symmetrical, more functional shape. You'll trim your waist, expand your chest, build up your arms and legs, increase your stamina, and incidentally, look better in clothes as well as on the beach.

You can shape your body much more easily than you think. While it takes a tremendous amount of effort to produce the physique of a Mr. Olympia, only a moderate amount of weight training is required to shape up, become stronger, get in top condition, and look terrific. What's more, it's fun—not boring, like most forms of exercise—and it's cheap.

So let's shape up!

INTRODUCTION

•

Since the publication of Butler and Gaines's *Pumping Iron* and the movie based on the book, bodybuilding has slowly emerged from the small subculture that nurtured it for the last fifty years into a full-fledged popular movement. No longer are "musclemen" looked upon with distrust and embarrassment. Instead, they have become the new folk heroes of an age in which more people are interested in being physically fit than ever before.

It's taken a long time to happen, and there have been ambassadors from the bodybuilding world to the world of ordinary mortals since a time before Arnold Schwarzenegger was born. Bob Hoffman, our Olympic weightlifting coach, founded *Strength and Health* magazine in 1931. John Grimek won the Mr. America contest for the first time in 1941. Steve Reeves made all those Hercules movies in the fifties. Superstars like Bill Pearl, Dave Draper, and the current Mr. Olympia, Frank Zane, have been around since the early sixties. Arnold was a latecomer, as was Franco Columbu and Louie ("The Incredible Hulk") Ferrigno. Mike Mentzer and Robbie Robinson, the top contenders for Zane's crown, are today's entries for the title of "world's best-built man."

All of these men have one thing in common: they began with a strong dissatisfaction with the way they looked, and they used a consistent, scientific approach toward their bodies to change themselves into the men they wanted to be. It took an enormous amount of work, discipline, and dedication. They made it, and thousands of other men across the world are trying to duplicate what they did.

All well and good for them. If they have the genes and the fierce determination required for such a transformation, then more power to them. But what about the rest of us? What about the average man, who doesn't want to become gargantuan like Arnold Schwarzenegger, but simply wants to be strong, healthy, and have a symmetrical physique? We're talking about every man who wants to be able to retain his youth and vitality through the years, who wants to lead an enriched, active life, and who wants to be able to look with a smile at the guy whose waist has gotten beyond control.

Bob Hoffman had the answer way back in 1931. The secret is simple, and it really works. A consistently followed weight training program will make you strong, will keep you young, and will make you retain the shape of youth and vitality. In fact, there is no activity known to man that will give you the results you want as fast, as effectively, and as permanently as weight training. Some people run. Some people play tennis. Some people climb mountains and some people play golf. But the overwhelming evidence—from everybody from the Houston Oilers to experts in exercise physiology—is that only scientific weight training will give you that combination of strength, agility, stamina, and shape that we all secretly want.

The only people who still want to argue the point are those who either are ignorant of the benefits of weight training or are still hanging on to the prejudices they had when most of us thought that bodybuilders were those "funny freaks from California." Weight training is on the way to becoming one of the most popular sports in the United States. The International Physical Fitness Association (an association of health clubs) alone boasts over 400,000 active members who train with weights two to three times a week. And some of them don't know that they're lifting weights: all of the modern clubs now have variable-resistance exercise machines, which are only a mechanical means of lifting weights.

This book is for all of those men who want to be fit, strong, agile, and vital; who want to look good in polo shirts as well as in three-piece suits; who aren't really interested in winning the next Mr. Whatsis contest, but want a fast, effective way to get in shape. The program we present will change your life, as it did ours, and very soon you'll wonder why you didn't get started a long time ago.

So let's get moving. And you'll learn what it's like to feel terrific all the time!

1

GETTING CRANKED UP

•

WHAT STRENGTH, STAMINA, SPEED, AND AGILITY MEAN TO A MAN

One of the great things about bodybuilding is that the change in your body's shape is a good indicator of the changes that have gone on inside your body. Although some would maintain that it is possible to have a solid, trim, symmetrical shape without being in good condition, those of us who have been in the weight training game for a number of years know better. Nobody achieves a trim waist, broad shoulders, rock-hard definition of muscle groups, and the light step that goes with strength and stamina without having done a lot of hard work to get there. It's possible to have big muscles and it's also possible to be extremely strong without having a great deal of endurance. But it's impossible to have the kind of shape we're talking about without having improved both strength *and* endurance. We'll talk more about this later.

When you're shaped well—when you have a trim waist, sturdy legs, well-proportioned arms, broad shoulders, and a deep chest—you know that several things have happened. First, you're getting stronger. You're able to do things that you couldn't do before you started weight training. You've begun to develop an explosive kind of strength that comes only from resistance exercises. It's no longer a problem to hop up the stairs, and tasks that once required a lot of effort now seem absurdly easy.

Second, and especially if you've raised your weight training program to the level of endurance exercise—complemented by a supplementary program of stretching, limbering, and the development of motor skills—you've become more supple and agile, and have greater stamina and speed in any physical activity that you undertake. You have strength *and* endurance. You are strong *and* supple. This is the combination that you want.

It will be a fountain of youth for you. If you've never participated in a regular, long-term physical conditioning program before, you will be astonished at the change it makes in your life.

Third, a hard look at yourself in the mirror in the morning will tell you faster than anything else how *out* of shape you are. Be honest with yourself. Are your shoulders broad? Is your waist narrow? Are your legs well formed, with good separation of the muscle groups? Do your latissimus muscles ("lats") form that sought-after "V" from shoulders to waist? Do your arms have that bulge front and back that denotes strength and assurance? Or do you have the kind of body that is best hidden under a three-piece suit? Can you see your abdominal muscles, or are they hidden under a layer of flab?

On the other hand, maybe you're not fat at all. Maybe you're like Ralph was when he was growing up: the archetypal skinny kid from the Charles Atlas ads. Maybe you got tired of having all that sand kicked in your eyes at the beach, and instead of going on a program to build yourself up you gave up the beach, put on a coat, and hid under layers of cloth. Maybe you think you're in shape because you aren't fat. Try running a mile in less than eight minutes, or bench pressing 150 pounds. Are you in shape or not? Maybe you're just shapeless in a skinny way instead of a fat way.

While your appearance will not tell you the extent to which your cardiovascular system is conditioned, it will give you a rough-and-ready guide to how far you have to go to get into the shape you want to be in. Get a copy of one of the top muscle magazines or any of the special-interest athletic magazines such as *Sports Illustrated, Runner's World, Strength and Health, Muscular Development,* or *Muscle Builder.* What do all the people in the illustrations have in common? They all look hard and lean. Even the bodybuilders. With all that muscle mass, they still don't have much body fat.

So let's lay down the first rule: what you want is to get into good, solid, lean shape. You want to get rid of all that fat you're carrying around. If you're a skinny person, you want to go the other route: you want to build some muscle size so that you won't look like a broomstick. Either way, what you want is the same. You want to look different from the way you look now. You aren't satisfied with the way you look, and you want to look good. What looks good? A symmetrical, lean, and muscular body. That's what you want, and there is no quicker way in the world to get there than through scientific weight training.

But, you ask, doesn't everybody who works out with weights wind up looking like Arnold Schwarzenegger? The answer is no. There are thousands of bodybuilders in the country who would love to think that such a statement is true. You can see them in any gym that attracts the heavy-metal boys. Few of them make it, because few people have the genes that made it possible for Arnold to build that massive body. When our book *Bodysculpture* was published, many women called us and asked if we were really telling the truth when we said that women can't grow big muscles. They all had visions of becoming huge like the muscle boys. If they had any idea of how hard it is for *men* to grow really massive muscles, they wouldn't worry. It takes years of grunting and groaning to achieve a physique like

Arnold's. Years of sweat and tears, plus a good set of genes that predispose your muscles to hypertrophy under extreme stress.

We make this point because the number of men who really want to look like Arnold are few. While almost everybody with any self-consciousness at all wants to look good and trim, there really aren't that many men who want to make such an impact on the crowds at the beach that they attract autograph hunters everywhere they go. Talk to the people at your local health club. How many of them really want to get that big? And remember, they are already working out. Think about all the millions of people who do not belong to a gym, and you'll get an idea of how unpopular herculean physiques really are.

The beauty of weight training is this: if you really want to grow to immense size, and if you have the genes to do it, you can go all the way. On the other hand, if what you want is simply to shape up and look better in a bathing suit and in your favorite clothes, weight training is definitely for you.

Indeed, there are strong signs in the bodybuilding world itself that the trend now is toward a leaner, less massive physique. Frank Zane's multiple victories as Mr. Olympia (the absolutely top physique title in the world) are proof enough. Zane represents a new ideal among muscle builders: symmetry and grace of movement instead of massiveness and sheer brutish bulk. It's not only a movement toward a saner brand of bodybuilding, it's a movement back to an older idea of the purpose of weight training: size isn't everything—shape and symmetry mean more. Steve Davis, Mr. California, calls today's bodybuilders the "new breed." A certain trend in bodybuilding has run its course and is being replaced with another one. The emphasis is now on shape. In at least that respect, your interests parallel those of the modern bodybuilder.

Of course, the best commentary on the new trend is Arnold himself. Since retiring from competition in 1975, he's trained way down from 250 to 200 pounds and has taken up running.

While the current trend among bodybuilders is seen as a step forward, it's really a step back to some ideas that have been kicking around for thirty or forty years. When Bob Hoffman first founded *Strength and Health* magazine, few men were as massive as almost all the top bodybuilders are today. As the name of the magazine implied, the emphasis was on strength and health, not mere appearance. Hoffman himself has been quoted many times as saying that you should train for strength and size will follow.

Further, the absurd size that some modern bodybuilders have attained has come as much through drugs like anabolic steroids (almost never with a doctor's supervision) as through hard work. In fact, you can usually tell when a bodybuilder has gone over to steroids. His eyes will become puffy from water retention, and his muscles will take on a bloated appearance. It's not healthy, and all of the major muscle publications have heartily condemned the practice of taking so-called growth-inducing drugs. Kidney, bladder, and cardiac problems are among the potential side effects, not to mention a strong suspicion among sports-medicine people of a link with cancer.

We go into all this because it's part of the milieu of modern bodybuilding. Despite the trend toward leaner physiques, it's impossible to pick up a copy of any of the bodybuilding magazines without being bombarded by admonitions to "bomb" and "blitz" your way to supersize, or to gulp your way through tons of protein supplements, mineral supplements, vitamin supplements, and strange foods. The muscle magazines abound with ads for everything from ginseng root to soybean shakes. The superstars will condemn steroids on one page and describe how they used them to win contests on the next. If you're dizzy when you've finished a quick survey of the magazines, it's not because you're losing your grip on reality. There are so many claims and counterclaims, it's hard to make sense of them at all.

Remember, the muscle magazines are special-interest publications, designed to cater to the interests of people who want to become a part of the bodybuilding world. Most special-interest magazines carry advertising and personal success stories about the superstars in the field. But while many people read *Road and Track,* few of them want to be the Formula I world champions.

Most of us live in other worlds vicariously. That's why we read and go to movies. While some people covertly want to look like Arnold, few of them are willing to put out the kind of effort he did to get there. While some men might secretly want to be as big as Mike Mentzer, for most of us it is enough to know that such people exist. What most of us want is to look good, to be healthy, and to have the strength and stamina required to allow us to do the things we want to do. That's all. And the good news is that we don't have to spend eight hours a day in the gym to get there.

Just the same, it's a good idea to buy the muscle magazines and to familiarize yourself with what they have to say. You'll want to know all the names, and who's on top at the moment. You'll also get a lot of good information about variations on favorite exercises and routines. You don't have to take some of the claims too seriously, and it will be fun to know about the subculture of bodybuilding when you defend yourself among your friends for being on a weight training program. Join the crowd. It's a lot of fun, and good for you besides.

The important thing to remember is that it is strictly up to you how far you want to go in weight training. If you want to be big, you can be big. If you want to be lean and muscular, you can be lean and muscular. It's up to you. But remember, you *can* change your shape. You can have that "V" shape that denotes a man in good condition. You can do it, and the methods that make it possible are available at your fingertips. All it takes is initiative and some work. But not as much work as you might think.

HOW TO GET IN SHAPE AND STAY IN SHAPE

As you change the shape of your body, you will change the "shape" of your life. Your "bodystyle" will be a good indicator to everybody that you have become a new person, that you have a new body and a new outlook on life. The change will be doubly rewarding, for not only will you feel good all the time, you'll look good, too. And since you can use weight training to shape your body into pretty much any shape that you want (within the limits of your genes), you can literally become the person that you want to become.

As you do the work required to bring your new shape into existence, you'll also be "getting in shape"—you'll be getting into better physical condition. The inner and outer changes go together, especially if you work for the cardiovascular conditioning you probably need so much. The change in your physical habits will show up in improvements in both the way you look and feel and in the way you look and feel about yourself. You'll have a more positive attitude, you'll handle yourself better in any kind of situation, and you'll exude the confidence that goes with being in shape.

But before we go any further, let's talk for a little while about what getting in shape is really all about. Let's talk about getting in shape as "getting in condition," instead of building ourselves into a particular shape. Let's talk about what goes on inside our bodies as we work out instead of the bodystyle we're ultimately after. In the same way that Bob Hoffman's admonition to "train for strength and size will follow" works for the person wanting to get big and strong, another adage will work for those who want to look good and have the right shape: "train for *overall* strength and stamina, and shape will follow." In short, if you train for strength and stamina, the kind of shape you want will begin to form. In fact, it will be impossible for you *not* to become more shapely if you follow a progressive, well-rounded weight training program.

Of course, there is always controversy when you begin to talk about the best way to get in shape—especially if you are among a group of people who each have a favorite way to achieve conditioning. The runner will tell you that only running gives you the kind of aerobic conditioning you need to be really in shape. The cyclist will tell the runner that *his* sport is at the top of all sports in making the kinds of demands that yield conditioning. You friend from next door will wave his racquetball racquet at you and tell you that the boys in the weight room don't sweat as much as he does. And the physician who runs will tell you that weightlifting is not aerobic and gets no points whatever on his conditioning chart.

Let's jump right into the middle of this crowd and make a few distinctions.

In the first place, weightlifting is not the same as weight training. Let's back up even a little further. There are three distinct activities that utilize the principles of weight training as a foundation. The first is Olympic weightlifting, which consists of lifting heavy poundages overhead, in two recognized lifts. One of them is the two-hands clean and jerk, in which the barbell is brought from the floor to the top of the chest in one movement, and then overhead in another movement. The second is the two-hands snatch, in which the barbell is brought from the floor to a position overhead in one lightning movement.

The second activity is powerlifting, a relatively new sport; as in Olympic lifting, the goal is ever-heavier poundages. The powerlifter does three lifts. In the first of these, a barbell is taken from a rack by a person lying on his back, brought down to the chest, and then pushed back up again. In the second lift, called the squat, the person takes the barbell from a rack and squats with it on his shoulders until his upper legs are parallel to the floor; then he returns to a standing position. In the third, the deadlift, the barbell is lifted from the floor with two hands to a position in front of the thighs.

Each of these two activities requires a specific type of training designed to build maximum strength in the arms, legs, back, and chest. Olympic lifting and powerlifting are specific sports, in the same way that rowing or running are specific sports, and you would expect athletes in these sports to train in such a way that they would be able to perform well in their specialty. No mystery here.

Consequently, the lifter trains for strength and does not specifically train for endurance. His performance is limited to lifting an exceedingly heavy weight as quickly as he can. Contrary to popular opinion, weightlifters are not slow at all. Indeed, they are extremely fast, as they have to be to lift such heavy poundages overhead.

The third activity that uses weight training as a foundation is bodybuilding. The bodybuilder is not particularly interested in the amount of weight he can put over his head or lift off the floor to his waist. He does not train specifically for strength, but instead trains for shape, size, and general health. While it is frequently the case that weightlifters will lift even when they know that an injury might occur, the bodybuilder rarely takes such risks. His goal is to have a physique that is sculptured in such a way as to approximate the ideal form for the human body. That's why a bodybuilder sometimes talks about Greek sculpture as his ideal. He uses his own body as the medium, and he utilizes whatever exercises are necessary to sculpt his body into the shape he wants.

As mentioned above, the current ideal is a moderately muscled body, with perfect proportions between muscle groups and overall symmetry between arms, legs, upper body, and lower body. While the lifter has his poundages as the product of his labors, the bodybuilder has his body. Consequently, he takes exceptionally good care of it. Now that the popularity of drugs is waning, bodybuilders are more than ever interested in issues of health as well as shape. It's a good sign, and one that all of us are grateful for. Lest we condemn the bodybuilders for their affection for steroids, we should remember that they got the idea from athletes in more popularly recognized sports such as football and field events.

How does the bodybuilder train? Well, not like his heavy-lifting counterparts. Since his goal is not to lift heavy weights but to shape his body, the bodybuilder spends more time on exercising all the muscle groups than does the lifter. He concerns himself with symmetry. In order to do that, he must go through a routine that is in some ways more extensive than the one followed by the powerlifter or the Olympic lifter.

In the first place, the bodybuilder must learn to work his muscles in such a way as to maximize growth and shapeliness. There are many ways to do this, but they all boil down to a simple principle: you have to perform a certain number of repetitions of a certain exercise, and you must repeat that exercise in the form of multiple sets in order to put an amount of stress on the muscle sufficient to trigger growth. Muscle growth comes about in two ways. First, a certain amount of muscle fiber is damaged when you stress the muscle. Second, muscle fibers previously "dormant" will be triggered into use by intensive exercise and will increase individually in size. As a result, the muscle will "grow" although the number of muscle cells you have is pretty well what it is going to be by the time you are twelve or thirteen years old. This "growth" is further made possible by the presence of testosterone, the male sex hormone. It is the absence of high levels of this hormone that makes huge muscles in women impossible.

Second, the bodybuilder is interested in making his body into a sort of factory for the development of muscle. Consequently, he will supplement his diet with all the nutrients that he should have to remain healthy while he is training. Most beginning bodybuilders overdo it and fall for the hype that sells protein supplements and other nutritional products. But they are right to take special care with diet, because they know that muscle growth does not occur if they aren't providing themselves with the right kinds and amounts of fuel.

Third, and as a byproduct of the kind of exercise program the bodybuilder must undergo, he will develop a great deal of stamina. When Dr. Kenneth Cooper, the author of *Aerobics,* said that he would give weightlifting no points for aerobic conditioning, he should have gone on to explain that he was talking about the kind of training program followed by people who wanted to lift heavy weights. He wasn't describing the program that the serious bodybuilder follows, because it is impossible *not* to get aerobic conditioning in such a program, even using Dr. Cooper's definition of how and why such conditioning occurs.

Dr. Cooper states his case simply. Aerobic conditioning occurs when the pulse rate gets up to at least 150 beats per minute and is sustained at that rate for a period of over five minutes. If the pulse rate does not reach this level, it will take longer than five minutes for the aerobic effect to occur. The best aerobic exercise is one in which it is possible to sustain the 150-beat-per-minute pulse rate for a long period of time without building up such an oxygen debt that you will have to stop before the aerobic effect is achieved.

Consequently, running wind-sprints will not condition you aerobically, but sustained running at a pace that will elevate the heart rate to 150 beats will. The reason? Wind-sprints (for example) establish such a terrific oxygen debt that it can be paid only by stopping and resting. In other words, you'll become so winded, you'll have to rest until you catch your breath. The exercise doesn't last long enough for the aerobic effect to get started. At the other end of the scale, strolling through the park won't do it either, because you never get your pulse rate up high enough.

Weightlifting involves explosively fast movements in which you push barbells overhead in defiance of gravity. A movement is done as quickly as possible, because that is the only way that inertia can be sufficiently overcome for the lift to be completed. As a consequence, *weightlifting* is not an aerobic exercise.

Weight *training,* or bodybuilding, on the other hand, is a different story entirely. In bodybuilding the goal is not to lift the weight, but to lift weights in many ways, during a large number of repetitions and sets, in order to stimulate muscle growth. This is the key to shaping the body successfully.

In order to do this, the bodybuilder must work out a systematic program that makes sufficient demands on his body to achieve his goals. Look for a moment at the most popular bodybuilding exercise, the squat. There are many ways to do the squat. The lifter will go through a small number of repetitions with as much weight as he can handle. The bodybuilder, on the other hand, will probably use a relatively lighter weight and do as many repetitions as his body has told him he needs to do to stimulate muscle growth. He will also combine his squats with other leg exercises in order to get the maximum "flushing" of the muscle with oxygenated blood. This is the vaunted "pump," and without it muscle won't grow. Squats are usually combined with (for example) leg extensions, in which the leg is brought from the position it would be in if you were sitting on a bench to a position that is straight out from you. This exercise works the muscles around the knee as well as the lower quadriceps muscles of the outer thigh.

Here is a typical routine. The bodybuilder will do ten repetitions ("reps") of the full squat, in which the barbell is held on the shoulders behind the neck and the body is lowered until the buttocks rest on the backs of the calves. With no more than ten seconds' rest, he will go to the leg extension machine and grind out ten repetitions on it. Then, with fifteen seconds' rest, he will go back to the squat rack for another set of full squats. This will go on until he has performed four to six sets of ten repetitions of the squat and four sets of ten repetitions of the leg extension. The total time spent resting between sets will be a product of how carefully he has marshaled his stamina. The between-sets rest period will increase as he nears completion of the exercises, but he will pace himself so that he will be able to finish. Each set will be a maximum effort, and each repetition, especially toward the end, will be agony. He will spend approximately ten to fifteen minutes doing the full squat and the leg extension before going on to other exercises. If he is working on a high-repetition routine, he may spend twenty to twenty-five minutes at such activity.

Then, with a minimum rest so as not to lose the "edge" that he has established, the bodybuilder may combine calf raises with leg curls so as to "superset" them, alternately doing ten sets of twenty reps of the calf raise with ten sets of twenty reps of the leg curl.

According to the advocates of aerobic conditioning, the secret is to get the pulse rate up to 150 and keep it there for over five minutes. When a bodybuilder really puts himself through a workout, he will be in aerobic territory for as many minutes as he wants to be. If they overexert themselves, bodybuilders "hit the wall" in exactly the same way as runners: they reach the point where the muscles no longer work. They "bonk out" the same way that runners do: their brains suffer loss of oxygen when they push themselves too far. The bodybuilder's training program can be aerobic with no trouble at all. All he has to do is get his heart rate up to 150 and keep it there for over five minutes.

After you've read the descriptions of these exercises (in Chapter 4), try the squat and leg extension routine as we've described it above. Since it is the demand on the cardiovascular system that makes aerobic conditioning physiologically functional, it doesn't make any difference how you constitute that demand as long as it is made and sustained in the way Dr. Cooper describes. Although weightlifting is not aerobic (and who ever claimed that it was?), weight training certainly can be and usually is aerobic.

The reason for this long dissertation is simple. Detractors of weight training usually cite the literature, and the literature often states that weight training will grow big muscles but won't get you into condition. Nothing could be further from the truth. The truth is, if you do it correctly weight training is far superior to other forms of exercise in a large number of ways. It makes it possible for you to achieve aerobic conditioning while at the same time building strength and speed. You get double value for the effort you expend.

Another point should be cleared up, too. Muscle fibers are usually divided into two kinds: red, slow-twitch fibers and white, fast-twitch fibers. The fast-twitch fibers are the ones we use when we do sudden, powerful movements. The slow-twitch fibers carry us through sustained movements. Consequently, it is popularly believed (even by some physicians) that weight training works only the fast-twitch fibers, while we have to turn to running (for example) to work the slow-twitch fibers. Since the slow-twitch fibers use more oxygen than the fast-twitch fibers, it would appear that we should perform only those movements that utilize the reds in order to build endurance.

In the first place, it is impossible to stimulate *only* the red or *only* the white fibers in any specific movement. In fast, strong movements, most of the cells that are triggered are white. That's what they are for. In the endurance movements, such as sustained running, mostly the red cells are triggered. But they all get triggered more or less, and it is not the case that intensive, progressive-resistance exercises—weight training exercises—provide no endurance conditioning.

On the contrary, ten sets of calf raises supersetted with ten sets of leg curls, each set containing twenty repetitions, results in two hundred repetitions of each movement. The sets are done with maximum strength over a period of fifteen to thirty minutes, with the heart hitting at 150 beats per minute or more halfway through the second set. When you do that many repetitions, your strength movement becomes an endurance movement because the red cells are stimulated along with the white. In fact, the latest fad in bodybuilding is the development of exercises that utilize both types of cells, in the hopes of building ever-larger muscles.

All of the requirements for aerobic, cardiovascular conditioning are there. To say that you can't get into shape with weight training is to reveal simple ignorance or prejudice. Don't worry about it. When Valerie went on the program presented in *Bodysculpture,* one of our best friends (a physician) advised her to wise up to the fact that she would never be thin. She's thin now, from head to toe, and she did it with weight training. It peels fat off and (at least for men) it builds the muscles up. It gives you cardiovascular conditioning, and it makes you strong to boot. Almost all of the top physique stars are runners, too. Not because they have to turn to something else to get them in condition, but because the natural exuberance that weight training gives you will lead you into other forms of physical activity.

It's one of the greatest sports you can do. Take it from us.

I guess this is as good a time as any to tell you how Ralph got into weight training in the first place. It's relevant, because his motives were essentially the same ones that made you buy this book. He wanted to look better, and he wanted to be stronger and healthier. He had a long way to go.

Ralph had rheumatic fever when he was a child. It went undiagnosed for three years, and when he was nine years old he had the dubious distinction of being one of the youngest cardiac patients in Atlanta's Henrietta Egleston Children's Hospital. He suffered the usual valvular damage that accompanies rheumatic fever, and he was put in bed and told to stay there.

Stay there he did, for six months in 1938 and for a whole year in 1940–41. By 1944 the prognosis was poor, and Ralph was told by an eminent cardiologist (now dead) that he shouldn't even sweep a floor with a broom—the violent exercise would kill him. When Ralph was fifteen, he was his present height (five feet ten inches) and he weighed eighty-four pounds. He hated the ninety-seven-pound-weakling ads that Charles Atlas put into the backs of all the comic books, because he was thirteen pounds below the kid with sand in his face.

It was not until he visited his father at the Guantánamo Bay naval base in Cuba that Ralph found a doctor who advised him to do what he had always wanted to do anyway: eat, exercise, and stop worrying about the enlarged heart. He took the advice reluctantly, since all the other physicians had said that such activity would kill him, but his father, Randal Carnes, an old-time weightlifter, goaded him into it. The summer of 1947 was a summer of sun, fun, and the first feelings of life that he had experienced since he was seven years old. By the summer of 1948 Ralph was almost forty pounds heavier, and he no longer had to put up with bullies in the schoolyard.

That all sounds a little silly now, but it was serious business then. In an age when you were either a sissy or you stood and fought, having a chronic illness was no fun at all. Being able to stand up for your rights meant the difference between being accepted by the rest of the kids or being relegated to the sidelines with the other cripples.

In 1948 Ralph bought a York 110-pound barbell set from Karo Whitfield in Atlanta. Karo died last year. In 1948 he was the only person in Atlanta who knew anything about training with weights. When Ralph bought the barbell set, he had to get his stepfather to help him lift it into the car. In two years he had exceeded the "normal" body he was after. Had he not suffered a severe back injury from high diving in 1952, there would never have been a break in training.

As it was, the back injury put him out of weight training for several years. Then college and graduate school took over his time, and weight training was shoved back into the corner. It wasn't until his fortieth birthday, when he thought he saw an old man walking out of a shop and realized that he was looking at his own reflection (!), that he pulled out the barbells and started back to work.

Because of the benefits of weight training, Ralph has overcome a debilitating childhood disease and a serious back injury. He has lived a full, active life, and has participated in athletics long past the age when most men give up and let it sag. He founded the Karate Club at the University of North Dakota in 1966, and taught the club under the supervision of the All-America Karate Federation for three years.

Ralph got Valerie interested in weight training as a means to solve a chronic fat problem (it wouldn't go away, even with starvation diets). She solved the problem, and that's how *Bodysculpture* came to be written. Today both of us go though three heavy workouts a week: Monday, Wednesday, and Friday. We're constantly experimenting with new methods and new exercises. We wouldn't dream of giving it up. It makes us feel good, it makes us healthy, and it keeps us strong. It makes us look good, too. Who could ask for more?

What weight training did for both of us was to provide us with the strength and the conditioning needed to lead the active lives we wanted to lead. In Ralph's case, it helped him to overcome the restrictive effects of a chronic illness. In Valerie's case, it helped her to win her fight with the "Fat Demon."

Did weight training help us improve ourselves in other sports? Most sports-medicine professionals say that the only way to excel in a particular sport is to practice that sport. All of the evidence indicates that the best way to train for a particular sport is to do that sport again and again until you get good at it. If you want to be good at tennis, play tennis. If you want to be good at karate, then do *kata* and *kumite* and hit that *makawara* board 400 times a day with each fist.

But what if you are so out of shape and lacking in strength that you don't even have the musculature to get into the sport of your choice? What if you are so gangly (on the one hand) or fat (on the other) that you are lacking in fundamental motor skills such as coordination and balance? Or what if you are so embarrassed by the way your body looks that you won't even get out there and try the activities you would really like to try?

Let's make another distinction. Football is a sport. Baseball is a sport. Swimming, running, shot putting, cycling—these are all sports. Weightlifting is a sport. But *weight training* is not a sport in the sense that ball games or track-and-field activites are.

Instead, weight training is strength-building and speed-building *exercise* that helps you to improve in certain sports, especially those that require strength and speed. In the same way that weight training will improve your performance as a weightlifter, weight training will improve your performance in other sports. The trick is this: if better performance in a particular sport is a product of increasing strength and speed, then there is no logical reason why weight training cannot be employed to achieve this increase.

Which weight training movements should you do? The answer's easy. Take an example from karate. It wasn't for nothing that the All-America Karate Federation's *Samurai* magazine advised in an early issue that *karatekas* perform weight training movements to improve their karate techniques. For example, take the front snap kick. In this movement you bring your leg up, bent at the knee, until the knee is about in line with your midsection. Then you "unfurl" the coiled lower leg, while rotating the foot at the ankle until the ball of the foot is at the end of a line of bones that begins with the ankle and ends with the hip.

What's the movement? The same as a combination of the leg extension and the front leg swing. Which weight training movements will give you more strength and speed? The leg extension and the front leg swing. Do them with as much weight as you can handle, and do them as fast as you can.

Then put on your karate uniform and practice that front snap to make sure that the increase in strength and stamina doesn't throw your timing off. That's the key. Supplement your sports activities with weight training exercises that duplicate the movements called for by the particular sport, and then practice that sport to make the fullest use of the increase in strength and speed.

But, you say, doesn't everybody know that weight training makes you move slowly and ponderously under all that muscle? Well, a lot of misinformed people have made statements to that effect, but the truth is just the opposite. Why? Because it is the *fast-twitch* muscle fibers that are chiefly developed in weight training movements unless you do high repetitions and many sets.

Remember, you can build endurance with weight training by doing lots of repetitions and lots of sets while using relatively light weights or you can build strength, size, and speed by using heavy weights for a few sets of low reps. Again, the beauty of weight training is its versatility. It's strictly up to you how you train. Whatever your goal is, you can reach it more effectively through weight training.

Will weight training make you a black belt? No. And it won't make you a champion tennis player, soccer player, footballer, or cyclist. But it will help you in these sports if what you need is increased strength and speed, or, if you train the other way, increased strength coupled with endurance. Let us make the point again. Weight training per se is not a sport. It is a form of constructive exercise that can help you in certain ways to improve your body. Running is both a sport and a form of beneficial exercise. It is a sport when the object is to run a certain distance in a certain length of time. It is a form of exercise when you use it to achieve the aerobic effect that comes from sustained activity of more than five minutes that produces a pulse rate of 150.

In the same way that running can be both sides of the coin, weight training has two faces. On one side, it is a sport that involves lifting heavy weights off the floor. On the other, it is a form of exercise that builds your body. When people say that weight training will not condition your body, they are confusing the sport of weightlifting with the exercise form called weight training.

Again, weight training is the best all-around form of exercise, because of its versatility. There are no other kinds of exercise that will build muscle size, give your body the kind of symmetrical shape you want, build strength, stamina, and speed, provide cardiovascular conditioning, and supplement other physical activities. All this and enough variety to keep you from becoming bored with the same old routine every day.

And not only will weight training do all this, it will help you to fight the Fat Demon too. The next section tells you how and why.

FIGHTING THE FLAB

All right, let's face it. You're not in the best of shape. You're plump, "a little flabby," "about five pounds over." Or you have a "pot," a "beer belly," or some "love handles on the sides." Forget the euphemisms. Let's face it: you're just plain *fat*.

Never mind how you got there. Maybe you're an ex-school athlete who maintained the athlete's eating habits without his expenditure of energy. Or maybe you're a new VP, a new director of marketing, a new department head who finds that you're sitting more and moving less as you work your way up the organizational ladder. Or you're on the road a lot, and suddenly the business lunches and dinners and happy hours and breakfast meetings add up to too many unwanted pounds and inches.

Whatever the cause, there they are—the extra five or ten or twenty pounds, the extra inches on the waistline. The question is, What to do? There's only one answer: go on a diet *and* exercise. There's no royal road to weight loss, no easy way out.

Why diet *and* exercise? you're probably asking. Can't I just eat less—fast, maybe—and forget the workouts? Or can't I just work out extra hard and eat anything I want? Wrong on both counts. You've got to combine the two before you hit a winning regimen.

Let's talk a little about fat first (helps to know the enemy). Your body is composed of muscle, fluid, bone, and fat. Fat is stored in the muscles, around the vital organs, and under the skin. *Internal fat* is the fat that surrounds the organs, and this is what we're talking about when we say that excess fat puts a strain on the heart. *Subcutaneous fat* is the "visible" fat which is stored just beneath the skin. When this fat disappears, friends begin telling us how marvelous and slim we suddenly look.

The principle behind dieting to lose weight is simple. There is only one way to lose weight, and that is by eating less. You need to cut roughly 3,500 calories to lose one pound of body weight. If you eat 350 calories less per day, you can lose a pound in ten days; if you eat 700 calories less, you can lose a pound in five days or two pounds in ten. And so on.

It all sounds simple enough, and it is. The complicating factor is exactly *what* is lost. Body weight, as you remember, includes muscle and fluid as well as fat. Dieting alone results in a loss of muscle and organ tissue and a tremendous loss of body fluids as well as fat. Dieting in combination with exercise results in a loss of fat (and some fluid loss) without the loss of muscle and organ tissue. That's why we speak of weight loss from a combination of diet and exercise as a "higher quality" loss than loss from diet alone—more of the loss is real fat loss, and because of improved muscle tone you avoid the flabby, loose-skinned look that the once-heavy, newly thin person otherwise has.

Also remember that there are three groups of foods which we all need: protein, fat, and carbohydrates. Protein, much touted as "the food of bodybuilders," is the building block of body tissue but is *not* a source of immediate energy and cannot be stored for energy—any excess is either stored as fat or excreted. Fat (as a food) is a good source of *secondary* energy during athletics, but carbohydrates furnish the primary fuel for exercise. The body stores carbohydrates in the muscles and in the liver as glycogen. So a great plus for exercise as a means to "burn off" fat is that frequent glycogen depletion teaches the muscles "to burn a greater percentage of fat during all stages of exercise and thereby spare muscle glycogen. Burning fat with muscle glycogen is up to thirteen times more efficient than burning glycogen alone" (Gabe Mirkin and Marshall Hoffman, *The Sports Medicine Book,* Little Brown & Co., 1978, p. 41). Moreover, for several hours after you stop exercising, your body continues to burn calories—which means that your metabolic rate continues to be high even after the exercise period itself is over.

Let's talk about some other facts and some myths connected with fat. One popular view holds that men have an easier time losing fat than women. Well, yes and no. Men don't have the monthly menstrual cycle and its fluid-retention problems to plague them, but they do have some peculiarly male cultural and physical problems: the macho traditions of beer, booze, and beef; the difficulty of finding man-sized dietetic meals, and the general unavailability of good diets for men. Your lady may exist on three salads a day, but you need some protein in the form of meats, fish, or fowl to sustain your greater body mass while you lose.

On the other hand, it *is* true that men and women collect fat in different places. The average overweight woman is a pear or an ice-cream cone, but the average heavy man is a tub or barrel. Most of his weight is concentrated in the center of the body—in the abdomen, in the upper part of the midriff (the "spare tire"), or on the sides as "love handles."

This is not to say that men don't have other problems. Occasionally, for some reason, a man will collect excess weight in his hips, upper arms, shoulders, neck, calves, or thighs. But this is rarer in men than in women; the male weight distribution is typically more above the waist and less below, while a woman's is just the opposite.

Let's look at another popular conception: "If you exercise and build muscle, then stop, the muscle will turn to fat." Wrong. First of all, muscle is muscle and cannot "turn to fat." The football player or championship tennis player who "goes to fat" continues his old eating habits after his energy demands have slacked off and as he grows more sedentary starts packing on the pounds.

By the same token, you can't "turn fat into muscle" either. If you lose fat, you lose fat, and a corresponding drop in weight and inches will result. What you can do is to build muscle, which weighs more than fat, and at the same time develop more shapely contours as you lose those pounds. Technically, "spot reducing" is also impossible. Weight loss takes place at roughly the same rate all over your body. Hence if you have "3*x*" fat all over the body and go on a low-calorie diet combined with exercise, you will lose "1*x*" fat all over your body in, say, one month. But let's suppose that on your waist you have "5*x*" fat, whereas on your legs you have only "2*x*." The decrease will be most dramatic and noticeable on your waist, less so on your legs, and you will *appear* to have practiced "spot reduction." High-repetition progressive-resistance exercises will help the process along, too (more about that later).

And now, on to the matter of diets. Women seem to diet for one reason: to lose weight. Men, however, diet for a variety of reasons: for overall weight loss, for greater definition, or for building strength and increasing muscle size. Each goal requires a specific kind of diet with specific do's and don'ts.

First, some general facts about diets. Remember that there literally are no "miracle" diets. There are some diets which are more effective than others, certainly, and they are usually safe, reasonable, health-conscious regimens, as opposed to those that are dangerous, faddish, silly, or unnecessarily gimmicky. The dangerous ones include no-carbohydrate diets, extended fasts, no-protein diets, and most single-food diets. Although diet fads vary greatly and come in and out of vogue with the speed of last year's hottest fashion or disco step, the basic categories of good and bad diets remain the same. Let's look at some of the most popular types of ineffective diets and see why they don't work.

Zero-calorie or mini-calorie diets: These diets are usually some variation on the theme of fasting—either total fasts, juice-only or liquid-only fasts, or 500-calorie (or less) diets. The advantage: rapid weight loss, which is encouraging and also is helpful in reducing fluid retention. The disadvantages: overly rapid weight loss; loss of potassium, salt, bodily fluids, and necessary minerals; tissue loss. Fasting has been touted as "the ultimate diet," which it might well be for you if undertaken without strict medical supervision. Stand warned of those who claim instant detoxification or mystic experiences will accompany your fast—your visions may be accompanied by ketosis (a state in which ketones are present in the urine), dizziness, weakness, and dangerous potassium depletion.

High-protein, no-carbohydrate plans: Let's make a useful distinction at the very beginning. *Low*-carbohydrate or carbohydrate-counting diets are fine, with medical supervision; *zero*-carbohydrate diets are not. That means OK for levels 2 and 3 of the Atkins super-energy diet, the Scarsdale diet, the Adrian Arpel "sacred cow" plan, and all other carbohydrate-restricted regimens which permit thirty to sixty grams of carbohydrates per day. Verboten are level 1 of the Atkins diet, the Stillman diet, the famous water diet, the "doctor's quick weight-loss diet," and various liquid-protein diets circa 1977–78. The dangers include ketosis, potassium loss, fatigue due to carbohydrate depletion, and an excess of protein and fat. It's a great dietary myth that "you can't eat too much protein." An average-sized man needs about a gram of protein for every two pounds of body weight. The excess is stored as fat or excreted. And everyone, man or woman, cardiac patient or not, should beware of a diet too high in fats. You simply *can't* eat all the whipped cream, nuts, cheese, egg yolk, bacon, and marbled steak you want.

High-carbohydrate, protein-poor diets: Equally dangerous are regimens like the rice diet, the inches-off diet, the salads-only diet, and many vegetarian diets that claim if we'd only drop animal protein the excess pounds would melt away. It's true that American diets are heavy on protein and fat, that we eat far too much saturated fat and red meat, and that generally whole grains, fruits, and vegetables are healthy fare. But vegetable protein is incomplete protein, and at least a small amount of animal protein is needed to digest your tofu-sprouts-and-yogurt dish. Even if your major source of protein is vegetarian, plan to average thirty-plus grams of animal protein a day (eggs and dairy products are fine) in order to assure that you get the so-called essential amino acids, which are needed to aid digestion and other vital processes.

Single-food diets: There are almost too many of these to name: the drinking man's diet, the bananas-only diet, the grapefruit diet, the junk food diet, the fast food diet, the pizza diet, the nibbler's diet, the hamburger diet, the cucumber diet, the yogurt diet, and so on ad nauseum. Their effectiveness is based mainly on boredom—how much of anything can you eat before acute distaste sets in? And most have the additional danger of being terribly unbalanced from a nutritional standpoint. There's no magic food, whether it's alcohol, grapefruit, mangos, cucumbers, yogurt, or Big Macs, that will allow anyone to exist on it alone for very long.

"Head" diets: These have nothing to do with drugs; rather, it is claimed that you can eat all you want as long as you eat from one bowl/take no seconds/think yourself thin/want to get rid of your protective covering of fat/relax/use hypnosis/try acupuncture. While all these tricks are fine and perfectly legitimate ways to motivate yourself, they do *not* help you cut calories, reduce your intake of fats or simple sugars, or expend more energy—which is, after all, what the whole process is all about. Only a reduction in the total number of calories you ingest, plus an increased output of energy, will make those unwanted pounds come off.

As for the good diets, not surprisingly most are simple, gimmick-free, and low-calorie. Weight Watchers, the Diet Workshop, TOPS, and Overeaters Anonymous have excellent programs. So do the various spas and "fat farms" like La Costa and the Greenhouse. One good plan is outlined in a U.S. government report published as *Dietary Goals for the United States* (available in pamphlet form from the U.S. Office of Consumer Information). Its goals are simple but right on target: reduce refined-sugar, salt, and cholesterol consumption; increase complex-carbohydrate intake (fruits, vegetables, whole grains), and maintain adequate protein levels. Another good plan is the "prudent diet," originally designed by Dr. Norman Jolliffe for his Anti-Coronary Club. So is that old standby, *Harper's Bazaar*'s "nine-day wonder diet," reprinted annually for women, but men can use it as well.

So what is the best diet for a man who wants either to build muscle or to slim down? In general, the same basic rules apply for any man's diet: balanced nutrition, moderate caloric intake, higher than the average American diet in protein and long-chain, *unrefined* carbohydrates (fruits, vegetables, and whole grains), lower in fats, salt, and refined carbohydrates.

The chief difference between the building and reducing regimens is the number of calories ingested. The man who wants to build and increase muscular size will ingest 3,000-plus calories a day, perhaps; the man who wants to slim down or who is interested in "definition" (the bodybuilder's technical term for more visible separation of muscle groups attained through a reduction in body fluid and subcutaneous fat) will want to cut down to 2,000 or less (with medical consent, of course). The muscle builder will also take in substantially more complex carbohydrates in the form of raw or steamed vegetables, fruits, nuts, and whole-grain breads and cereals. The man who is dieting for weight loss or for definition will go for a diet slightly lower in complex carbohydrates, with more protein and lower-carbohydrate fruits and vegetables (salad greens, melon, berries). If he wants high-quality protein, he will probably choose chicken, water-packed or fresh fish, and extra-lean beef rather than heavy, fat-marbled steak.

To develop your own diet for whatever your goal is, first see your doctor to check on the number of calories you need for maximum performance. If you are trying to lose weight, check on the drop in calories your body can safely take before fatigue, muscle and tissue loss, and mineral depletion set in. Then develop your own eating patterns according to the following general guidelines.

For muscle building or endurance athletics: multiple small meals each day, plenty of complex carbohydrates, a moderate amount of protein, reduced amounts of saturated fats, plenty of fluid, adequate intake of dairy products (chiefly low-fat yogurt, skim milk or buttermilk, and low-fat cheeses, including cottage cheese), limited salt and sugar intake, few refined carbohydrates, adequate caloric intake for the building process to continue.

For definition and weight loss: four to five small meals a day, with the heaviest one early in the day and the lightest one in the evening; only twenty to thirty grams of complex carbohydrates a day (chiefly from low-fat, skim-milk dairy products, raw low-carbohydrate fruits and vegetables, fresh fruit or vegetable juice, and plain wheat germ or bran flakes); a moderate amount of protein (preferably fish, chicken or turkey, egg whites, skim-milk yogurt and cheese, sprouts, tofu, and soybean products); controlled amounts of fluid (to prevent water retention), and limited salt, sugar, and fat intake. Both calories and carbohydrates should be controlled for best results—but do not attempt a zero-carbohydrate diet no matter how strong the temptation.

The May 30, 1979, issue of *New York* magazine carried a cover story entitled "Why Diets Don't Work." The conclusions are simple but disheartening. Of the total number of Americans who lose substantial amounts of weight, 95 percent regain it (and sometimes gain more) within a year. Diets, clearly, are effective in the short run but not in the long run—at least not for most of us. The reason for their long-range ineffectiveness is that we look on them as short-term deprivations, not as complete changes in long-established eating habits. We go "on" diets and "off" diets, try one, compare one to the other, looking for the miracle that will let the pounds melt off effortlessly. And we're invariably disappointed when there's no miracle forthcoming.

The secret to successful dieting is reeducation of your self—your *whole* self: head, stomach, mouth, eyes, muscles, psyche—concerning food and eating. In a very real sense, the only way to assure that you'll never have to "go" on a diet ever again is to *stay* on a diet of some kind the rest of your life. And that diet should not be a fast, killing no-carbohydrate and high-fat plan or a tasteless menu of cottage cheese and carrot sticks. The dieting process should not be a two-week crash followed by a two-week binge, but a total, thoughtful, lifelong examination of the way you eat followed by a decision to eat less of the wrong foods and more (in smaller quantities) of the right ones. That's all. Sounds simple, but it works. Best of all, it's good for you and gives you the extra energy and stamina to sustain hard work, play, travel, exercise, and even occasional partying. Try it—we guarantee you'll like it!

2

GETTING READY FOR THE STARTING LINE

•

ASSESSING THE DAMAGE/ ESTIMATING REPAIRS

The first step toward shaping your body is to take a good honest look at the shape your body is presently in. No matter how much you may talk about getting in shape, it is still a painful thing to admit how out of shape you may really be. As in fighting alcoholism, drug abuse, or a host of other problems, the first move toward recovery is admitting that there is a problem.

If you don't already have a full-length mirror at home, go out and buy one. Almost any home repair/household goods shop has inexpensive mirror panels that can be mounted on the wall or on the back of a door. Get the mirror, put it up, and use it.

Strip down out of those protective clothes and take a good look. What do you see? If you're naturally heavy, let us make a few guesses, starting from the top and working down.

First, your shoulders will slope right into your upper arms. There will be no separation between deltoids and trapezius muscles, and the upper arm will show no break from the shoulders. Your collar bones will be buried, and your pectorals won't have any definition. In fact, there will be no line beneath the "pecs," and fat will have accumulated to the sides and under the nipples, indicating that the weight has shifted down and toward the armpits.

Rising directly under your flabby chest will be a bulging curve that will culminate in a pear shape at the belly, with stretch marks both in the chest and in the lower abdomen. Your sides will also bulge, and your waist will show the line made by your trousers and your belt. Poor subcutaneous circulation will have been worsened by an attempt to "hold it all in" with tight pants and belts, and your love handles will rise out of your back and sides like slabs of dough.

Your underbelly will all but hide your genitals, and your hips will be cocked backward to compensate for the weight in front. Your buttocks will be flabby, with some overhang at the bottom over the backs of the thighs, and your legs will bulge on the insides while showing no underlying musculature on the outsides of the thighs. Your knees will be overshadowed by fat hanging down from the upper legs, and your calves will be swollen not only with fat but with fluid. Your ankles will be thick with fluid, and your feet will probably be a little redder than the ankles that connect them to the calves.

Not a very shapely sight, is it? How about the naturally lean person? Let's take a look at him.

A lack of subcutaneous fat will give the superficial appearance of muscularity, but the appearance will be deceiving. The muscles will look more like ropes or strings than muscles, and again there will be no sharp separation between muscle groups. Arms will stand out from the body like sticks, and the chest will probably be concave instead of convex. A scrawny neck will lead down to a scrawny upper back, with the shoulder blades the most prominent feature of the upper body. In front, you'll be able to see the collarbones, but only because there is neither muscle nor fat to cover them up.

If a person is lean and really out of shape, there will be no definition in the abdomen, and there may even be a small belly accentuating the sway-back condition that sometimes accompanies a fundamental lack of lower back and abdominal development. The legs will look more like arms, and the calves will be practically nonexistent. It will be the body of a skinny boy instead of a mature man.

Even worse than these two bodies is the one that the ex–high school athlete finds in the mirror. The physique that once turned on the entire cheerleading section of Sylvan Hills High School now looms balefully in the mirror, coming loose at the seams.

The first body is that of hundreds of thousands of American men in their twenties and thirties, who have good appetites, sufficient money to buy the food and booze they want, and a tendency to pack it on rather than use it up.

The second body belongs to the same group of men, except these are the people who do not naturally collect fat. Both types are out of shape. The fat one knows he's in dangerous cardiac territory. The thin one probably thinks that just because he's thin he's healthy.

The third body is a familiar sight. When people see him on the beach they always say, "There goes what's left of a good build."

Now let's get down to business. This is not a pleasant subject, and few people really have the nerve to look at themselves with an unprejudiced eye. Nobody really wants to admit that he is fat, skinny, or merely a ghost of what he once was. It's bad medicine, and it reminds us of our mortality. If we allow ourselves to remember our fathers and uncles, we have to admit that we look much like they did just before they (choose one or more) developed cancer, had a coronary, had a stroke, gave up and hit the long boozy trail to old age.

We're serious about this, because this is serious business. If you look like any of these three men, you're in rotten shape and you need to get hold of yourself and your life and make some changes. Compare yourself with photographs of men in sports. You don't have to drag out pictures of bodybuilders. Look at the guys in *Sports Illustrated.* Look at the professional athletes. Look at their faces. That's the element we left out. Look back into the mirror and this time study your face.

Do you have a pallor, the result of a completely sedentary life? Are there bags under your eyes, the result of a mild kidney dysfunction due to the kind of life you lead? Do you have jowls? Or are your cheeks so thin you worry about cutting yourself every time you shave? Are your eyes rheumy from too much booze and too little sleep? Is your hair dull instead of glossy? How are the lines in your face coming? Stick out your tongue. What color is it?

Again, we're deadly serious. This is no joke, this condition you've let yourself get in. You should see a doctor, to make sure that nothing is organically or structurally wrong. You should have a complete physical, get a grip on what your real situation is, then come back to the mirror and take another look.

Now you're ready to start doing something about yourself. Many people ask how they should build up their arms or legs. Others want to know how they can learn to lift 200 pounds over their heads. Let's ask a more fundamental question, one that has to be answered before we can start developing a corrective program.

The question is "How the hell did you get in this shape?"

The answer holds the key to getting yourself out of the shape you're in and back into better shape. Think back for a moment to high school. Did you take phys ed? Did you like it? If you weren't a jock, you probably didn't. In Ralph's high school, you either played football or you were nobody. The phys-ed classes were geared to produce football players, and everybody who couldn't make the team was weeded out and relegated to the football band.

This is no criticism of the football players, God love 'em. If Ralph could have made the team, he would have been right out there. Instead, it's a commentary on the way in which athletics were taught in high schools in the fifties, and it's one of the clues to why there are so many "average" people walking around today who never got into exercise on a long-term basis. Until recently high school athletics were strictly team-oriented. If you weren't particularly interested in sports, you didn't learn much about how to take care of your body or about the benefits of exercise. Exercise always served as an adjunct to the teams. Also, if you weren't very good at physical activities, oftentimes you took so much abuse from people who were good at them that you got out of phys ed as soon as you could and never went back.

There's another reason you're out of shape, too. Only in the last five or six years have we really begun to think of exercise and health, strength and stamina, as being within the grasp of and beneficial to the nonathlete. All too often there was a kind of snobbery on the part of nonathletes that rivaled the prejudices of the jocks. If you were really smart, intellectual, sensitive, creative, etc., the last thing you did was exercise.

Instead, and especially if you attended college and graduate school, it was *de rigueur* to affect the pseudo-bohemianism of (what we conceived to be) the life-style of the Left Bank expatriate of the 1920s, with its attendant booze, tobacco, narcotics, late hours, and heightened sense of melancholy.

If you were *really* an intellectual, it was *obscene* to look healthy. It meant that you weren't really serious about sacrificing yourself for your art.

Of course, all of us now know that this is the most refined kind of bullshit imaginable. The mind works better when it gets enough oxygen. Tobacco doesn't do much for the lining of your lungs. Dope leaves holes in your mind (as Norman Mailer put it), and late hours merely make you sleepy. People who drink too much over too long a time are called drunks. They slobber a lot and are boring after the first couple of drinks.

During the sixties, there was a sort of eschatological essence in the air: a feeling that everything was going to end. Arlo Guthrie, on "Kup's Show," said that he had visions that the buildings along Lake Michigan were going to fall over into the lake. When Kup asked if he was speaking figuratively, Arlo replied, "No. Like I really mean really fall off into the lake."

Thousands of young people actually believed that Jim Morrison, Jimi Hendrix, Janis Joplin, and other pop stars were deliberately sacrificing their health by overdosing because it was the only way they could play their music the way that the kids wanted to hear it played.

In an atmosphere like this, it was hard to develop any kind of sustained interest in prosaic things like strength, stamina, endurance, and being healthy. To be healthy was to be . . . to be *straight,* man. An outright betrayal.

Paradoxically enough, the current health movement grew directly out of the "back to nature" movement that evolved from the hippie ethos. And now we've come full circle, back to where Bob Hoffman started in 1931 when he founded *Strength and Health* magazine. We're looking for ways to be strong, healthy, and happy and to enjoy life.

We're wiser now than we were in the old days, thanks to research done by exercise physiologists, sports-medicine M.D.'s, and trainers and coaches all over the world. We know more about diet, rest, sleep, exercise, and all the things that go into being healthy than we ever did before. Whatever the reason you are now in rotten shape, you can probably reverse the process that got you there. There's no time like the present to start.

Why such a long digression? Well, it's not really a digression. We said earlier that the first step to doing something about a problem is to admit that there is a problem. One of the best ways to get yourself started in the right direction is to look back to see how you got where you are in the first place. More often than not, you've recently asked yourself just that: "How did I get into this mess?" And then the other question: "How do I get myself out?"

You can get yourself ready to act by discovering the elements in your life-style that put you where you are today. When you find out what these elements are, then you've got to make a decision to change things. Nobody can do that for you. You've got to do it yourself, for yourself. That's why so many people fail to stay on diets and exercise programs. They don't go through the process of self-discovery that is required to turn themselves around toward the right track.

Recently we were in Dallas promoting *Bodysculpture*. A young lady at a TV station asked us, "How do I get rid of this little pot I've got here in front?" Ralph responded with a word about diet and abdominal exercises. Before he could finish his sentence, the girl interrupted with a loud "Naw, I don't want to do exercises! Don't tell me I gotta stop eating. You're the experts, tell me how to get rid of this the easy way."

It wasn't good PR, but Ralph told her that if that was her attitude, she would just have to get used to being sloppy around the belly.

Tough talk, but necessary. If you want to change your shape and get into shape, you can do it. Weight training will do it for you faster than anything else. But you've got to do the following things:

1. Make an *honest* assessment of the shape your body is in.
2. Make an honest assessment of the elements in your life-style that put you where you are.
3. Resolve to change those elements in your life-style that are self-destructive, and replace them with life-enhancing ideas and activities.
4. Get off your duff and go to work!

Now that we know where we stand, let's talk about how to develop a personal program that will get you moving in the right direction.

The best way to start an exercise program is to get into it gradually. This keeps down the incidence of injuries, and it also makes the transition from a sedentary life to an active one easier to take. In the following sections of this chapter, we'll describe the equipment you'll need to do the job, and we'll also give you some advice on how to get the kind of support you'll need from those around you. In chapter 3 we'll give you a variety of stretching, limbering, and toning exercises that will get you in shape for the heavy stuff that will follow. Chapters 4, 5, and 6 will describe in detail all you'll need to know about gaining strength, developing stamina, changing the shape of your body, and using weight training as a springboard for other physical activities.

You should begin with the stretching and limbering routines. Choose the ones that suit you best. You'll know by the difference in the way you feel which routines are doing the job for you. Then move into a general conditioning routine, using the weight training exercises described in chapter 4. After two months of general conditioning, you can move on to variations on the program, suited to the specific problems that you have.

For example, if you have pretty good upper body and arm development but are lacking in leg development, you'll want to follow your general conditioning routine with emphasis on squats, leg extensions, Jefferson lifts, hack squats, and calf work.

If the opposite is true—if your legs are your best feature but your upper body is lagging behind—you'll want to emphasize work for the arms, the pectorals, and the back, and some extra work for the shoulders.

As you'll see when you finish chapter 4, the exercises described can be combined into hundreds of different routines, each directed toward a specific problem area. Further, if you want to use the basic exercises for strength training instead of shaping, the right combinations and methods will be easily put together.

You'll see results almost immediately. In three months, you won't believe it's you.

Now, take another look in the mirror. Tell that droopy guy good-bye. You'll never see him again.

GETTING GEARED UP

You're going to need some equipment in order to do the exercises described in this book. None of it is very expensive, and most of it will last a lifetime. The first thing you will need is proper attire. That means footwear and an exercise suit. Don't scrimp at this point, because exercise clothes can make the difference between getting a good workout and not being able to concentrate on what you're doing.

Let's start at the feet and work our way up.

Go down to your local sports store and buy a good pair of jogging shoes. They will provide you with excellent support as you do weight training exercises, and they will double for the purpose for which they were designed. Ralph has a pair of Adidas shoes that he bought in 1975. He works out three to four times a week, and he's used them extensively for running. They show no significant signs of wear. They'll cost you about $30, but you'll never make a better investment. If your feet hurt, you won't be able to concentrate on your workout, and concentration is one of the keys to success in exercise. So go out and get a good pair of jogging or gym shoes.

While you're buying the shoes, you'll discover that there is a great deal of lore not only about what kind of footwear you should buy but about socks as well. Many stores have huge bins full of cheap "tube" socks (socks made with no reinforcement in the toe and heel, and not shaped to fit the foot—they're elastic enough to stretch into shape). Other stores don't have tube socks, but offer a wide range of thick, thin, cotton, nylon, white or colored socks. Professional runners advise against thick cotton socks, since they make it impossible for the feet to benefit from the snug design of the shoes. On the other hand, many people feel that they need a thick pair of socks to cushion the feet and absorb perspiration.

Remember why you are buying the shoes in the first place. You're going to wear them in the gym or at home while you do weight training exercises. Buy several pairs of thick cotton socks. They're cheap, and they'll give you all the support you need. You can throw them into the washer when you've worn them. If you decide to run after you exercise, you can always change into a thinner pair of socks.

Now, how about exercise suits? Again, the most important things to look for are comfort and support. If you are going to work out at a gym or a spa, there may be dress codes. Check about this when you join. If you are going to work out at home, you can wear whatever you like as long as you remember that it is sometimes psychologically supportive to get into your exercise gear when you do so.

A psychiatrist friend once told us that scientists have a built-in "prop" that the humanities people don't have, which makes it easier for them to knuckle down to work. The prop is the lab smock. Once the scientist puts it on, he or she has made a sort of rite of passage from ordinary life to a different life. Humanities professors have only the books they plan to read or write. So even if you are planning to do all your working out at home, get an exercise suit. It will strengthen your resolve while the exercises strengthen your body.

Most people at the gym wear some form of jogging warm-up suit, without the jacket. They'll wear a tee shirt, or if the rules allow it, a tank top. I prefer the tank top because you can see the effects of the workout immediately and you can mark your progress. The gym owners have a simple reason for not wanting you to wear tank tops. Your perspiration rots the padding on the exercise machines and costs them money. Hence the regulation requiring shirts with shoulders or sleeves. If you are going to work out at home, wear a tank top. It's less restrictive anyway.

Don't spend a lot of money on a jazzy suit to wear when you exercise. There'll be some wear and tear, and there is no use wasting your money. Get a suit that is fairly loose-fitting and that doesn't get in the way of the movements you are doing. Try to find a lightweight suit, because the really heavy ones become too hot during a workout. You may want to sweat, but you don't want to become overheated. During the summer (and if you work out at home) you'll want to stick to gym shorts instead of a full-length suit. They're more comfortable and you can watch the progress of your legs, too.

Many men use an athletic supporter, or jockstrap, when they work out. It's supposed to provide "support" to the "vital organs" while you are zooming around the gym. Most good brands of gym shorts have a built-in jockstrap, but jogging suits do not. Ralph has never been able to take jockstraps seriously as a necessity for workouts. Over the years, he's seen many men grinding away in the gym in discomfort, their crotch strangled by a heavy elastic jockstrap. It restricts your movements, and it chafes, especially if you're doing high-repetition leg work. Ralph's Japanese karate instructor, Takayuki Mikami, never used a jockstrap, and he was the all-Japan champion in *kumite* (free fighting) and *kata* (formalized fighting movements) for three years. What you want is freedom to move. If a jockstrap restricts your movements, don't wear one. Jockey shorts will provide the same degree of support without the disadvantages of chafing elastic.

If your hair is long or if you sweat a lot, you might buy a headband. It's made of terrycloth and other absorbent materials, costs only a few quarters, and will keep your hair and your sweat out of your eyes.

That's about it in the way of personal equipment. One reminder: if your wristwatch is not stainless, you should take it off when you work out. The perspiration will corrode the case.

Now that you're all outfitted and ready, you have two places to go: home or to a gym. Let's talk about gyms first, then about working out at home. You may be surprised at the advantages and disadvantages of both places.

Over the last five years, a new type of gymnasium has come into existence in America. It's called the "family fitness center," and it has been created for the purpose of providing exercise facilities for the whole family—at a profit for the owners. Many of these gyms (or "spas," as they are usually called, although they are not actually spas) are beautifully designed and equipped, are staffed by people who know about exercise physiology and sports, and are bright, cheerful, dynamic places to work out.

Other spas are poorly staffed, are put together by people who know nothing about the fitness field, and are smelly, dirty, unsanitary down trips for the members. Many clubs are built solely for profit, and the number of scams being run by fitness centers makes it hard for the legitimate clubs to compete. Here are a few things to look for when you think about joining a gym.

1. Is it equipped with free weights as well as exercise machines? If it is not, then you can be assured that the owners are not really serious about providing weight training equipment, since free weights still

constitute the core of any genuine weight training routine. The machines have their function, but you can't do a complete training routine with machines alone.

2. Is the gym clean? Look at the locker room. Check out the showers. Gym owners usually make the exercise area itself the showcase and spin you through the locker and shower areas too fast for you to get an idea of the real conditions there. When you get the guided tour, make sure you see what you want to see.
3. Is the equipment in good repair? Check out how many machines are not in service. Do the barbells have collars? Are the barbells Olympic Standard sets, or are they merely cheap little sets bought at the local department store? Are the cables frayed on the pulley machines? Do the machines bind in their movements? Is the padding rotted and smelly? It won't take you long to get a clear picture of what it's like to work out in a particular gym. All you have to do is look around and know what to look for.
4. Do the instructors really know anything about exercise? Take a good look at the instructors. Are they better-than-average physical specimens? Ask them about their training. After all, they are supposed to provide you with tips about the best ways to work out for maximum progress. More often than not, the gym instructors will be former high school athletes, with no genuine training in exercise past what their coach taught them on the football field. The reason they're there is they are a cheap labor supply, especially during the first summer after graduation. If they tell you that all you have to do is whirl through the machines for fifteen minutes a day twice a week, then head for the door. They're merely trying to make a sale.
5. Make sure you understand the fee structure before you sign the papers. If you get a special deal, remember that there really aren't any "special" deals. The fee structures in modern health clubs are determined not by individual salesmen but by the owners and the factoring or financing firms with whom they do business. When you pay your initial check and sign on the dotted line, the club has all it needs to get all of its money. After the first check, you will be dealing with the "X" Acceptance Company, and it will go after you if you are late in your payments. If you find out that the club is a rip-off and that the facilities are really abominable, you can't stop paying. Your "deal" is not only with the club; it is with the "X" Acceptance Company, which couldn't care less whether or not the club delivers what it told you it would.
6. You should also understand that in many states a "lifetime membership" has nothing to do with *your* lifetime. Many clubs make lifetime-membership offers as a come-on in their membership drives. Make

sure whose lifetime they are talking about. It is usually the lifetime of the corporation, not yours. That means that when the corporation takes a dive, you've simply paid out all that money for nothing.

7. Make sure that the hours of the club allow you to get the workouts you need. Some clubs, in order to advertise as family fitness centers even though they maintain only one workout room, will alternate days between men and women. This means that half the time you can't get into the gym. It also means that if you and your lady both work out, you won't be able to do it on the same day. It's a hassle, and it will be a deterrent to working out. Some small cities will have two gyms in the same chain, one on one side of town and the other on the other side. They will both alternate between men and women, and you'll have to drive all over town every time you and your lady want to work out. If the club alternates and such a schedule interferes with your schedule, don't bend. After all, they need your business. Go out and look for another club.

With all these caveats, you may get the idea that the clubs are all out to separate your cash from you. To an extent that is true, but no more than in any other business. The good clubs are so good that they don't have to worry about profit margins to the point of driving away members. They provide cheerful, well-planned workout areas, and they are staffed with people who really know what they are doing. We belong to the Presidents/First Lady Club (a part of the same chain as the Chicago Health Club), and the machines are in good repair, the staff is expert, and there are plenty of free weights along with the machines.

In some ways, a health club is like a marriage. If it's a good one, then life with it is a joy to behold. If it's bad, then you have to get out before you can begin to do anything constructive. If you've got the money and you need the supportive atmosphere of a health club, spa, or gym, by all means join one and go to it at least three times a week. But before you leap, take a look at the things we've mentioned above. It'll save you money as well as grief.

What about working out at home? Can't you do all of this bodyshaping at home, without the expensive equipment and the lush trappings of a health club? Of course you can.

One of the many beauties of weight training is that you *can* do it in the privacy of your own home, with equipment that is practically indestructible, at a cost that is really peanuts.

To begin with, the basic unit of weight training, the barbell set, costs as little as $39.95 at almost any sporting goods store in the country. You can buy sets with vinyl-covered plates that won't clank, rust, or chip your furniture. You can buy chrome equipment that will make a terrific high-tech addition to your living room. There are dozens of manufacturers of weight training equipment all over the United States, and they make not only barbells and dumbbells but benches, racks, and all kinds of safety equipment as well. For less than a year's membership in a posh health club, you can outfit a home gym with all equipment you need to make whatever changes in your shape you want to make.

Remember, Valerie transformed herself from a 185-pound fatty to a sleek 110-pound fox with an ancient York 110-pound set, working out in the living room of a high-rise apartment. Ralph did the same thing in reverse with the same 110-pound set, working out in the bedroom of his parent's house.

Get a copy of *Strength and Health, Muscular Development, Muscle Builder, Iron Man, Muscle Digest,* or any of the host of muscle magazines presently on the market. They're chock-full of ads for equipment. And if the full-fledged chrome and ball bearings Olympic Standard is too rich for your blood, you can always hop down to Sears and pick up a 110-pound set for under $40.

While we're on the subject of costs, let's make a few comparisons. For forty bucks you can own a barbell, two dumbbell handles with collars, and enough plates to make up 110 pounds of weight. For another forty bucks you can get a good solid bench to do pullovers and bench presses with. For $350 you can buy a safety bench that includes pulleys for lat work; a bench-press bench with foolproof construction so that the bar won't wind up on your neck if you can't make that last repetition; a built-in squat rack, and pins to hang the plates on when you're not using them.

That means that for about $400 you can have a complete home gym, with all the weight you'll need to start your program, plus a workout suit and this book. All for less than you would pay for a year's membership in one of the better health clubs. And the nice thing is that once you've bought the equipment, it's yours. It doesn't wear out, because the only moving part is you.

If you want to go the whole route, if you have the funds to indulge your whims all the way, companies such as Dynacam in Houston, Paramount in Los Angeles, Universal, or a score of others can provide you with machines, barbells, benches, racks, and all the pulleys you could ever want to pull. Get ready to spend anywhere from ten to sixty thousand bucks and you, too, can have a gym like Clint Eastwood's.

On the other hand, if you're like we are, you should be happy to know that you can accomplish all you need to accomplish with an expenditure of about $40. Don't forget that giants like John Grimek, Steve Reeves, Bill Pearl, Dave Draper, Arnold Schwarzenegger, Frank Zane, and Steve Davis all work out primarily with our old friends the barbell and the dumbbell. The next time you're in a health club, look around at the members. If the club has free weights, compare the people working out with free weights with the members on the machines. The serious guys are all over at the squat rack or the bench press.

As far as space is concerned, a barbell set doesn't take up much room.

When Ralph started working out back in the forties, he rolled the barbell under the bed after each workout. When Valerie fought the Fat Demon in our twenty-fifth-floor apartment, she set up the weight training equipment in the same room that held the bookcases, the piano, her typewriter and desk, and a huge poster collection. The room was eleven feet by twelve. That should give you some idea of how much room you need. I doubt that Valerie had more than a six-by-eight-foot square to work out in. For twisting movements, she usually migrated into the living room.

Many people set up the equipment in the garage. If you do this, make sure that you have adequate ventilation in the winter as well as the summer. If you heat your garage with a gas space heater, you'll need some way to get rid of the fumes. During the summer, unless your garage is air-conditioned, you may become overheated. Don't believe all the stories about it being better to work out in the heat. That's just some more macho bullshit. It's better to work out in a well-ventilated place that is kept at around seventy degrees or a little lower. The purpose of weight training is to put intensive stress on the muscle fibers, not to cook them.

Whether you're working out at home or at a health club, your workouts will affect those around you. You'll need some support in this undertaking, and unfortunately wives, girl friends, and other well-wishers don't always know enough about what it takes to work out to be supportive. Rather than having to put up with complaints and misunderstandings, do a little missionary work. It'll enhance your workouts and it'll make it easier for you to stay on a long-range program. Further, when you really get into your program, you are going to become a new person. You should prepare the way for this new person from the beginning. Working out on a regular basis is going to make a significant change in your life. It'll be a permanent change if the people around you understand what you are trying to do and why.

EXPLAINING IT ALL TO THE LADY IN YOUR LIFE

So you're all geared up, ready to go with your new exercise program. You've got your new warm-up suit, the brand-new Adidas and striped socks, a roomy carryall, and a weightlifting belt for the heavy stuff. It's early Sunday morning and you're raring to go. Over your healthy, low-cal breakfast you break the news to Her: "I'm off to the gym for a workout with the weights. Want to come along?" She lights her third cigarette of the morning and sputters into her coffee and Danish, "Yuk! No, thanks. I don't want to look like big Arnold. What's more, I don't want you looking that way either. All those big bulgy muscles don't turn *me* on!"

And so you go off to work out alone while She sits sulking at home, or worse still, sips and noshes her way through the morning at the friendly little corner pub with a guy who hasn't a muscle in his body. Or maybe She tags along to the gym to lounge in the sauna and laugh and point at the weekend athletes. At dinner that night, there are numerous innuendos about muscle-bound meatheads and men with more brawn than brains.

How to get through to her that what you're doing is healthy, demanding but rewarding business? It's a tough assignment, but there are a few ideas to get you going:

1. Get across the idea that you are serious about your workouts and about fitness in general. Stress the health-related aspects of your new program. Quote or show her some statistics on the alarming death rate of American males—even comparatively young ones—from cardiovascular disease. Convince her that overweight and poor fitness are unhealthy, that you're prolonging your life (and her happiness) by what you're doing.
2. Don't be a stick-in-the-mud or a fanatic about your program. She probably fears that you will become a total health nut—no more nights at the disco, no more restaurants, no fun. She envisions a mostly bare refrigerator stocked only with spring water and organic vegetables instead of Dom Perignon and chocolate mousse. Put her fears to rest by finessing an occasional workout and splurging on a night on the town. Take her to an elegant restaurant that specializes in vegetarian dishes or *cuisine minceur* so that she can see the most appealing side of healthful eating.
3. Try to get her to join you. This is easier if she's either overweight or imagines that she is. (Few women are ever totally satisfied with their bodies!) Remind her of her dissatisfactions—flabby upper arms, thin calves, big hips—and then suggest that she could reshape her body through exercise. Invite her again to join you for a workout. Arrange for her to take a tour through the gym or health club. If you've picked one with shiny chrome machines, lots of plants, and an attractive women's locker room and dressing area, so much the better. Help her design a program or have one of the instructors do so. Also buy her a copy of *Bodysculpture* or any of the other exercise books designed for women.
4. Buy her a magazine with articles on fitness for women. Point out the annual and semiannual fitness guides published by *Vogue, Cosmopolitan, Redbook, Woman's Day,* and many other magazines. Buy her a subscription to *Self*. Whenever one of the fashion magazines carries an item on fitness, call it to her attention. One of her secret fears is of turning into an unlovable "female jock." She *wants* to be strong, healthy, and athletic in a golden-tan-California-girl sort of way, but she does *not* want to be a powerlifting champion. Show her that she's not alone. Remind her that many women are now into all sorts of fitness activities and remain attractive, sexy, intelligent, and successful.

5. Don't be condescending toward her efforts. Tell her when she starts to lose inches off her hips or when her upper arms firm up noticeably. Tell her *she* looks great instead of drooling over every ninety-pound model in the disco. (You *like* firm, trim women with some muscular definition, remember?) Don't give her pastel pink barbells or make fun of her doing the bench press with thirty-five pounds. Don't joke about "the little lady getting big muscles" while she huffs and puffs with five-pound weights. Her gains and losses are just as important and represent just as much hard work as yours, although the poundages she is handling will be less.
6. Stress to her what weight training will do to and for her. It will *not* make her grow big muscles (she hasn't got the hormones for it). It *will* make her firmer, trimmer, stronger. It *will* help her lose inches in areas where women collect the most fat: hips, thighs, midriff, waistline, and tummy. It can also help to shape and slim her knees, calves, upper back, and arms if she happens to collect weight in those places. And in the meantime, remind her that an hour of steady weight training can burn from 300 to 500 calories, depending on the speed and intensity of the exercises. If she's on a strict diet at the same time, she can't help losing both pounds and inches.
7. There are some fairly complex psychological problems involved in any drastic change in body image, male or female. She may make fun of your new regimen, but secretly she's afraid that you're getting a little too slim of waist and broad of shoulder to stick with a little dumpling like her. If you suddenly start paying a lot of attention to yourself—new haircut, bronzers and colognes and skin products, sharp new clothes—she'll be all the more fearful. Her worst fear is that she'll get dumped for some foxier-looking lady. Reassure her, and she'll stop laughing at your efforts to look better.
8. The whole thing works in reverse, too. As she turns from plain little Jane into a reasonable facsimile of FFM or Wonder Woman, you may find yourself becoming a bit anxious. If you do, fight it! Don't undermine her efforts by playing Jealous Lover. Praise her. Tell her how good she looks in the new tight jeans, the clingy tube top or leotard or maillot. She worked hard to get in shape to wear it. So be supportive! And be specific in your praise. "Honey, you look great tonight" is *pro forma* praise. But to remind her that she's lost two or three inches in her hips and that the new (or old) jeans look sensational on her now means that you're observant. Show that you do notice, that you like the results, and she'll love you for it.
9. Don't sabotage her diet by insisting that she pig out in restaurants. It's perfectly OK to substitute a salad or appetizers for the entree if they are the only diet foods available. Better yet, pick a place famous for its broiled seafood, dinner salads, or vegetarian dishes. Try

a salad bar or health food restaurant for a change of pace. Investigate ethnic places with imaginative salad entrees. Go out for brunch or lunch instead of dinner—prices are lower, dishes are lighter, and she can have a plain omelette or salad for her entree.

10. Get involved in low-calorie cooking together. Buy a book on the new *cuisine minceur* (classic French cookery without all the heavy sauces, creams, and gravies) and whip up a diet gourmet feast. Buy a wok and try your hand at Oriental dishes. Learn to steam vegetables lightly or eat them raw, skipping the butter and hollandaise. Try diet recipes or alter standard ones with substitutions (cottage or ricotta cheese for sour cream, Sweet 'n' Low for sugar, etc.). Be supportive of her diet at home and remind her to do the same for you.

11. Don't undermine her morale by going into ecstasies over every eighteen-year-old ectomorph on the beach. If she's even a pound or two overweight and anxious about those pounds, it will only make her feel fatter and unlovelier and more defeated. Start rethinking exactly what you admire in a woman's body. Don't you really prefer a trim, athletic-looking flesh-and-blood woman to a wire sculpture or a figure like a preadolescent boy's?

12. Substitute other activities for eating to keep her mind (and yours) off food. Take in an art gallery, a street fair, a movie, a disco (drink Perrier instead of booze), a carnival, or a baseball game instead of going out to eat. When she loses ten pounds, reward her with a piece of jewelry or a good book, *not* a meal out in the Pump Room. Walk, play tennis, go to the beach, build something, go jogging on weekends. Keep your collective minds off food and watch the pounds come off.

13. As she advances in her program, start doing some serious workouts together. Remember that you can do the same exercises (we do) and follow the same routine. Her poundages will be lighter and she may do more reps, but the formula for the workouts is the same. If you can find a coed gym, so much the better. Do couples' exercises at home on weekends, travel exercises on the road together. Jog or run together in the evenings. Swim or do water exercises in the pool together. Take your bikes out for a Saturday spin. If you make fitness a regular part of your life together, you'll both be equally involved and you'll keep each other motivated.

Now let's look at some facts and some common misconceptions about women and weights. Weight training is a relatively new fitness movement for women—in fact, only in the last five years or so is it "coming out of the closet." Until the mid-seventies, there were no books on the subject; now there are *Bodysculpture, Getting Strong, Starbodies,* and *The Zane Way to a Beautiful Body*. There are also numerous articles in women's magazines, from the now-defunct *Viva* to *Ambience, Self,* and *Cosmopolitan.* Joe Weider's *Muscle Builder* now has an extensive section on women and weights, and plans are afoot for an entire magazine devoted to weight training for women. It's clearly an idea whose time has come.

Yet it's an idea that still meets with plenty of resistance. Women themselves are afraid to try weight training, either because they think they can't handle the poundages or because, as mentioned earlier, they fear it will make them grow big muscles. Both fears are unfounded.

First, the matter of the poundages. We are not talking about powerlifting or even weightlifting. These two sports both involve lifting heavy weights—working for maximum poundages in order to build strength. The aim of the powerlifter, male or female, is to increase to the maximum the amount of weight he or she can handle. The look of the body or the form of the exercise is less important than the amount of weight one handles.

Bodybuilding, by contrast, is the (primarily male) sport which focuses on the body itself as the end result. The bodybuilder's real product is himself. He builds, slims, tones, "bulks up," "rips up" (works for definition) in order to achieve precisely the look he is after. Fashions in physiques, as in clothes, come and go. Right now the current look for men is massive chest, shoulder and arm development, high definition in the midriff and waist area, massive thighs and calves. The bodybuilder goes for maximum poundages in certain lifts in order to build muscle mass, but also uses lighter weights in order to achieve more definition and get the "ripped," chiseled look.

Certainly most women don't want to build massive muscles. But there are many parallels between what bodybuilders achieve and what the average woman wants to do with her body. She wants a leaner, more defined midriff and waist area, less fat and more definition in her upper arms and back. She may want to slim down heavy thighs and calves or build up skinny ones. In other words, she wants to use weight training to build, slim, tone and define certain areas of her body—just as a professional bodybuilder does! And that's the secret advantage that weight training has over any other method of shaping the female body. The woman who trains with weights can literally sculpt her body into the shape that most satisfies her—within the confines of her own skeletal structure, of course.

Let's talk about that whole question of body types for a moment. The body type we happen to admire at any given moment in history is a matter of popular fashion very much like the clothes, movies, soft drinks, or discos that are In or Out. In the mid-sixties, thanks to the impact of Mod clothing styles and the Twiggy-like shape it took to wear them, our ideal female type changed from a curvy, well-padded Marilyn Monroe or cuddly Doris Day to an ectomorphic preadolescent with polelike arms and legs, flat boyish hips, and no bust or abdomen. Even the men's magazines (with a few exceptions) switched to this type in their centerfolds. It was the heyday of the fashion-model as popular icon, and our culture held that women ought to look this way *naturally*—no fair running, weight training, jogging, or swimming to whittle yourself down to the Twig's proportions!

Now popular taste is changing again, and the stick-thin figure as ideal is on its way out. The up-and-coming ideal shape of the eighties is the lean, trim mesomorph with plenty of muscular definition and a healthy, fit, but unmistakably female shape. Now we enjoy seeing a definite curve to a calf, a well-developed arm, a ripple of muscle in the shoulder and back. We don't expect women to be cuddly sex objects or starved-to-near-perfection clotheshorses, but functioning, strong, vital human beings. And if the lady has to work *hard* to achieve that shape, well, so much the better!

There's been a lot of talk in the past decade about women's liberation from male standards of beauty. We went through a phase in the early seventies when women spurned makeup, hair styling, clothes, and even diet and exercise because these things were thought to "enslave" women and make them the toys of boardroom and bedroom. But now the pendulum has swung back again, and women are realizing that looking good, feeling good, and being healthy are things that they do, not for the men in their lives but for *themselves*. Women still value good looks and good health—but as the marks of caring about themselves first and others secondarily.

It's a healthy and liberating attitude, this new freedom to want to look and feel good. And it's the only motivation that works. A woman who diets or exercises to satisfy a critical or demanding friend/lover/husband, to get a better job, or to fit into a certain social group is a woman who will eventually give up on the whole thing and backslide to her old ways. But the woman who does these things *for herself* will keep up the regimen and probably stick to it for the rest of her life. She's a true self-starter, motivated by inner satisfactions rather than other-directed impulses.

The greatest help you can give the lady in your life, then, is to give her the support she needs while she's doing this program for herself. The worst thing you can do is to nag, criticize, or imply that she doesn't look good enough for you. Ditto for her—you deserve the same treatment! If each of you can furnish the support the other needs, you'll both be much happier and healthier as a result.

As for expectations: we hear a lot these days about "getting results" from various kinds of exercise programs. Health clubs and spas promise "fast results," and some even sign money-back guarantees if you don't reshape yourself within a certain time period.

If the lady in your life goes on a weight training program she will get results, and fairly fast—but *only if* she stays with the program on a regular basis and *only if* she is also on a rather strict, low-calorie, balanced diet. If dieting alone has failed to do the trick before, weight training will supply just the right amount of progressive-resistance exercise to get her metabolism in high gear and start the fat-burning process. But she can't continue to nibble or sip pastries, pastas, breads, desserts, colas, or rich creams and sauces—such self-defeating indulgence will only slow down her program to a discouraging snail's pace. At the same time, she can't starve herself or she will suffer from general weakness, fatigue, and potassium depletion, and simply won't have the stamina to finish her workouts. Probably the best possible combination is for both of you to go on essentially the same diet. You can consume a few hundred more calories, but you both will eat the same foods at the same times, and most important, give each other the moral support you need to stay with the diet.

Also, remember that she isn't going to reshape herself totally through the program. Some things are givens, and no amount of twisting, squatting, stretching, rolling, or lifting is going to (1) make her legs four inches longer, (2) increase her bust measurement, (3) change her pelvic structure, or (4) turn an Audrey Hepburn type into Wonder Woman. But she can shape her legs with hack squats so that they appear longer; she can chisel out her pectoral area with flyes; and she can shape her hips so that her rear view is trim and tight instead of saggy and spreading.

As to how long it takes: individual metabolisms and skeletal structures respond to exercise in very different ways, so it's impossible to predict exactly. But results are usually visible at the end of three to four weeks, encouraging after six to eight weeks, and dramatic at the end of three months. In *Bodysculpture* we recommend a ninety-day (three-month) program for best results in a fixed time period.

All right, let's sum up. Let's say your lady is dissatisfied with the shape she's in—what woman isn't?—and wants to join you in your workouts. If she wants to trim down, get rid of the fat, and firm, tone, and generally condition herself, she should stay on that balanced, low-cal diet and work out three to four days a week on a ninety-day program much like the one you're using. Same exercises, just different poundages and more reps. And since she's a woman with a woman's genes and hormones instead of a man's, her muscles will remain essentially the same size and will increase in density and strength. But the fat surrounding the muscle will burn off, resulting in higher definition and a shapelier, more chiseled, leaner look. She'll love herself—and you for introducing her to the program. And if the two of you continue to enjoy getting and staying fit together—well, that's what it's all about, isn't it?

3

TUNING THE SUSPENSION: EXERCISES FOR STRETCHING, LIMBERING, AND RELAXATION

•

No serious exerciser goes directly into a heavy workout without some kind of warm-up. There are a number of good reason why this is so, and we ought to explore these reasons before we launch into our program.

First, if you've gotten into a sedentary rut, your muscles are probably stiff, weak, and unused to stress. Further, if you want to get the most out of each exercise period, you'll want to avoid overdoing it when you first start out. Consequently, it's a good idea to stretch and limber up your muscles before you start a full-fledged weight training program. You should do some stretches as a warm-up at the beginning of each workout. You can use stretching and limbering exercises in two ways: to get yourself ready to begin a strenuous, long-range exercise program; to get the muscles ready to be stressed at the beginning of each exercise period.

Second, if you swing right into a strenuous program without any preliminaries, you'll probably pull something, which will simply set you back a couple of weeks in getting started. So take it easy at first, and slide into heavy exercise slowly. The gains will come soon enough, and you won't be haunted by aches and pains during the ensuing months.

Even stretching exercises can be strenuous, as many a person has learned trying to keep up with the advanced *karatekas* as they go through the stretches that mark the beginning of any karate workout. For many people, a good stretching routine is exercise enough while they make the passage from a sedentary life-style to an active one. Stretching done in this way becomes a form of calisthenics, and while it doesn't earn many points as a cardiovascular conditioner, it will go a long way toward showing you how out of shape you really are.

There are other reasons for taking it easy at first. If you've never done strenuous exercise, preliminary stretching and limbering can serve as a sort of shakedown cruise, to see if you are going to float or sink. Most people start an exercise program with a visit to their physician. Not a bad idea, especially if they have any idea that something may be wrong that would preclude an exercise program.

A general physical is a good idea anyway, a bit of preventive maintenance for the body machine. You might balk at the idea of things like stress tests, however, because they not only show you what your limits may be but can also take you beyond your limits and into dangerous territory that could have been avoided if you had simply started a slow, sure routine of exercises. A dear friend of ours, recovering from a heart attack, was given a stress test to see how far he had progressed. It popped him right into another heart attack. Ralph was given a stress test (by error) less than twenty-four hours after surgery several years ago. In addition to the premature atrium contractions that started when his pulse reached 190, fifteen minutes on the treadmill without adequate footwear permanently damaged his left arch. No more running for him.

What we're saying is this: if you want to get a checkup before going on a strenuous program, be sure that you go to a doctor who knows something about the effects of systematic exercise on the human body. Go to an exercise physiologist or an expert in sports medicine. Call up the physician who looks after the local pro ball club, or who specializes in the treatment of amateur athletes. Doctors are specialists and just as you wouldn't expect the rocket ceramic throat liner specialist to understand the electronic circuitry on your Apollo spacecraft, you shouldn't expect precise and comprehensive knowledge of exercise physiology from someone who specializes in the diagnosis of internal medical problems.

Sports-medicine experts such as Dr. Gabe Mirkin constitute a new breed of physicians, and we can't applaud their efforts enough. So if you have problems, or if you think you might have problems, see a physician. If you want sound advice on the benefits and avoidable hazards of exercise, see a sports-medicine physician.

Given a clean bill of health, you are then ready to start some exercises. Before you swing into the heavy stuff, start with some sensible stretches. Here are some of the stretching and limbering exercises used by the Japan Karate Association and the All-America Karate Federation before their workouts. They are among the best possible exercises of their kind. If you keep them up, you'll become more supple, have better timing, and lay the foundation for the weight training exercises that are to follow.

MARTIAL-ARTS STRETCHES AND FLEXES

NECK ROLLS

As you will learn from your workouts, your neck is probably a lot stiffer than you thought. Many of the lifts, such as the shoulder shrug and squats with the bar behind the neck, will make the neck feel even stiffer. Let's begin by loosening it up.

Front and Back Roll

Stand erect, hands resting on the hips, and bow your head to the front as far as you can. Try to touch your chin to your chest. Now slowly move the head backward and try to touch the upper back with the back of the head. Of course, you won't be able to move your head that far in either direction, but these are the directions you should move in. As in all stretches, move slowly and don't bounce (you'll pull something if you do). Do ten repetitions, with each full movement constituting one rep.

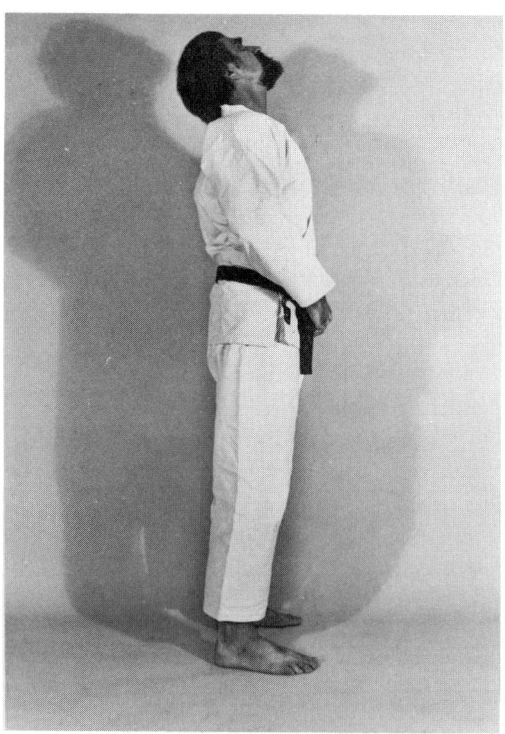

FRONT AND BACK NECK ROLL

Side-to-Side Roll

While continuing to stand erect, move your head from side to side as far as you can. Try to touch your ears to your shoulders. Don't lean the torso, but instead do all the movements with the head. Be especially careful on this one, because if you bounce or if you jerk your head over too far before the muscles get warmed up, you may spend tomorrow with a "crick" in your neck. Do ten reps.

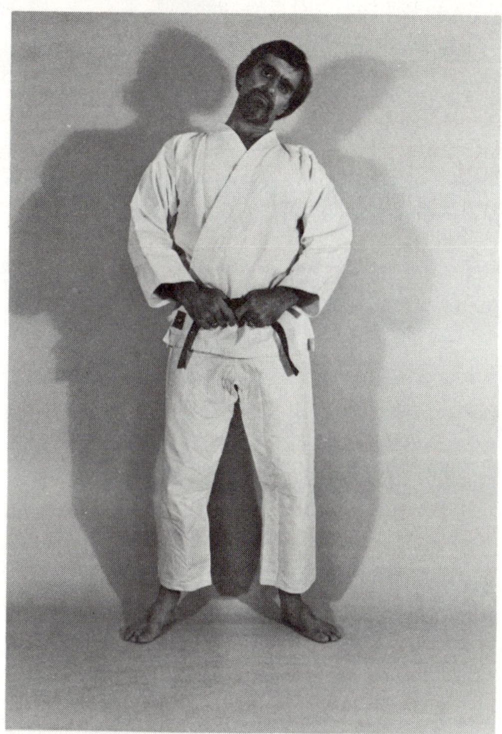

SIDE-TO-SIDE NECK ROLL

Revolving Roll

We were told recently by a TV performer that this one is injurious to the spine because of the way the neck bones are formed. Hundreds of thousands of *karatekas* have been doing this exercise for decades with no ill effects. It may make you dizzy at first, but that is an indication of how out of shape you are. Here goes. While staying in the same erect stance, imagine that your head is a ball attached to your chest by a thick cable. Start with the chin on the chest, and roll the head around to the right, keeping the chin down. As you round the shoulders, lift your chin as if you were going to describe a circle in front of you. Keep the head back as far as it will go throughout this portion of the movement, and bring the chin down to the left shoulder as the head rolls around to that side of the body. Continue until the chin reaches the chest again. Do five repetitions to the right, and then reverse and do five repetitions to the left. Do each repetition slowly, and with as much relaxation of the muscles as you can muster. You'll hear some crackles and pops, but no snaps. Ralph has arthritic spurs in his neck, and the movement helps him to prevent the stiffness that usually accompanies such a condition.

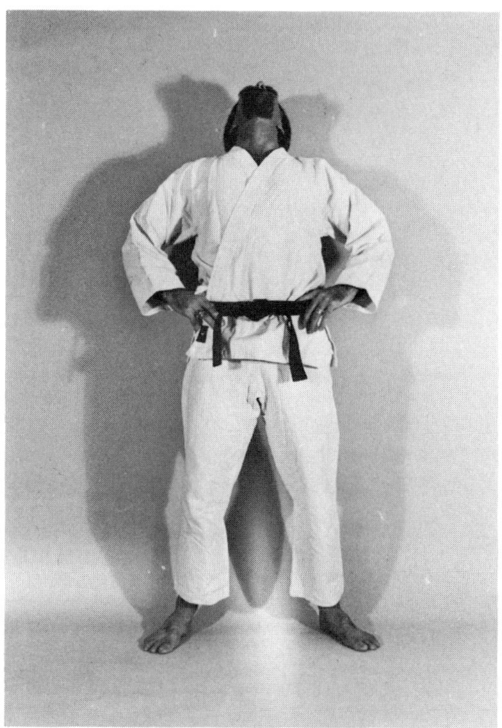

REVOLVING NECK ROLL

UPPER BACK AND PECTORAL STRETCHES AND FLEXES

Now, let's get the upper back and chest limbered up. Stand erect for these exercises.

Straight-Arm Stretch Overhead

Extend your arms overhead, and clasp the hands together. Keep the elbows straight but not quite locked. Now arch your back and lean backward as far as you can, while pulling your arms back in the direction of the movement. You'll feel your latissimus (underarm) muscles stretch on this one, and you will also feel the muscles bunch up at the base of the neck. Do ten repetitions.

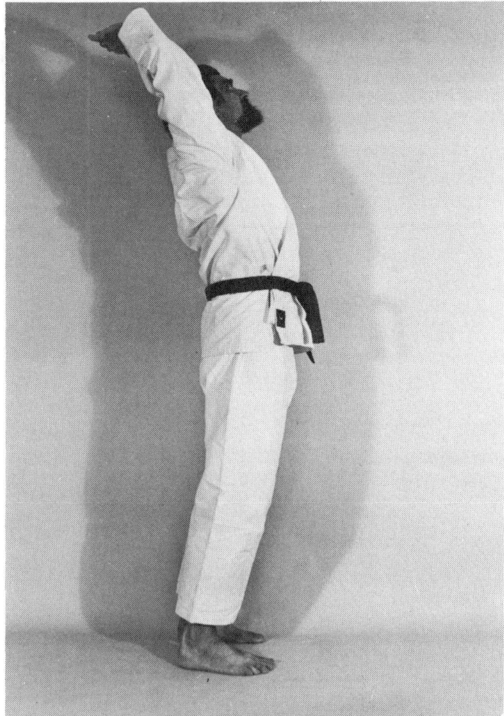

STRAIGHT-ARM STRETCH OVERHEAD

Straight-Arm Stretch to the Sides

Extend your arms in front of you, palms facing each other. Then bring the arms back, elbows almost locked, until the arms are at the sides as far as they will go. The arc made by the arms should be parallel to the floor. In this exercise, you will stretch the chest muscles while at the same time flexing the upper back muscles.

Bent-Arm Shrug

This is not one of the karate stretches, but is a good addition to them. Stand erect, with your arms down by the sides, palms facing the rear. Raise your arms straight up to the sides, while simultaneously bending them at the elbows. As you bend the arms, keep raising them as you shrug your shoulders and try to touch your deltoids to your ears. The forearms should be pointed toward the floor, and the elbows should come as high as you can get them. This exercise will flex the trapezius (upper back) muscles and the front and lateral deltoids (shoulder muscles), while stretching the latissimus muscles. Do ten reps.

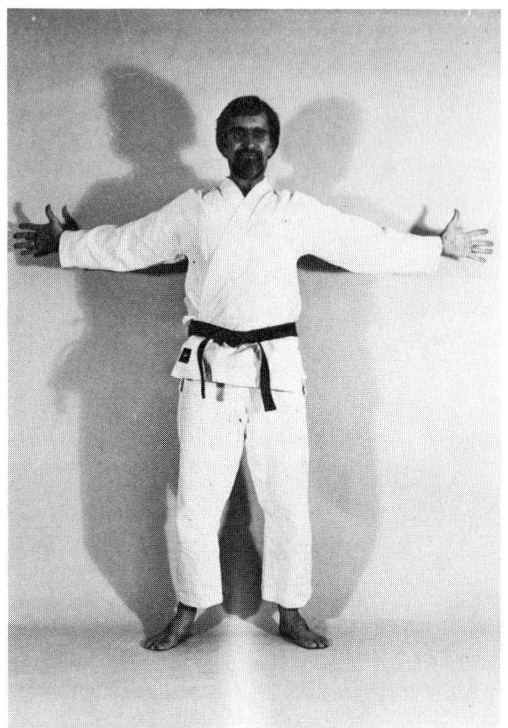

STRAIGHT-ARM STRETCH TO THE SIDES

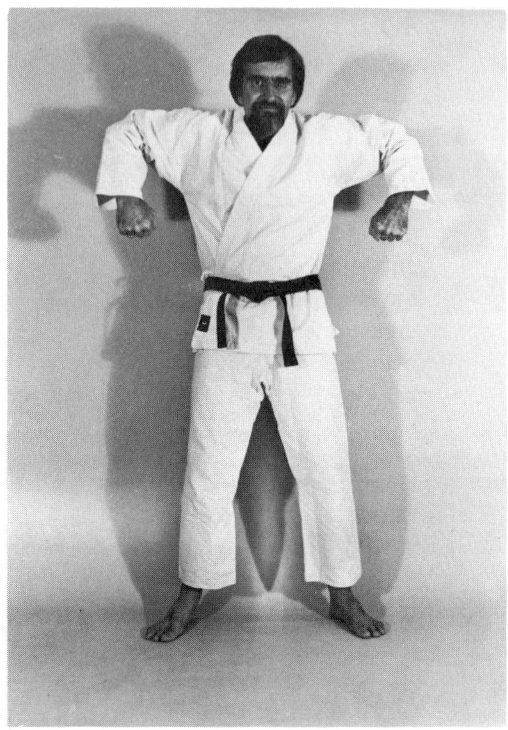

BENT-ARM SHRUG

Pectoral Stretches Lying on the Side

In addition to the pec stretch you get when doing the exercises listed above, you can get an even greater one this way: Lie on the floor on your right side and extend your arm toward the ceiling, stretching as far upward as it will go; then slowly move the arm back in an arc at about a forty-five-degree angle to the upper body. You'll feel the pectoral stretch as you do the movement. Do ten reps, then turn over on your left side and repeat the movement with the left arm.

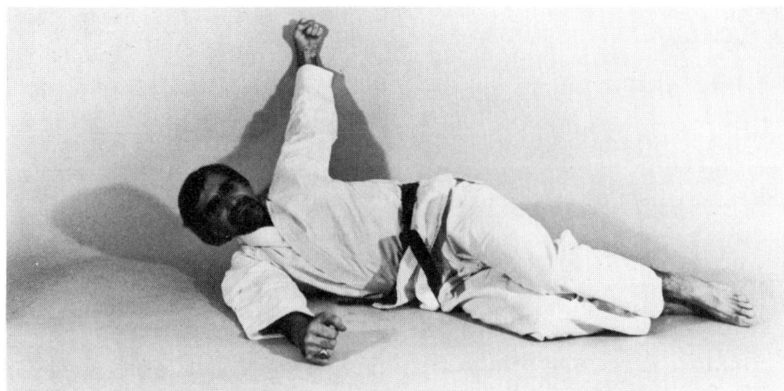

PECTORAL STRETCH LYING ON THE SIDE

SHOULDER SHAKERS

Your deltoids will already be slightly warmed up from doing the upper back and pectoral stretches. Now let's go after them directly.

Windmills to the Side

Stand erect, with your arms down by your sides. Start a propeller movement with the arms, keeping them in a plane perpendicular to the floor. Start by swinging the arms to the front, making a full circle. Start slowly, and increase the speed as you count up the reps. Do five reps; then reverse the movement so that you swing the arms in a circle to the back for five more reps.

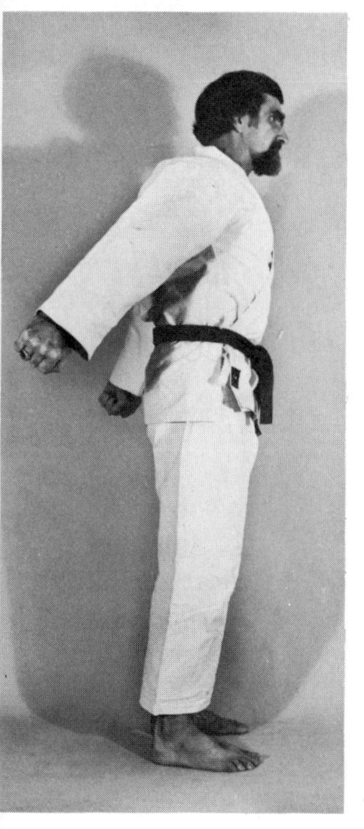

Step 1

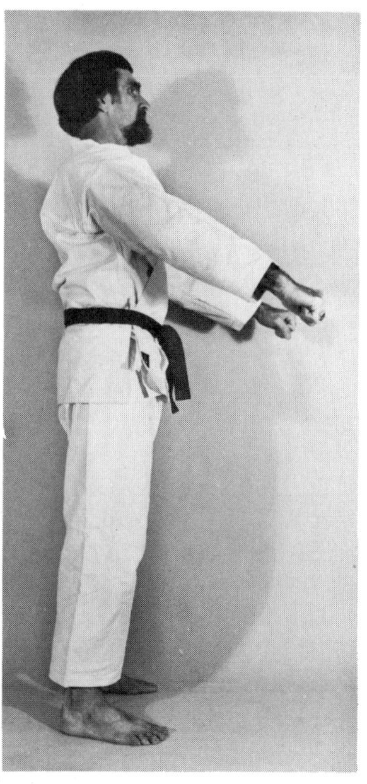

Step 2

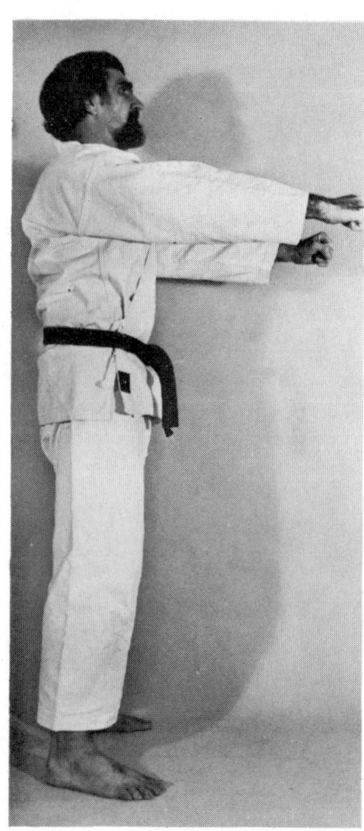

Step 3

WINDMILL TO THE SIDE

Windmills to the Front

Now swing smoothly into a movement where the arms cross in front instead of making their circles at the sides. Interleave the arms as they swing around. Do five reps, and reverse the swing for five more reps.

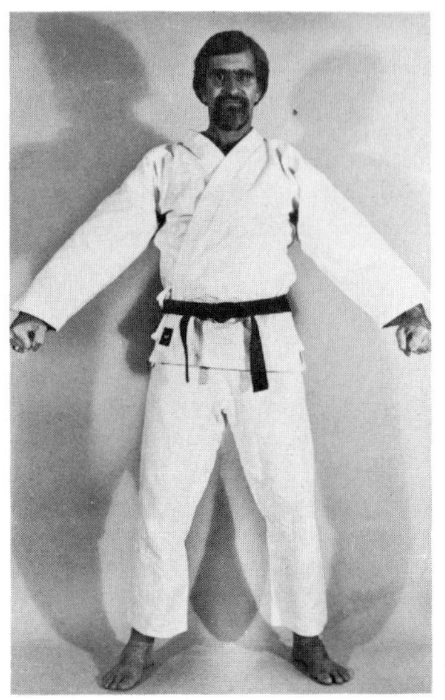
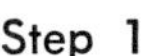

Step 1

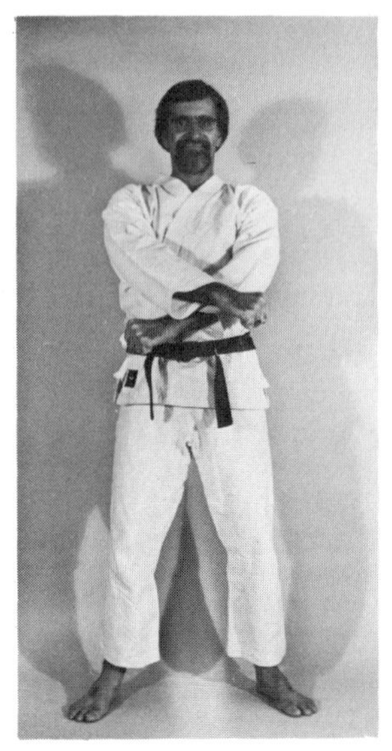

Step 2

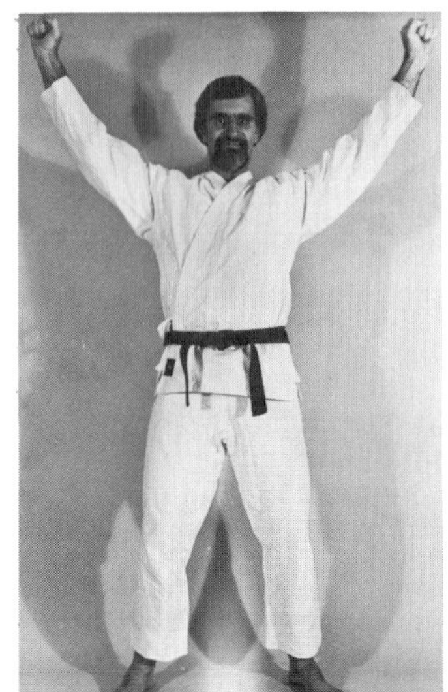

Step 3

WINDMILL TO THE FRONT

WAIST WRINGERS

You're warmed up to the waist. Now let's get the blood moving around your middle.

Front Slumps

Bend slowly at the waist toward the front, as if you were going to tuck your head in between your knees (which you will be able to do after a few weeks of this). Don't bounce, and do the movement very slowly. This is a good stretcher for the lower back, but if you have injured discs or pulled back muscles it will aggravate the condition. So take it easy and do the movement slowly. The point here is to stretch the lower back muscles without pulling anything. When you've gone as far forward as you can go, then pull yourself up to a standing position again. Do ten repetitions, pausing for a count of three at the bottom of the movement.

Side Leans

Stand erect; put your arms overhead with the hands clasped. Cock the right hip up, and then lean the upper body to the right. The point of cocking the hip up is to put more of a stretch on the opposite side. Lean as far as you can go, and return to the erect position. Do five reps, then five reps for the other side.

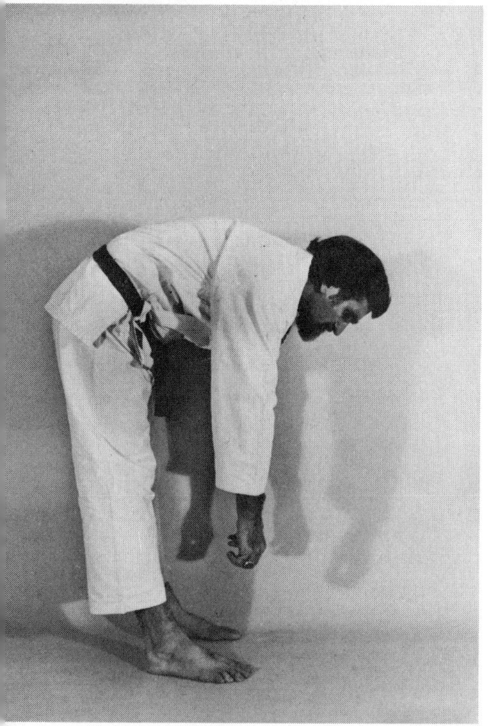

FRONT SLUMP

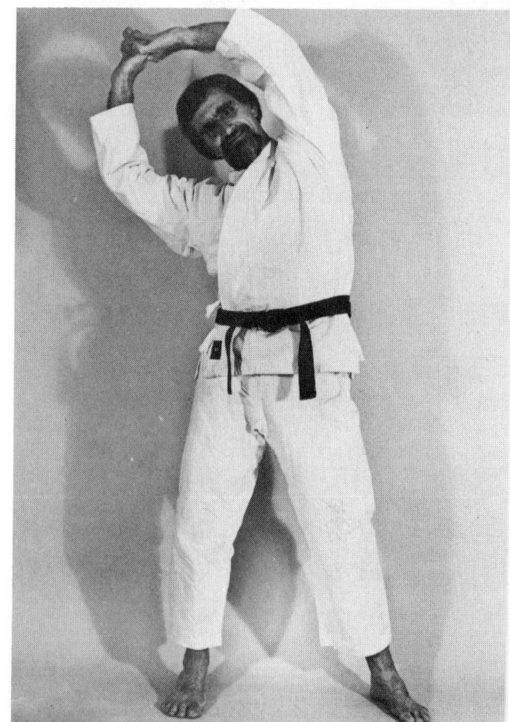

SIDE LEAN

Seated Twists

Place a broomstick behind your neck, and extend your arms out so that your hands clasp the stick toward the ends. Sit down on the floor or on a bench in order to immobilize your hips. Twist as far as you can in either direction, rotating the body at the waist. Work up to where you are doing these twists with considerable speed. This will stretch the intercostals in the front and sides under the arms, as well as the abdominals. Do thirty reps.

HIP UNHINGERS

The hip muscles are essential to full squats, and they should be stretched and flexed during a warm-up just like all the other muscles. They'll get some limbering from the front leg swings. Now try these exercises.

Front Leg Swings

Stand erect, and extend your right arm out in front of you, palm facing the floor. Bring your right leg up with the knee locked, until the toe hits

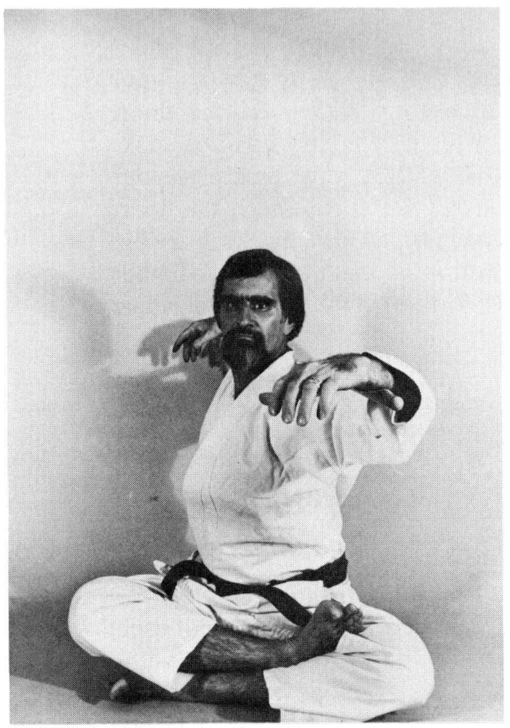

SEATED TWIST

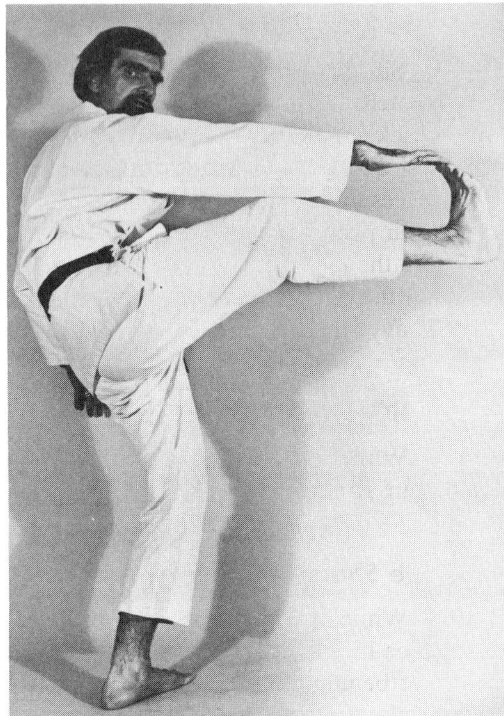

FRONT LEG SWING

the palm of the hand. Do ten reps, then try the other leg and arm for another ten reps. This will stretch the hip muscles while flexing the abdominals and the tie-ins between the pelvis and the thighs.

The Rocket Thruster

Lie on the floor on your back, with your feet pulled up as far toward the hips as they will go. Then thrust the hips high into the air while flexing the buttocks. Hold for a count of three, then go back to the floor. Do ten repetitions.

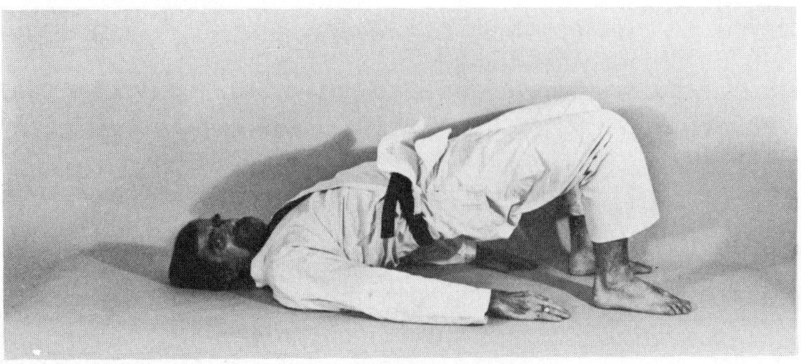

THE ROCKET THRUSTER

The Trailing Arms Suspension

Sit on the floor with your knees bent, feet pulled up toward your crotch, soles of the feet together, and sides of the feet on the floor. Tuck the feet in as far toward you as they will go. The knees will be sticking up at about a forty-five-degree angle. Now place your hands on your knees and push them down until the sides of your thighs touch the floor. You probably won't be able to do this movement at first, but keep trying. Do the movement slowly, and really push with your hands. This will limber up the whole area where the thigh fastens to the pelvis, and it will make heavy squats with weights easier. Do ten reps.

THIGH AND KNEE STRETCHES

While you're still on the floor with the hip exercises, you can finish off your stretching and limbering session with two final exercises.

The Shock-Absorber Stretch

While seated on the floor, stretch your legs out in front of you until each knee locks. That's the easy part. Now reach over and grasp your toes without bending your knees. Easy now, because this stretches both the lower back and the backs of the knees. Hold for a count of three, relax, then try it again. Do ten reps.

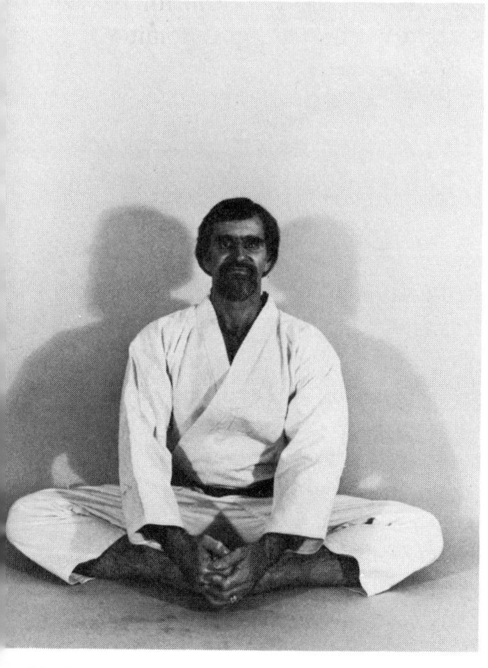

THE TRAILING ARMS SUSPENSION

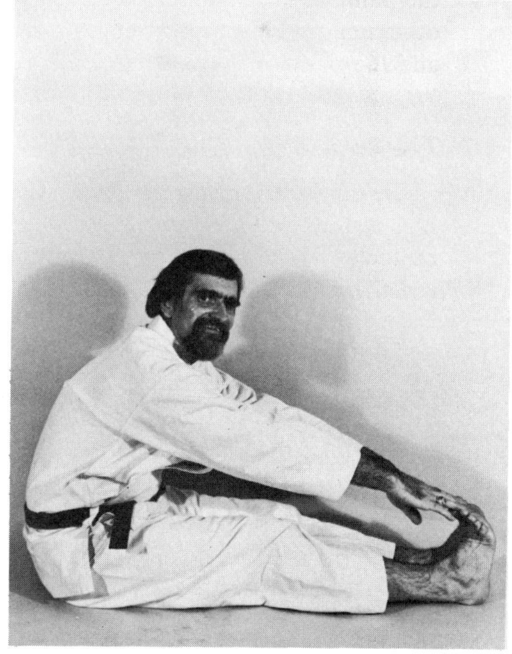

THE SHOCK-ABSORBER STRETCH

The Independent-Suspension Stretch

Stand erect, then go down on your right leg until the leg is fully bent at the knee and your right hip is resting on your right ankle. The left leg should be extended out from the body to the side—heel on the floor, toes pointed toward the ceiling. Your upper body should be upright, and your left hand should be on your left leg, just above the knee. You may have to rest on the ball of your right foot (few people can start off flat-footed on this one). Now rise up on the right leg, shift over, and come down on the left leg so that you are in the same position as before, but with the legs reversed. Shift from one leg to the other for a total of ten reps, each time coming up only far enough to make the shift. When you become able to do this movement easily and with some fluidity, you can count yourself among those who are really getting in shape. This one will develop your timing, improve your sense of balance, stretch the back of the legs, and build strength in the thighs and hips. It's an all-around fine exercise.

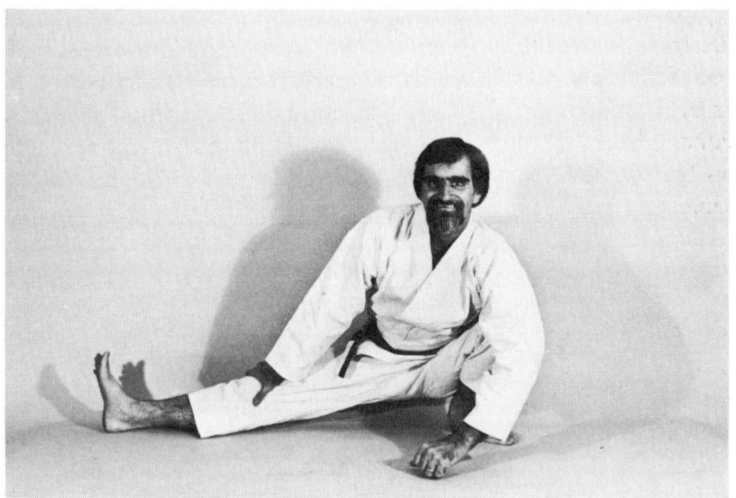

INDEPENDENT-SUSPENSION STRETCH

All the exercises in this section are one way to stretch out and limber up. In the next sections you will learn two more sets of exercises, some overlapping with the ones above. If you've done any yoga, you'll recognize some old friends. If you've ever done serious dancing, you'll be on familiar ground. Choose whichever method does the best for you, or develop a combination of all three types of exercises. They'll get you ready for the heavy stuff, and they'll also provide you with a fine repertoire of exercises to do when you are on the road and can't get to your weights.

YOGA MOVEMENTS FOR RELAXATION

The karate movements that you've just learned will help you become more agile and quicker. Now let's try some yoga movements to make you supple, limber, and relaxed. While yoga will not slim you or help to build muscle, it *will* help you learn proper breathing techniques, and make you more flexible, coordinated, and fluid in your movements. The positions also serve as instant de-tensers and energizers either in the morning, before the day's activities start, or in the evening, after a hard day's work. You can incorporate all or several of the positions into your regular warm-up before an exercise session, along with the karate and dance movements described in this chapter.

A few general words about yoga movements before we begin. First of all, remember that the object is not speed or lifting a heavy mass, but grace, flexibility, and coordination. Do each movement slowly, rhythmically, striving each time for a little more suppleness. Do each movement only to the extent that you don't feel pressure or strain. Don't force your back into a full plough position if it causes strain or pain. Settle for a simple half-shoulderstand and each day draw your legs back a little farther over your head until you can do the full movement easily. Remember: slow and easy is the key. You're not in competition with anyone, even with yourself.

Second, remember that regular, systematic breathing is very important. Always breathe through the nose, in and out, in a slow, deep rhythm. Try each time you inhale to expand your lungs and take in as much air as possible. Each time you exhale, try to empty your lungs completely. Never hold your breath during the yoga positions. The object is not merely to try to get your body into the correct posture, but also to learn to breathe properly—that is, deeply and rhythmically.

Third, try to practice your yoga positions under relaxed, unhurried conditions—no "three minutes of my yoga before I run for the bus." Wear loose, unconstricting clothing (lounging pajamas, a jogging suit or shorts, or a karate *gi* are ideal) and have the room properly ventilated. Better still, do the exercises outdoors if you can. The fresh air is an added plus and promotes relaxation.

Ready? Let's try some simple warm-ups first as a prelude to the more difficult postures.

1. *Breathing posture*: This exercise is a good overall warm-up. Stand with your feet about shoulder width apart. Now inhale deeply. Clasp your hands behind your back and arch backward. As you exhale, bend forward as far as possible without bending your knees and hold for three complete breaths. Relax and return to the standing position again. Repeat three times, remembering to move slowly and breathe deeply for best results.

2. *Meditation postures*: These three postures are traditional yoga positions for breathing and meditation. The first, the *easy posture,* is done sitting cross-legged on the floor, one ankle crossed in front of the other, hands resting on the knees. As you sit, maintain the posture and breathe deeply for five complete breaths, inhaling and exhaling slowly. As you become more "advanced," try the *half-lotus*. Cross the legs so that the right ankle rests on the left thigh. Palms should rest easily on the knees. Again, take five complete breaths. The most advanced of the postures is, of course, the *full lotus*. In this posture the ankle of each foot is resting on the opposite thigh so that the legs are literally intertwined. Palms can rest on the knees or on the floor. Save this one for a more advanced stage unless you're very supple and limber. And remember to count five complete breaths before going on to the next posture.
3. *The sun greeting*: This is not only a warm-up but also a complete series of exercises. It's an excellent combination of yoga positions and deep-breathing sequences. Here's a step-by-step guide:
   A. Stand straight with legs together, and hands together with fingers touching in "prayer" position. As you stand, exhale all the air in your lungs.

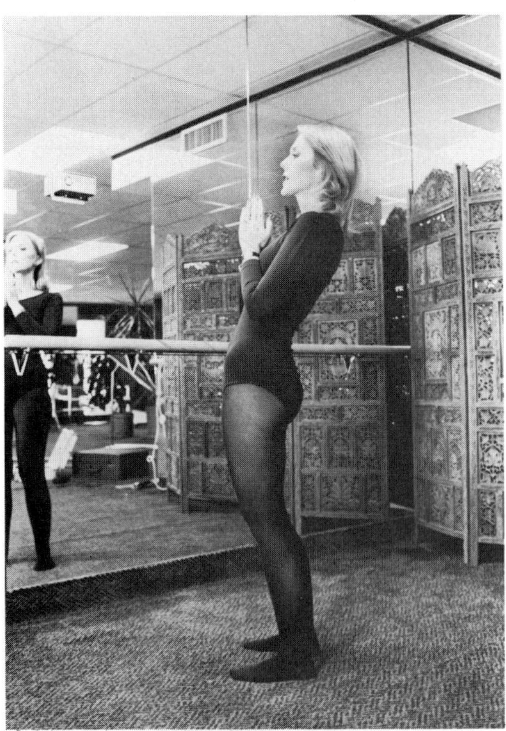

SUN GREETING

B. Now inhale deeply. Raise your arms high above your head and then arch backward as far as you can.

C. As you exhale, bend forward slowly, reaching down as far as possible. Keep the feet together and don't bend the knees. But don't strain your back by reaching back too far. The object is not to touch the floor but simply to bend forward as far as you can do so comfortably. Be sure you completely empty your lungs as you exhale.

D. Now place your hands on the floor and assume a partially kneeling position. Inhale and bend your left leg up toward your chest as you step back onto the right leg. Keep your head up and remember to inhale deeply, completely filling your lungs with air.

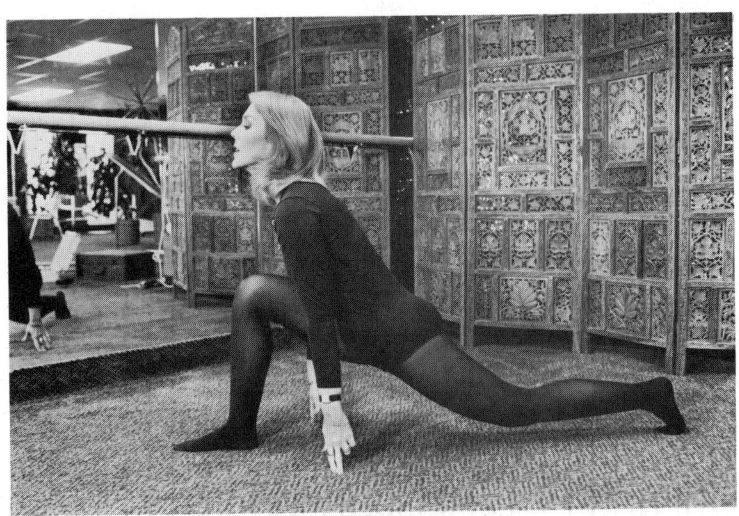

SUN GREETING

E. Now exhale as you step back into a "pushup" position. Stretch both legs out together so that your body is supported only by your hands and toes. Keep your body stiff and remember to exhale completely as you do so.

F. Now continue exhaling as you lower first your knees, then your chest and chin, to the floor. Try to keep it all one continuous motion. Arms should be extended on the floor in front of you.

G. Now slide onto your stomach with your legs extended fully behind you. Your chest and forehead should rest on the floor.

H. As you inhale, rise slowly into *the cobra position* by straightening your arms. Keep your head up and back. Toes should be pointed, feet together, thighs flat on the floor. Do the posture as fully as you can, but don't strain. Straighten your arms as far as you comfortably can and try for a little more each time.

I. Now begin exhaling as you lower yourself back to position G with legs behind you, chin and chest on the floor.

J. Continue exhaling as you raise your hips up off the floor so that your body forms a triangle. Lock your chin into your chest, look at your feet, and try to force your heels all the way down to the floor.

K. Inhale again as you step forward with the right foot, backward on the left. (This is the reverse of position D, in which the left foot was forward and the right extended.)

L. Exhale and bring the left leg forward beside the right leg. Bend forward as far as possible. Keep the feet together, knees straight, and make sure to empty your lungs completely as you exhale.

M. Inhale again and return to position B. Arms should be raised over the head and the back arched as far back as is comfortable.

N. As you exhale, repeat opening position A. Relax for a few minutes now that the whole sun greeting has been completed.

4. *The cat stretch*: Start this position on your hands and knees. Exhale so that you completely empty your lungs of air. Squeeze the air out with your diaphragm if necessary. As you inhale, lower your chin and chest to the floor, keeping the feet together and the toes pointed.

   Now exhale and arch your back like a cat. Bring the chin into the chest and keep the back bowed. As you inhale, extend your right leg back and upward. Arch your back and tilt your head back at the same time.

   Exhale and bring the right leg forward. Bring the knee up into your chest, lower your head, and try to touch your nose with your knee. Now repeat, this time with the left leg.

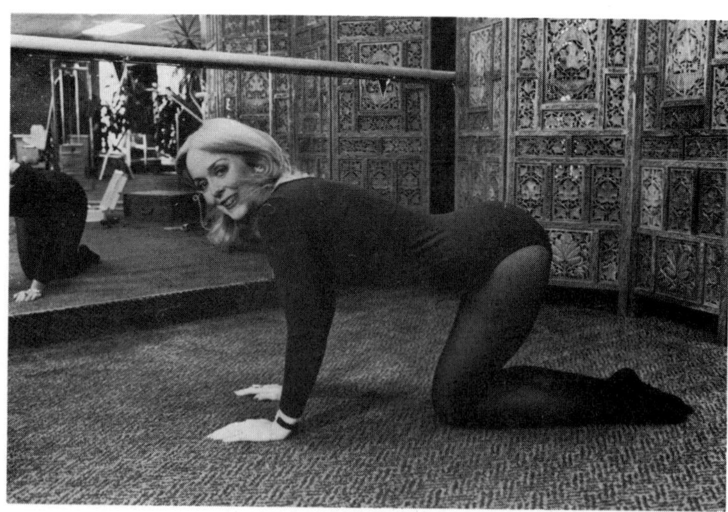

CAT STRETCH

After one repetition with each leg, relax into the *folded-leaf posture*: kneel on the floor, lower your chin to the floor, and extend your hands, palms up, behind you to either side. Hold this position for three complete breaths and then rise slowly as you inhale.

5. *Shoulderstand*: This is a basic posture and should be mastered before you try the plough position which follows. It's a fine all-purpose energizer and relaxer, aids circulation, and helps prevent fatigue and water retention. What more could you want?

   Lie on your back, with your arms to your sides. Exhale and then inhale, raising both legs slowly until they are perpendicular to the floor. Hold this position and exhale slowly as you hold it. Then inhale again, raising your hips all the way off the floor. Support them with your hands for added balance.

   This position is the *half-shoulderstand*. Hold the position for three complete breathing cycles and then try to straighten yourself to a completely vertical position (the *full shoulderstand*). Hold this position for five more complete breaths. Then come down very slowly. It helps to roll your back slowly onto the floor so that you don't hurt yourself by bouncing.

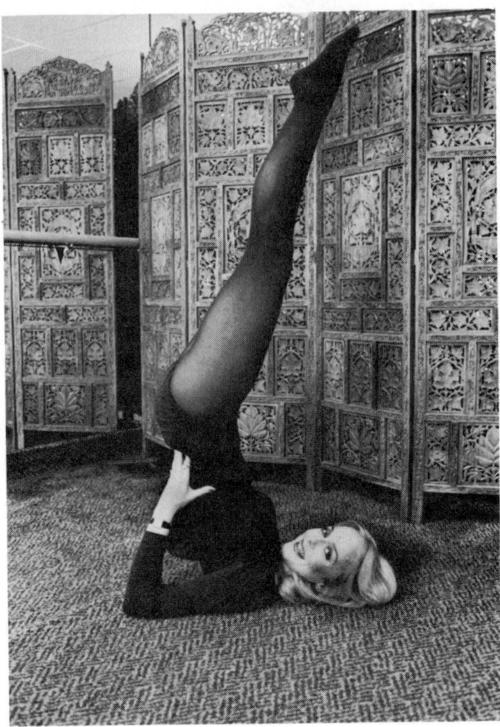

SHOULDERSTAND

6. *The cobra*: You should find this one easy since you have already incorporated part of this posture into your sun greeting exercise. Lie on your stomach with your arms by your sides and relax. Exhale completely. Then, as you inhale, lift your head up off the floor and bring your palms to a position just under your shoulders. Support yourself on your arms. Now arch your back as far as possible to attain a good stretch. Don't go any further than is comfortable—you should feel a stretch, but not a painful one. Inhale, hold for three complete breaths, and repeat the breathing cycle three times. As you become more supple, try arching your back even more until you are supporting yourself on your palms only. It's a great toner for spine and back muscles and is said to help digestion too!

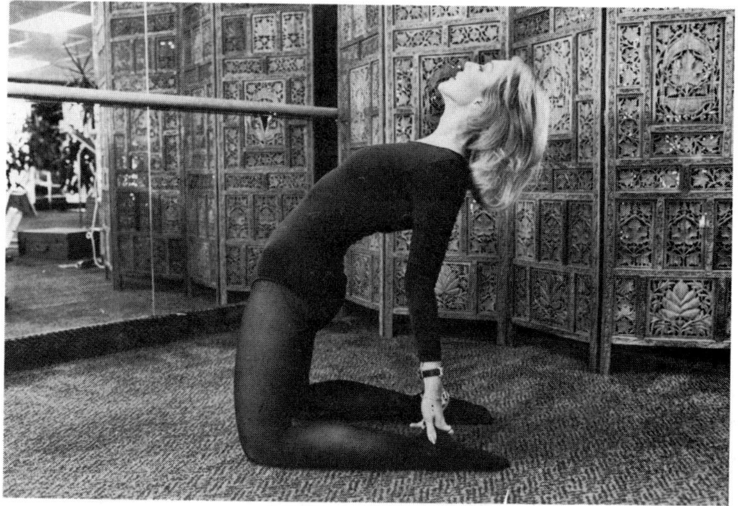

THE CAMEL

7. *The camel*: Begin by kneeling on the floor, sitting on your heels, in an easy, erect posture. Rest your hands on your knees. Exhale completely, and as you inhale rise up on your knees while swinging your arms behind your back. Stretch your arms as far back as they will go. Continue to inhale, and bring your arms up all the way behind your back and over your head. Stretch your whole body and gently start arching your back.

   Exhale and lower your arms down your sides so that they rest on your heels. Arch your back even further and let your neck relax. Hold the position for three complete breaths.

   Then relax into the folded-leaf posture for three more breaths to complete the exercise.

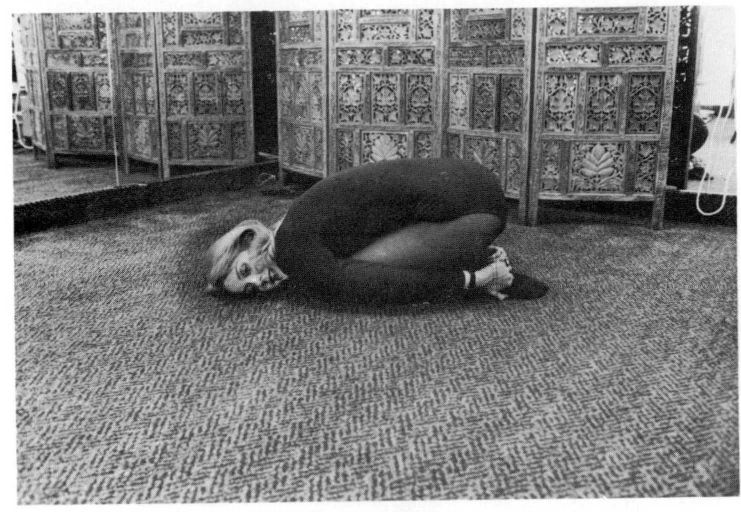

THE HARE

8. *The hare*: This posture is a counter-stretch for back-bending positions like the cobra.

Kneel on the floor, sitting on your heels, legs under you. Turn your toes down into the floor. First exhale, then inhale. As you exhale again, bend forward and pull your head toward your knees. Make sure your back is as rounded as you can make it. Hold this position while you exhale all the air in your lungs. Hold for five seconds, then rise slowly as you inhale. Repeat three times, and on the third repetition hold the head-into-knees posture for three complete breathing cycles.

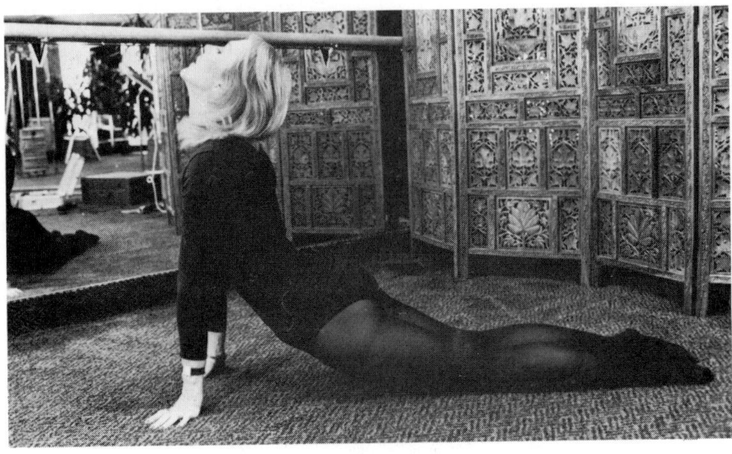

THE COBRA

9. *The fish*: This is a traditional counter-stretch for the shoulderstand and should be done immediately after either the shoulderstand or the plough.

   Lie on your back and prop yourself up on your elbows. You should be sitting on top of your hands, with the palms down. Holding this position, arch your back and throw your head back until you feel a stretch under your chin. Hold this position for five complete breaths. Then relax on your back again.

   As a variation, you can do the posture with your legs crossed, or in a half or full lotus. You'll find this position makes it easy to take those slow, deep breaths.

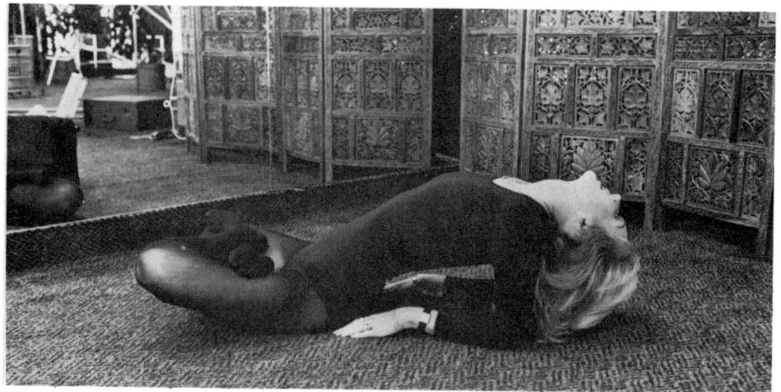

THE FISH

10. *Forward bend*: Sit on the floor with your legs stretched out straight in front of you. Exhale, and as you inhale stretch your arms high over your head. Exhale and bend forward slowly. Don't bend your knees, and keep your feet together. Repeat three times for three complete breaths. When you are finished, inhale and rise up slowly, then exhale and lower your arms to your sides again.

    This is a great stretch for the spine, calves, and thighs. It's also a good warm-up or cool-down after running or jogging.

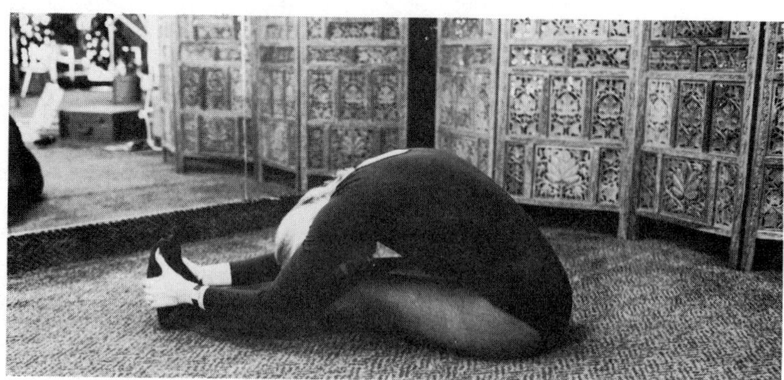

FORWARD BEND

11. *The twist*: Sit on the floor with both legs stretched out in front of you. Put your right leg over the left knee and rest your foot on the left side of the knee on the extended leg. Then twist your whole body to the right side, making sure both arms are on the right side of the right leg.

    Try to keep your left arm against the outside of your right leg for the maximum stretch. Hold this position for three complete breaths. Now repeat the whole twist with the left leg over the right. Isn't this a good stretch for the vertebral column?

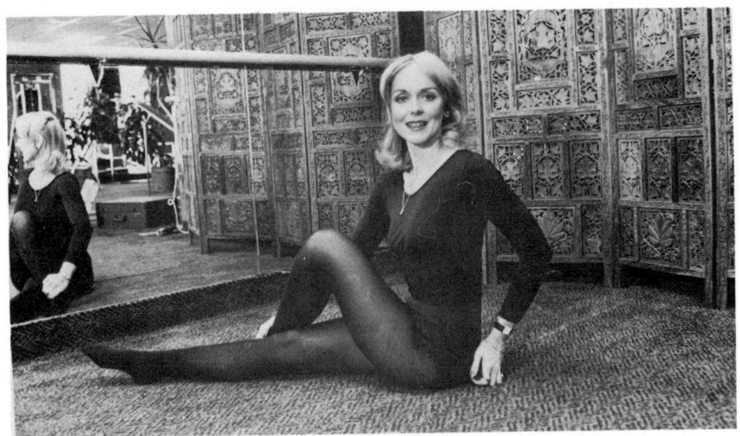

THE TWIST

12. *The boat*: Sit on the floor with your hands at your sides. Stretch your legs out in front. Exhale, and as you inhale lift your legs together to a forty-five-degree angle. Keep your arms extended out to the sides of your legs but not touching the legs. Hold for five complete breaths and return to the lying position. Repeat twice for maximum effect.

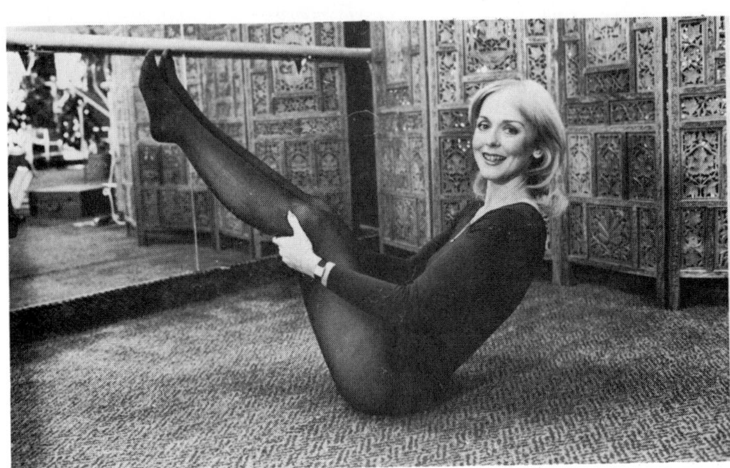

THE BOAT

13. *The recharge*: This is a breathing exercise rather than a "position" and is a good way to end the yoga workout. Sit on the floor in an erect posture—perhaps the easy posture or one of the lotus positions. Inhale and exhale a few times through the nose only. Exhale forcefully, pulling in the abdominal muscles as tightly as you can and driving the air out from your lungs. Make sure you do *all* breathing through the nose. Repeat four or five times, with all the emphasis on the exhaling motion. The inhalation should be just a fraction of a second.

When you have finished, close your eyes and relax for three complete breaths. Sit quietly in one of the three meditation postures, with your hands resting on your knees.

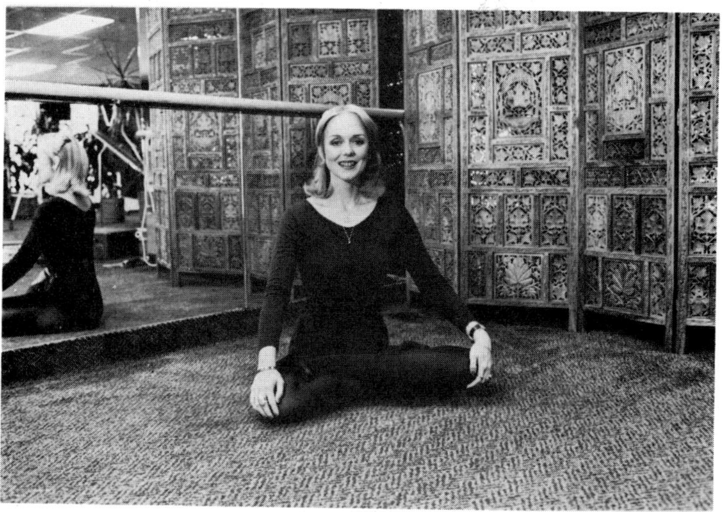

BREATHING POSTURE/RECHARGE AND FULL LOTUS

DANCE MOVEMENTS FOR STRETCHING AND LIMBERING

"What? Me dance?" you're probably saying. You're thinking Baryshnikov/John Travolta/José Greco/Nureyev. Then you visualize your own two left feet, your lack of coordination, and fall into a black funk.

Don't worry. There's no need for you to turn yourself into the world's greatest male disco/ballet/modern dancer in order to enjoy the benefits of this delightful and time-honored form of exercise. Dr. Leonore Zohman, director of cardiopulmonary rehabilitation at Montefiore Hospital in New York, recently put male cardiac patients on a dance routine and found that their fitness vastly improved after six months of steady dancing! She cites, in the June 1978 issue of *House and Garden,* the following benefits of dancing: increased heart rate for general conditioning; the possibility of pacing yourself to your own individual fitness level; increased joint and muscle flexibility, and increased coordination.

Add one more ingredient: dance is *fun,* and so you're less likely to become an exercise dropout than with a less varied program. Some exercises drawn from ballet, modern dance, and jazz dancing can all be incorporated into your personal fitness program.

SOME BALLET STRETCHES

1. *Grand plié*: For this exercise, and most of the ones to follow, you'll need a barre (use a chest top, sofa or chair back, or tall stool if there's no barre available). Stand with your feet together, toes pointing out (you'll feel awkward until you get the hang of it). Now slowly bend your knees, holding onto the barre for balance. You'll notice that your knees are pointing outwards if you're doing the motion correctly. Now go down even farther, letting your heels come up until you're touching the back of your hips with the heels. Don't "sit" and don't bounce. Rise by pressing your heels down and pulling yourself up with your thighs. Repeat eight to ten times.

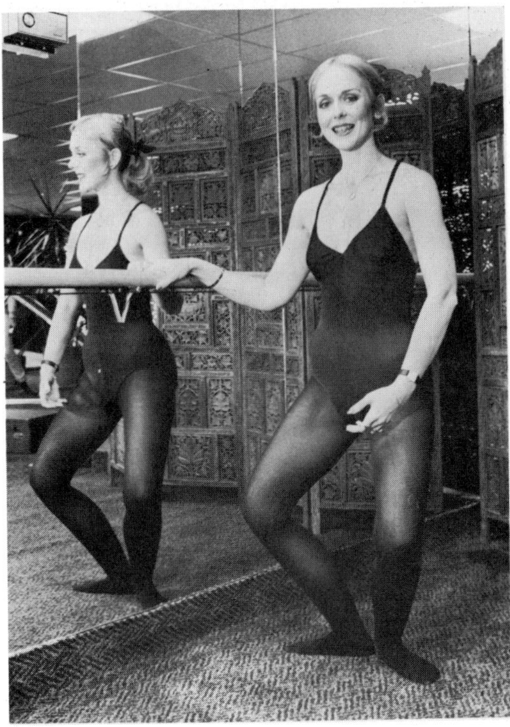

GRAND PLIÉ

2. *Port de bras*: Stand at the barre sideways—one hand on the barre, the other overhead. Now stretch out and over from the hips, making a huge arc with your body until the whole torso hangs down loosely. Touch your free hand to your toes and come sweeping outward. Your free arm should be overhead. Support the stretch in the torso from the abdominal area.

   Now bring yourself up straight again, stretching up and back at the same time. Focus on your hand to keep your balance. Arch back and stretch. Arch from above the waist and come up waist-first. "Roll" to the center, stretching up and out to avoid swaying your back. Now slide back to first position (feet together and turned out). Repeat eight times for each side.

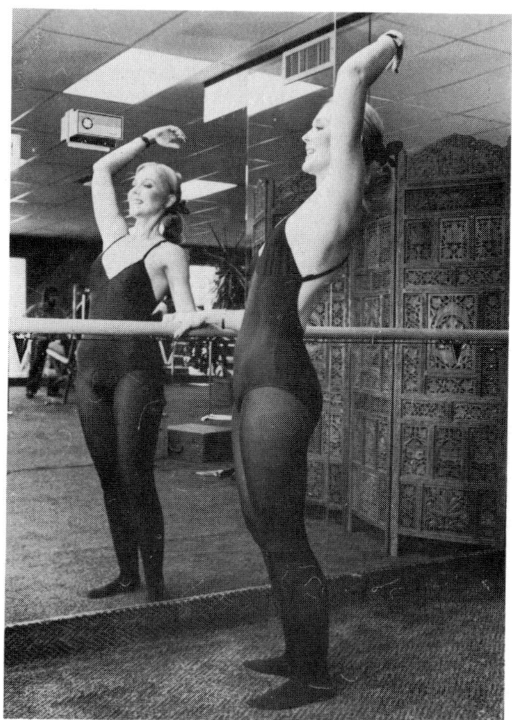

PORT DE BRAS

3. *Battement tendu*: Stand facing the barre, feet turned out in first position. Now slide your foot along the floor with heel forward, stretching, until only the toe touches the floor. Close (that is, return to your starting position) and repeat. Do eight repetitions for each side.
4. *Dégagé*: Stand facing the barre with both hands on it. Now lift ("disengage") your foot from the floor, starting with a *battement tendu* and stretching out even farther until the foot is just up off the

floor. Slide back to your first position and repeat eight times for each foot.

5. *Grand battement*: Begin by facing the barre, hands on the barre as if you were doing a *dégagé*. Now slide your foot along the floor, pointing and stretching until it leaves the floor and swings upward. Don't kick—swing it upward and control the movement. The lift should come from the foot, then from the back and inside of the leg. Stretch up on the supporting leg to keep your hips straight (you don't want them to shift). Close by sliding back to first position. Do eight to ten movements for each side.

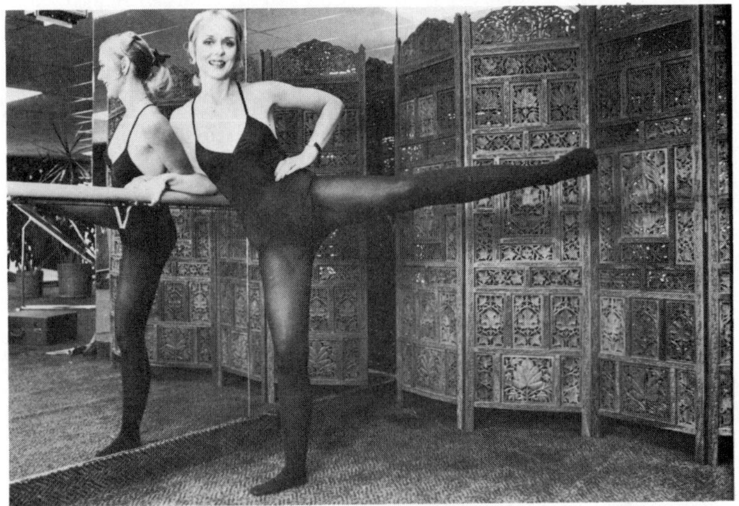

GRAND BATTEMENT

6. *Développé*: Stand facing the barre with your hands on it, and your feet in first position. Now pick up your foot by pointing the toe and touching it to the heel of the standing leg. Draw your foot up along the inside of the calf of the supporting leg until your toe touches the knee. Now bring the foot outward and up, keeping the heel forward to maintain the turnout. Extend the leg forward fully so that you feel a good stretch in the inside of the thigh and the back of the knee. Close with both knees straight (try to control the leg until you've lowered it completely). Repeat eight to ten times for each side.

Now for a change of pace. Forget the formality and precision of the ballet movements, the French names and the barre. Now your balance is your own, your movements freer and more improvised. Try these movements from modern-dance routines and feel those muscles stretch!

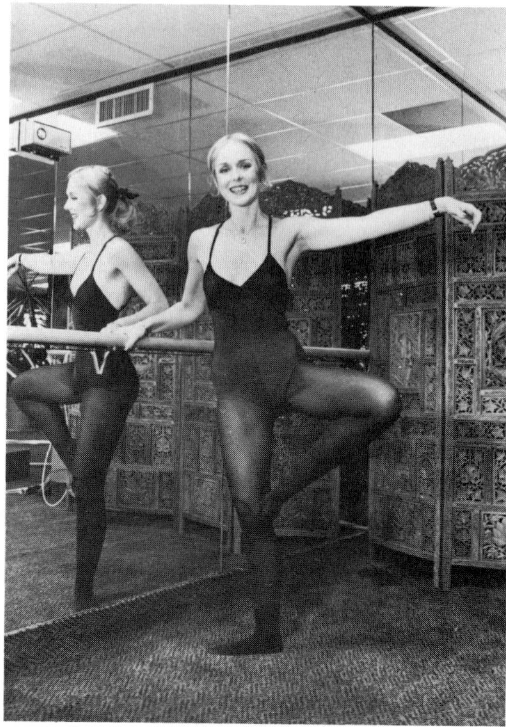

DEVELOPPÉ

SOME MODERN-DANCE STRETCHES

1. *Torso stretch*: Sit on the floor—one foot in front of you, the other behind. Sit up straight and raise your arms. Stretch out from the waist—first to the sides, then around and down to the floor in front of you, over to the opposite side, and back up again. Do this in one continuous sweeping motion. Keep your shoulders down and feel your arms move as part of your back. Try to keep the movement smooth and fluid. The stretch should be in your sides. Your abdomen should be doing all the "support" work; tuck it in as you move. Slowly lower your arms. Repeat six to eight times for each side.
2. *Lower abdominal and hip stretch*: Kneel on the floor on your hands and knees. Keep your back parallel to the floor. Now stretch one leg up and back while you lift your head and throw it back slightly. Next draw the leg in by contracting the abdominal muscles. Curve your back and tuck your head under. Bring your knee forward to your forehead so that you are curled up into a small ball. Now extend that same leg again, lift your head, and stretch. Return to starting position and repeat on the other side. Remember that the impetus for the movement always comes from the abdominal muscles. Repeat six to eight times for each side.

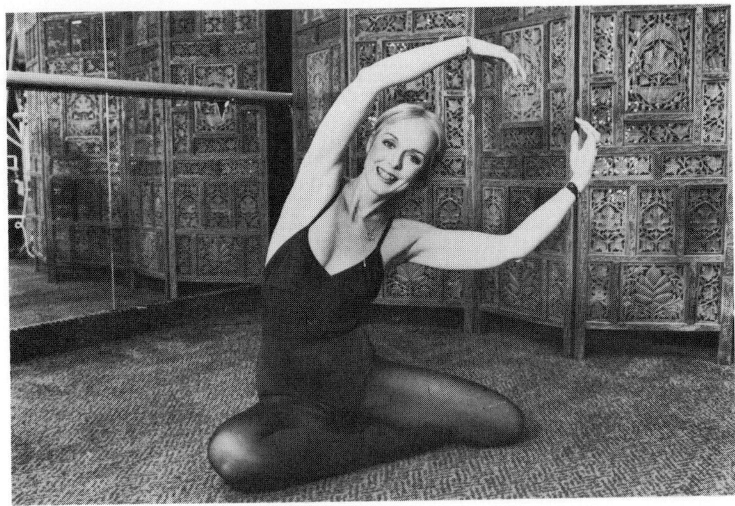

TORSO STRETCH

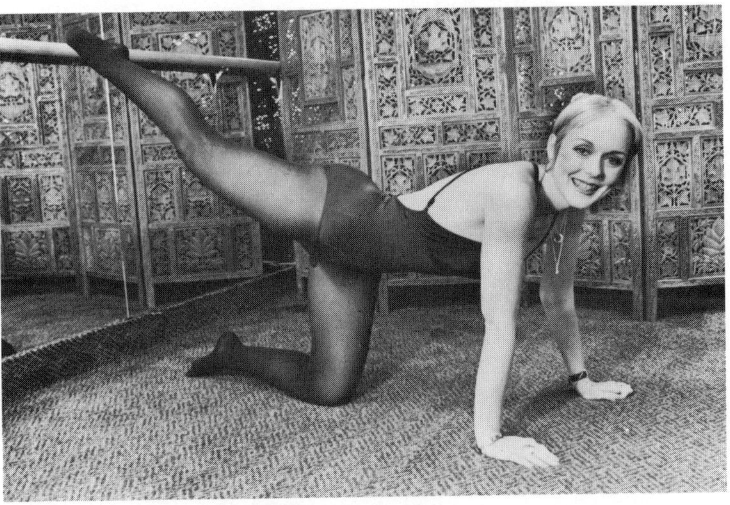

LOWER ABDOMINAL/HIP STRETCH

3. *Hamstring stretch*: Lie flat on your back on the floor with your arms down at your sides, palms against the floor. Draw one knee in close to you, touching your forehead with the knee. Now take hold of the leg just below the calf, holding on with both hands. Extend the leg as far overhead as you can. Feel the stretch in the back of the thigh and the knee. Slowly lower your neck and head to the floor. When the leg is fully extended, let go and slowly lower it to the starting position. Do this eight to ten times with each leg.

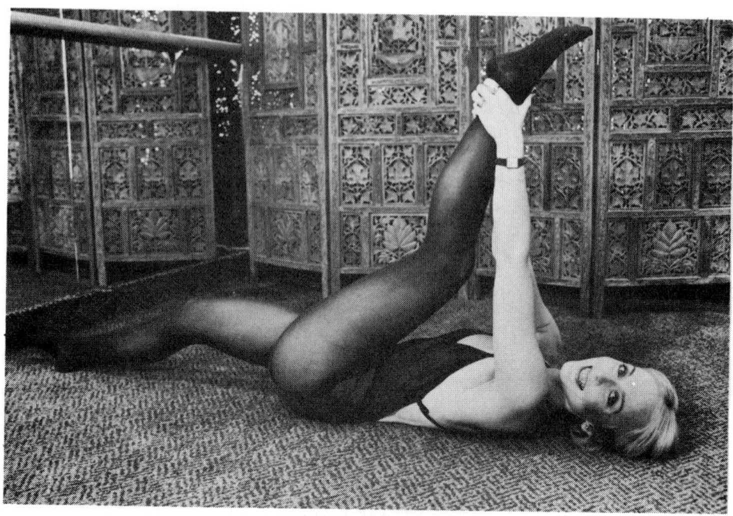

HAMSTRING STRETCH

4. *Buttock and thigh stretch*: Lie on your side and raise your top leg about a foot off the floor. Bring the bottom leg up to meet it, then down to floor again. Repeat ten to twelve times for each side.

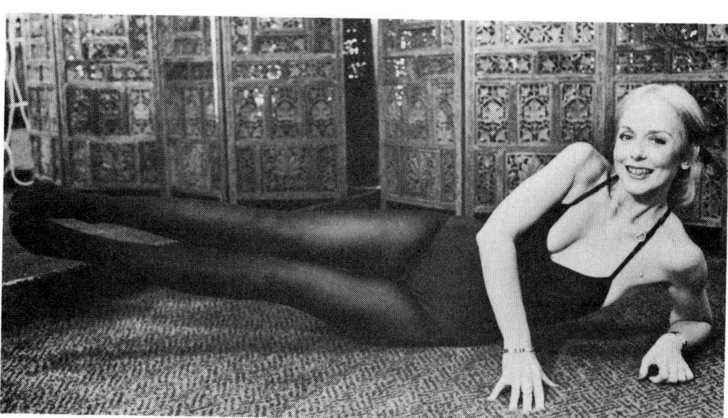

BUTTOCK AND THIGH STRETCH

5. *Waist and torso toner*: Stand with the feet apart about one shoulder width, hands on hips. Lean sideways as far as possible. Then lean forward so that both shoulders are parallel to the ground. In that position, sweep your upper body as far to one side as possible. Then twist up your front shoulder so that you're now leaning sideways. Straighten up and repeat in the other direction; do eight to ten reps for each side.

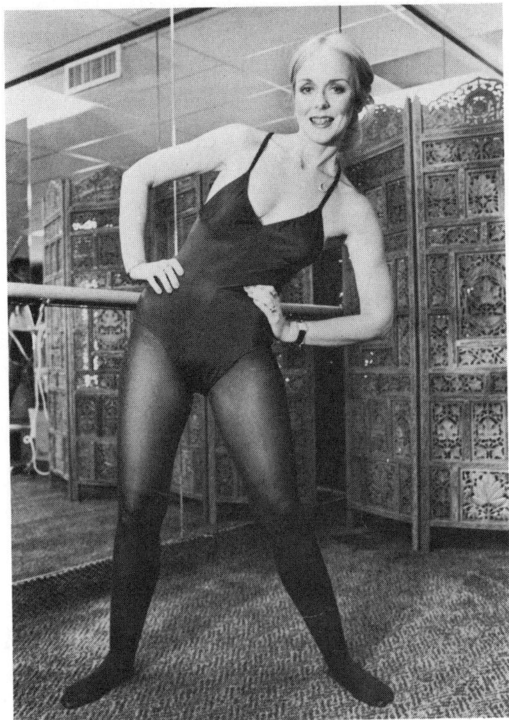

WAIST AND TORSO STRETCH

6. *Leg stretch*: Sit on the floor—knees bent, feet together, legs in front of you. Then straighten your left leg out and lift it high, grasping the ankle with both hands. Reverse legs and repeat. Then do the same with both legs raised together if possible. Begin with three to four reps for each side.

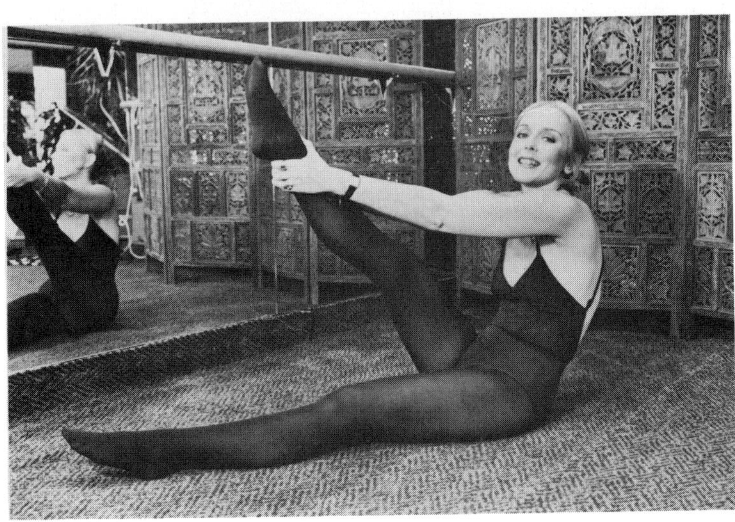

LEG STRETCH

7. *For your back and the backs of your legs*: Stand with legs spread about a shoulder width apart. Grasp one ankle as you bend over and lower your head to the knee of that leg. Switch legs and repeat. Do six to eight reps for each leg.
8. *Overall stretch*: Tuck one leg under you and extend one leg to the side. Then bend over and reach the toes of the extended leg. Straighten up and touch the bent knee (opposite leg) with your opposite hand. Switch legs and repeat six to eight times for each side.

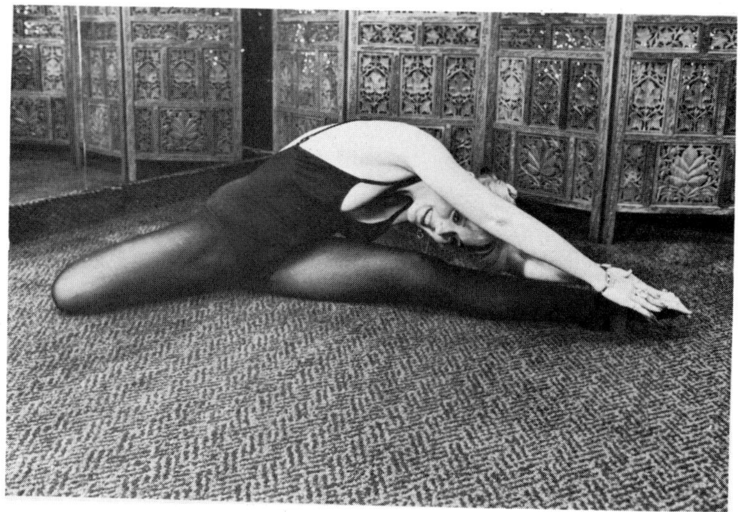

OVERALL STRETCH

9. *Thigh stretch*: Lift your left (or right) leg up in front of you onto a stool or chair back. Elevate onto your toes and push forward slowly until you feel the stretch in your thighs. Keep your back straight. Return to your original position and repeat ten times for each leg.
10. *Back-of-knee stretch*: Crouch into a knee bend and grasp your ankles. Then straighten your legs as much as you can, coming up slowly. Your aim is to touch your forehead to your knees. If you can't do this one completely, do it as well as you can and aim for the complete movement as your flexibility increases. Start with one rep and work up to five or more.

Finally, here are some basic movements from jazz and aerobic dancing. Some are just simple warm-ups and stretches; others are classy (and complex) enough to be incorporated into your latest disco routine. All are good stretches and will help you to tone, limber, relax, cool down, or warm up before your major training routine.

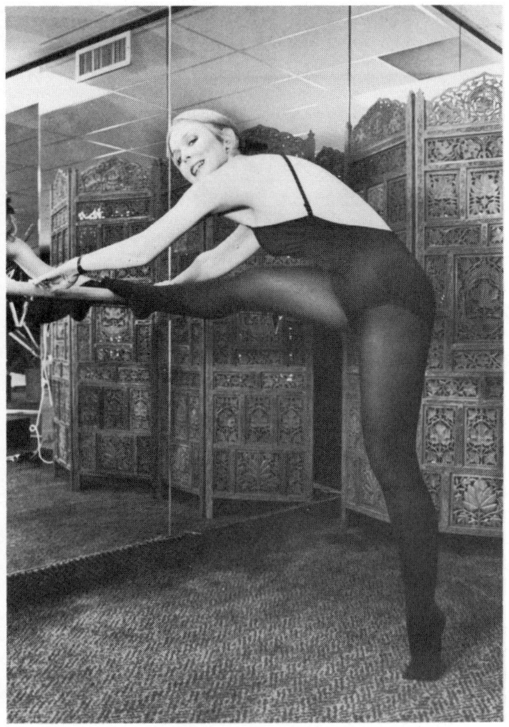
THIGH STRETCH

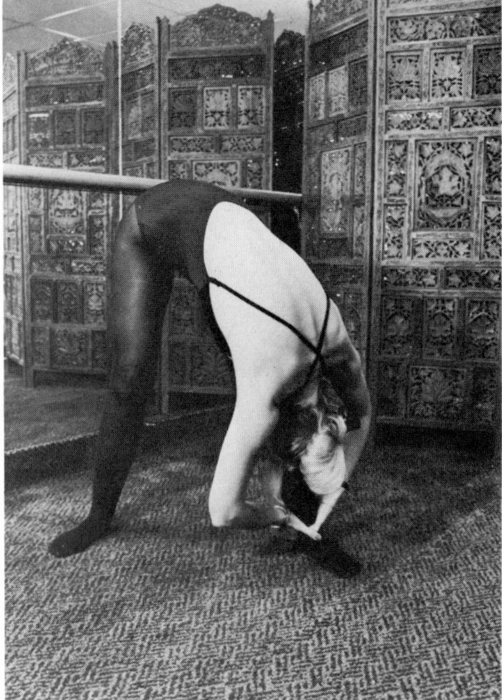
BACK-OF-KNEE STRETCH

SOME JAZZ-DANCING MOVEMENTS

1. *Aerobic/jazz warmup*: Start by stretching your right arm high up over your head. As you do so, lift your rib cage and feel it expand. Bend your right knee forward while you stretch your left leg back. (Keep both feet flat on the floor.) Repeat to left side.

   Now swing both arms to the back as far as you can stretch. (Your body should be parallel to the floor.) Bend at the waist as you do this. Then swing both arms high overhead and reach for the ceiling. Repeat entire movement eight to ten times for each side.

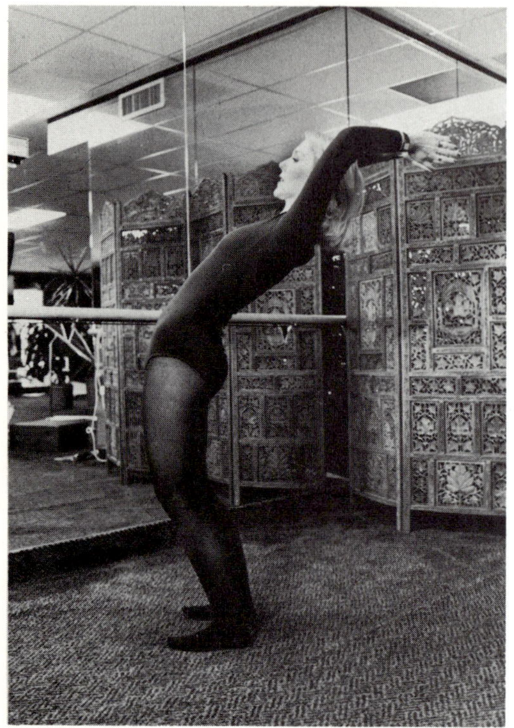

BASIC JAZZ WARM-UP

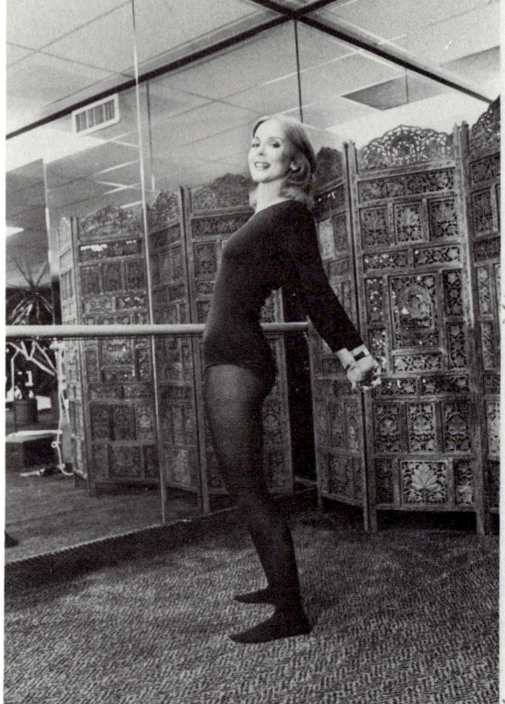

BASIC JAZZ WARM-UP

2. *Side Stretch*: Stand with your feet shoulders' width apart. Stretch your right arm to the right side and pull your rib cage to the right as you do so.

   Now reverse the movement to the left. Next, bend both knees and swing *both* arms over to the right. Exaggerate the motion and make the swing a pronounced one. Then repeat the motion to the left, and as you do it straighten both knees. Now bend the knees and swing back to the right. Repeat to the left. Do the full cycle of movements six to eight times on each side.
3. *Waist and midriff crunch*: Stand with feet about shoulders' width apart, with your hands reaching up toward the ceiling, palms facing in.

   Now bend to the left from the waist. You should feel a stretch to the right side as you do this. Try to do a side "crunch" as you bend so that the muscles on the left side are all contracted.

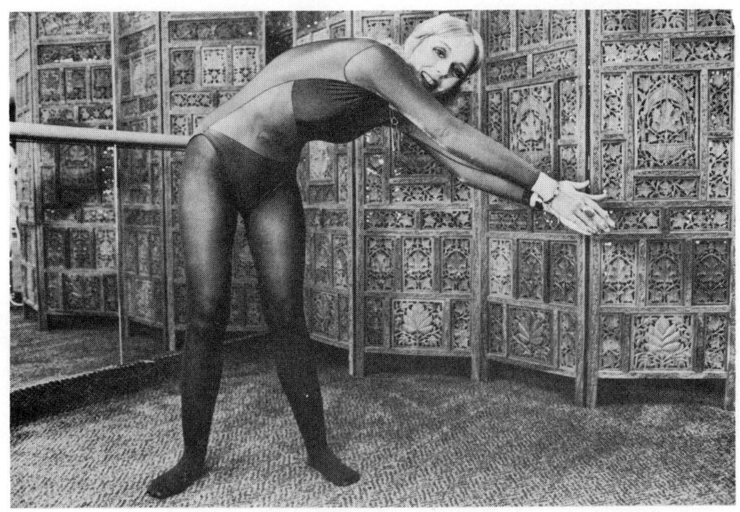

LATERAL STRETCH

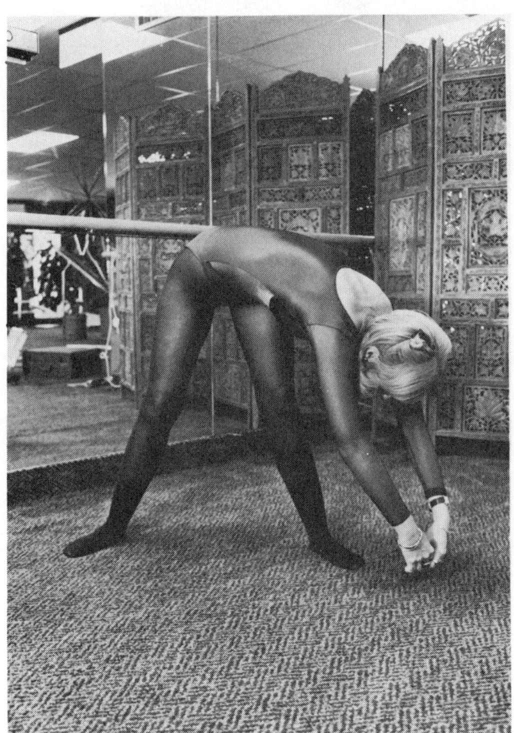

WAIST AND MIDRIFF STRETCH

Still in the bentover position, twist, pull in the stomach muscles, and flatten your back. Reach further out to the side as far as you can. Then *slowly* drop your body over the left knee. Control the drop as much as you can (don't just slump over—*drop!*). Grab hold of your left ankle with both hands and hold the position to a count of three.

Return to the starting position and repeat on the other side. Do eight to ten repetitions for each side.

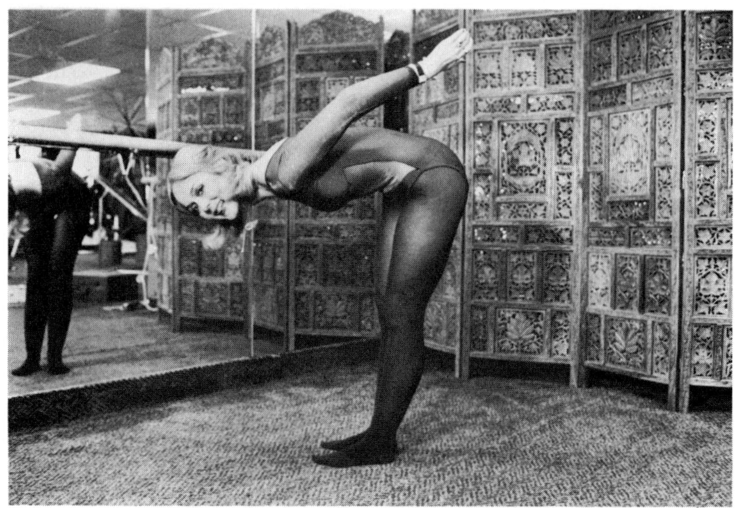

WAIST AND MIDRIFF STRETCH

4. *Jazz/aerobic walk*: Start this walking step with your hands on your hips, wrists resting just above the hip bone. Now lift your right knee up to about chest level. Point the right toe in an exaggerated "dancer's point."

   Step back and bring your feet together. Bend forward from the hips, keeping your back flat and straight. Try to keep your body parallel to the floor. Now pick up your left leg, point the toe, straighten up, and get ready to "walk" on the other side. Think of the movement as a stylized parade march or picture a jazz band strutting down Bourbon Street. You get the picture!

   For a variation, start with your feet together. Then bring your right foot forward, with heel tapping the floor (actually, just resting on the floor). Lean back, arms bent at the elbow, palms facing front.

   Then step back and bring your right foot back into line with the left one. Bend forward from the hips and swing your arms back until you feel the tension in the upper arms. (Clap at this point if you're working out to music or want to keep a rhythm to the exercise.)

Repeat this walk with left foot forward this time. Alternate left and right eight to ten times. By all means use music to keep your leans, bends, and walks in tempo for this one.

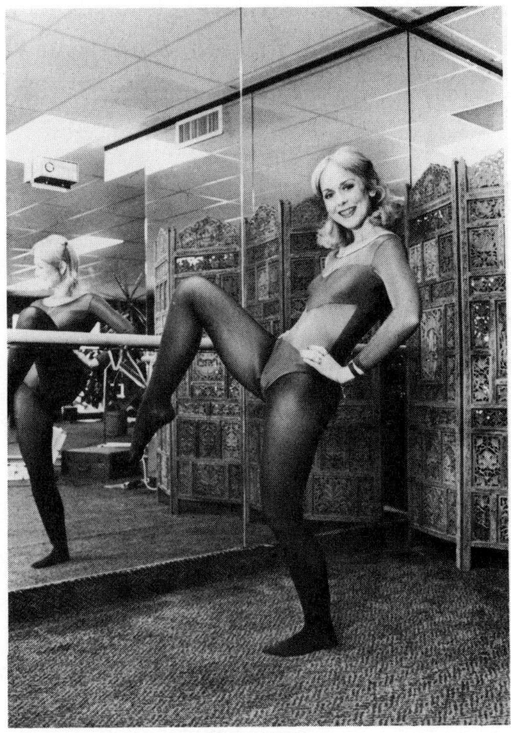

JAZZ STRUT

5. *Jazz arabesques*: These graceful movements are much like their ballet counterparts, but more exaggerated, free form, and more dynamic.

   Start by standing erect, with feet together, hands crossed in front of you at chest level. Now point the left foot to the left side and open your arms to the side, keeping the right arm higher than the left (the arms should form half of an "X").

   Now bend your right knee into a deep lunge like a fencer's stance and bring your left leg out to the side in an exaggerated stretch. Feel the stretch as you extend the leg and try to make it as "long" as possible.

   An alternate way to do it: lift the left leg up and out straight to the side, not allowing the foot to remain on the floor as you did before. (These are simply two versions of the basic side arabesque; either one is a good stretch or warm-up.) Repeat to the right side, doing eight to ten reps for each side.

For the *back arabesque,* begin with the poised stance (feet together, arms crossed). Now point your left foot behind you, swing your arms back at the same time, and lean forward. Next lunge with your left leg behind you into a deep bend. Touch your fingertips to the floor in front of you to keep your balance.

As you raise up, swing your left leg up and away to the back. Return to the original stance and repeat the entire movement with the right leg. Do eight to ten repetitions for each side.

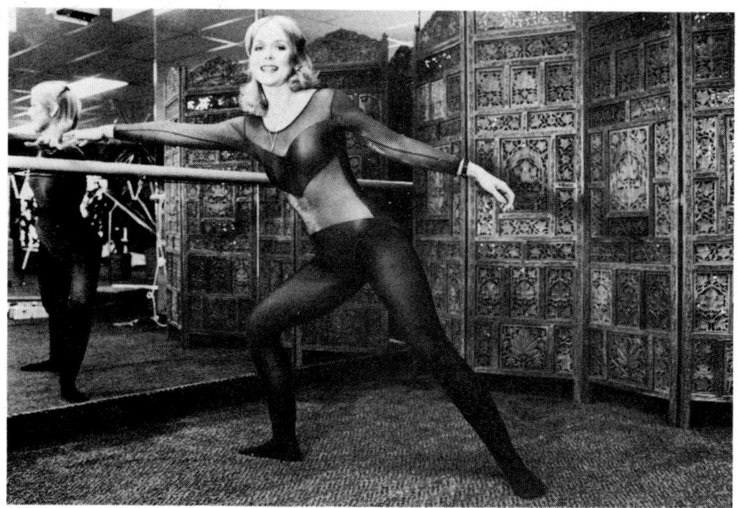

JAZZ ARABESQUE

There! Don't you feel better already? Obviously you can't do all the movements in one warm-up period, but you might try varying them—karate movements one session, yoga the second, ballet the third, and modern or jazz movements the fourth. Or pick one set of warm-ups and do them for two weeks, then switch to another for your next two weeks' worth of stretches, and so on. Or pick your favorites and combine them into one good, short routine that you can live with.

One last word: you don't have to "dress" for any of these warm-ups. Your jogging suit or warm-up suit or shorts will do just fine. But if you get in the mood to try the gear, too, a karate or judo *gi* that will also double for the yoga exercises can be bought at almost any good martial-arts store. Capezio, Danskin, Rudi Gernreich for Lily of France, and many other good dance design lines now have good-looking men's leotards, dancer's tights, and "body suits" that are also good for lounging, exercising, or relaxing. And if all else fails, your trusty old conventional gray sweatsuit will work for all the exercises. Happy stretching!

4

WEIGHT TRAINING EXERCISES: HOW TO MAKE ALL THE PARTS WORK TOGETHER

•

Earlier we said that weight training is a form of progressive-resistance exercise, used by bodybuilders to make their muscles grow larger and by weightlifters to make their muscles strong. Training for shape, on the one hand, and for strength, on the other, is a matter of emphasis. The bodybuilder concentrates on shape and size, while the lifter is primarily interested in how much weight he can lift off the floor.

Size doesn't necessarily mean strength. Many powerlifters and Olympic lifters have nowhere near the size of the champion bodybuilder. Yet, with exceptions like Franco Columbu or John Grimek in his heyday, few bodybuilders are as strong as the better lifters. The difference is in the way they train.

A lifter will do fewer reps and fewer exercises. The powerlifter will concentrate on the three lifts in his sport, and on those exercises that support high performance in these lifts. The Olympic lifter will concentrate on the snatch and on the clean and jerk, and on those exercises that support them. The bodybuilder, on the other hand, will work for symmetry in both size and shape, with no particular emphasis on one muscle or muscle group over another. As a consequence, the bodybuilder will usually have better *overall* muscular development than the lifter, and will have less fat both subcutaneously and within the body of the muscles themselves.

Further, while the lifter will certainly eat the kinds of foods that support the strength he must have for competition, the bodybuilder, since he is essentially in the business of sculpturing his body, will be much more careful about his diet. You can't have high definition while loading up on sugar, pastries, and fats! This is especially true if you are not going after a competition physique, but instead are trying to trim your waist and build yourself up so that you can look good as well as feel good.

While the lifter will do fewer reps and fewer exercises than the bodybuilder, the physique man will do many reps and multiple sets of those reps for each exercise. Before we go any further, let's describe both the language of bodybuilding and the concepts behind that language.

The basic unit is the exercise itself. There are many, and this section will describe most of them. For instance, a "curl" is an exercise for the biceps in which a weight is lifted toward the chest area. There are many variations on the curl, but they all involve flexing the biceps so as to crook the elbow and bring the weight nearer the chest or face.

If you are "doing curls," you will use a dumbbell, a barbell, or a machine. If you do a single curling movement, that is a "rep," or repetition. If you do ten reps and then stop for a rest, you have done one "set."

Most bodybuilders do multiple sets, with short rests in between. If you do a set of curls, for instance, and follow it with a set of bench presses without a rest period in between, you are "supersetting." Some advanced bodybuilders superset with three or four exercises, to achieve maximum intensity in their training.

If you do five, six, or seven sets without rest, then you are doing "giant sets." These are good not only for increasing the intensity of training but for cardiovascular conditioning as well. Another type of training which is gaining in popularity is "circuit training," in which the bodybuilder does one high-rep set (ten to fifteen repetitions) of each exercise, with no rest in between, until he has gone through an entire workout. This takes incredible stamina, and is not advised for the beginner.

In short, we have exercises, reps, sets, supersets, giant sets, and circuit training. The set system was popularized by Joe Weider, and the modern circuit training has been promoted by such exercise machine manufacturers as Dynacam. Whatever method you use, the time spent in the gym or health club is a "workout," and a gym is a place you go to "work out." To get a true workout, you need to work out diligently, without spending all your time between sets jawing about what a good workout you are getting.

Whether you work out at home or in a gym, it is up to you to make the workout worthwhile. If you rest for long intervals between sets, you will not receive the excellent cardiovascular conditioning available through weight training. If you push yourself too fast and don't rest for a sufficient length of time before going on to the next set, you will build up an oxygen debt that can be repaid only by stopping for a long rest. You must learn to pace yourself, so that you can get through the entire workout and come out feeling better than you did when you started.

The average workout should not take over an hour. At the beginning, thirty minutes is plenty, especially if you are really out of shape. One advantage of working out at home is that you can pace yourself more easily than if you were trying to fight for a place on the bench in a gym. However, for some people the psychological support of the gym helps keep up their dedication. Whatever works best for you, do it!

Now that we've got the basic language straight, let's get into the exercises themselves. After we've described all the exercises, we'll plan a program for you and show you how to develop your own program from the exercises listed, whether you are training for strength, size, shape, or all three.

Arm exercises should start at eight to ten repetitions, while leg and torso exercises start at ten to twelve reps.

INDEX OF THE EXERCISES

EXERCISES FOR THE LEGS

Almost everybody neglects his leg development, especially the calves. Your legs are usually covered up with a pair of pants, and as a consequence it's easy to get by in everyday life with poor leg development. Besides, the arms are always the "glamour" muscles. They're seen the most, and they are usually the pride and joy of every budding bodybuilder. But all the pros will tell you that the legs are the most important part of the body when it comes to building a solid foundation for any form of bodybuilding or lifting. If you don't have the legs, no matter how good the rest of your body is you will have neither symmetry nor strength.

Many bodybuilders catch on early, and concentrate on the squat. Tom Platz hated squats at first, but then developed his legs to a degree that few people in the history of bodybuilding can match. The squat became his favorite exercise.

Arnold Schwarzenegger had only mediocre calf development when he first came over from Austria, but multiple sets, supersets, and intense concentration on his calves eventually gave him the best lower legs in the world.

Frank Zane's legs may lack the massiveness of Sergio Oliva's, but their symmetry and deeply etched definition puts Frank in a class by himself.

Leg work also gives you stamina quicker than any other weight training exercise, because it involves the largest muscle groups in the body. If you can't get out of the house to run or jog, try substituting high-rep squats using a light weight, and watch the change. Your stamina will increase faster than you thought possible.

Rarin' to go? Here are the exercises.

THE SQUAT

This is the basic leg exercise. It is usually done with a barbell across the shoulders, although it can be done with the barbell resting in the hands at the top of the chest. If the bar is on the back, make sure that it isn't sitting on the neck, but is farther down. This way the trapezius muscles carry the load and you won't injure your neck. If you do squats with the bar at the top of your chest, make sure that you have enough arm strength to hold it there through the movement. Also, balancing will be different depending upon which of the two ways you choose. In any case, be sure that you have your feet planted firmly on the floor.

There are four basic ways to do the squat, depending on how far down you go. If you have trouble with stretching Achilles tendons, you will want to place a two-inch-thick board or book under your heels. In each case, begin the movement in an erect, standing position, eyes front, back slightly arched, hands gripping the bar a little more than shoulder width apart. If you have any doubts about the strength of your lower back, get a lifting belt at your local sporting goods store, and wear it fairly tight during the squats.

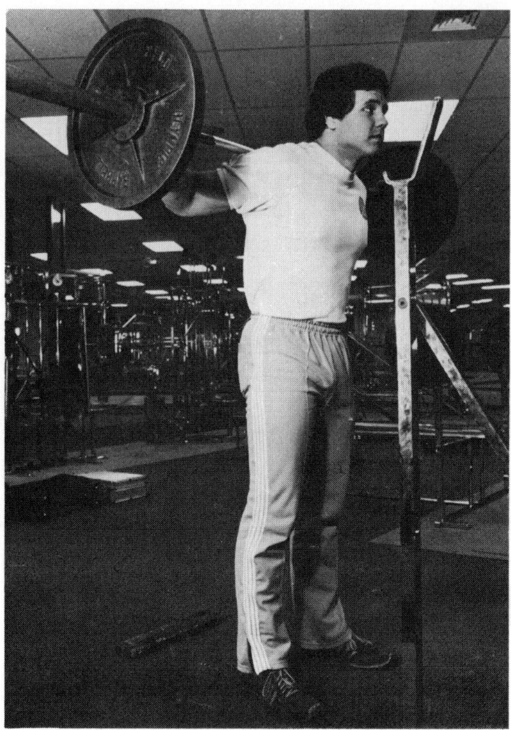

BEGINNING POSITION—SQUAT

Quarter-Squats

As the name implies, this version of the squat takes you only one-quarter down toward the floor. Do the movement in front of a mirror and you will see how far to go. If you have trouble with your knees, either from lack of strength or from old injuries, try the quarter-squat before going on to the other kinds of squats. Ralph had serious injuries in both knees, and had to begin with quarter-squats when he resumed training. You will be able to handle considerably more weight in this variation than in the lower squats, so don't get overeager and try it with too much, or you will find yourself unable to get back up (that's how Ralph injured one of the knees).

Half-Squats

This one takes you farther down toward the floor, and intensifies the workout of the muscles to the front and to the sides of the thighs. You will feel a hot, flushing sensation in the thighs on about the seventh or eighth rep if you do it right.

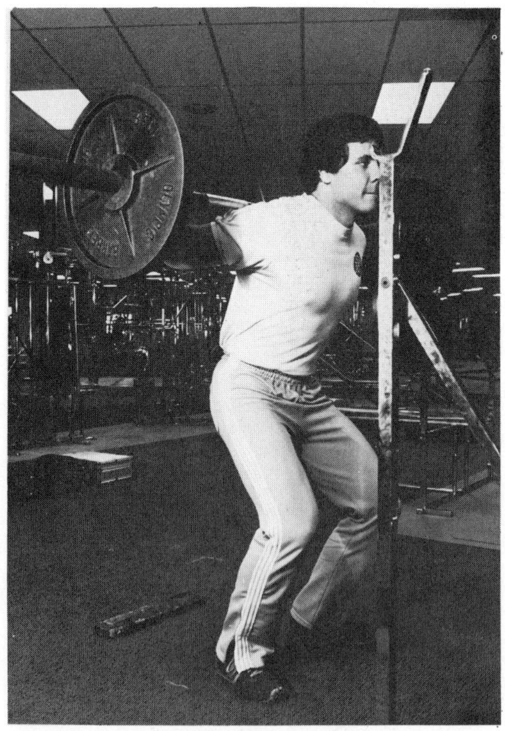

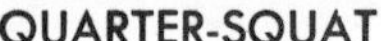

QUARTER-SQUAT

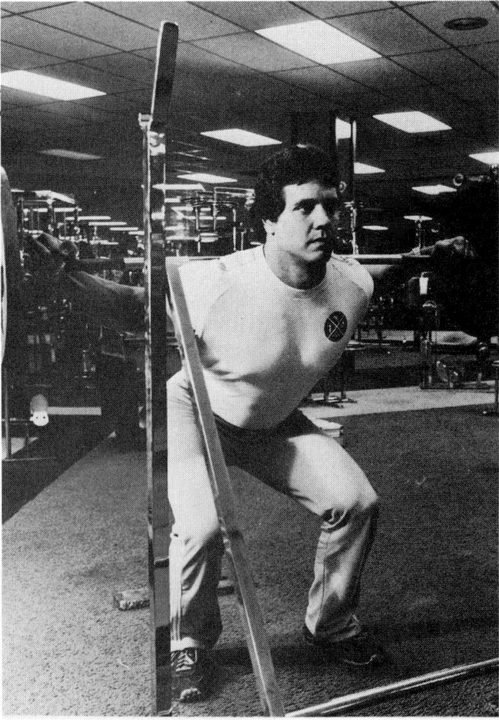

HALF-SQUAT

Parallel Squats

This is the most popular squat with bodybuilders. In this one, you drop slowly until the upper legs are parallel to the floor. Be careful not to let the back bend too much, or you will put undue strain on the lower back. Keep your eyes to the front and your back slightly arched. Keep that lifting belt tight. This exercise provides an intense workout along the full length of the front and outer thigh muscles, and when you get to the bottom of the movement, you will feel the gluteus (hip) muscles come into play.

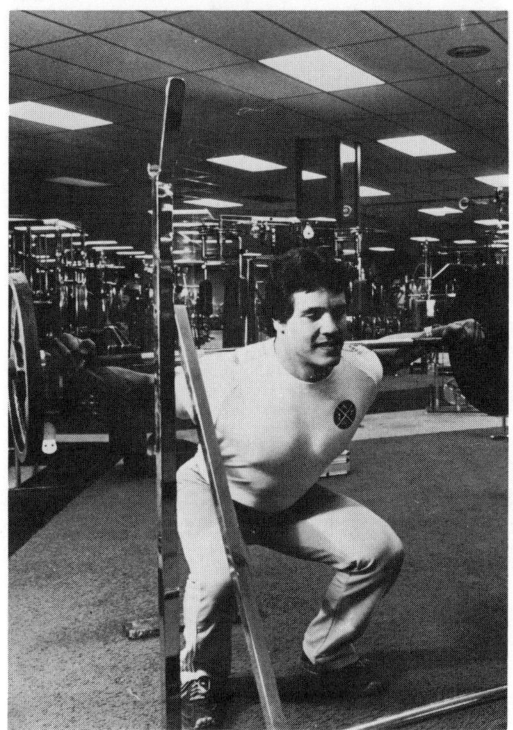

PARALLEL SQUAT

Full Squats, or Deep Knee Bends

For this one, you will certainly need a small book or board under your heels, since you go all the way down until the backs of your legs are against your heels. This is the most difficult squat to do, and requires the most strength to perform correctly. It not only works out the front and outer portion of the thigh but the buttocks and the back part of the thigh as well. It taxes your sense of balance the most, too, and you should be extremely careful to keep your back arched throughout the movement. Think of your entire torso as a cylinder that is keeping you together for this one. Keep it all tight.

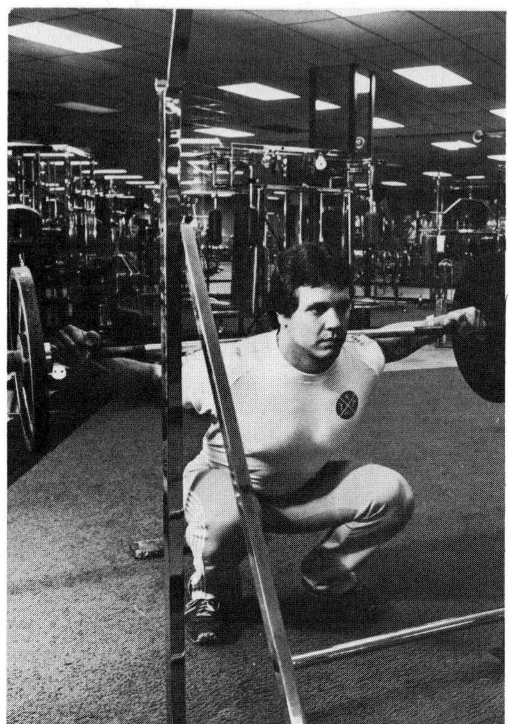

FULL SQUAT, OR DEEP KNEE BEND

There is some controversy about the full squat. Many people claim that it is bad for the knees, and puts too much strain on both the knees and the back. Granted, if you do the exercise incorrectly and bounce your way from the bottom of the movement halfway back up to a standing position, you will not do your knees any good. Also, if you allow your back to weave from side to side, you will eventually injure it. On the other hand, if the movement is performed in a slow, deliberate way—not increasing the speed at the bottom of the movement, but slowly rising up—you should not suffer any injuries. If knee pain or back pain develops, stick with the parallel squat or the half-squat, and add some lower back exercises (see the section on back exercises) to your program.

One further point: the position of the knees will determine which areas of the legs will be worked out in the squat. If you want to concentrate on the outer muscles, keep the knees close together. If you want to develop the inner portion of the thigh, do the movement with the knees spread wide.

The Hack Squat and the Sissy Squat

The hack squat is usually done on a machine, especially designed to isolate the muscles of the thigh. If you have access to a machine, you will readily see how the movement works. Most hack machines are built on sliding rails, and you do the movement by leaning back against the machine, gripping hand bars, and letting yourself down and up.

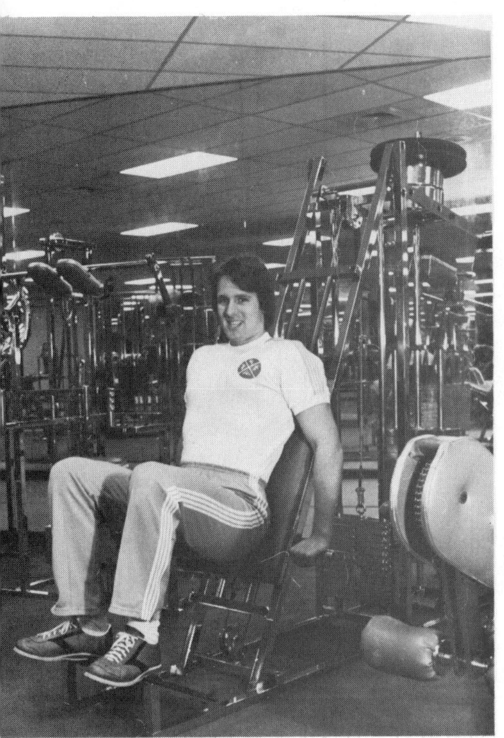

Step 1

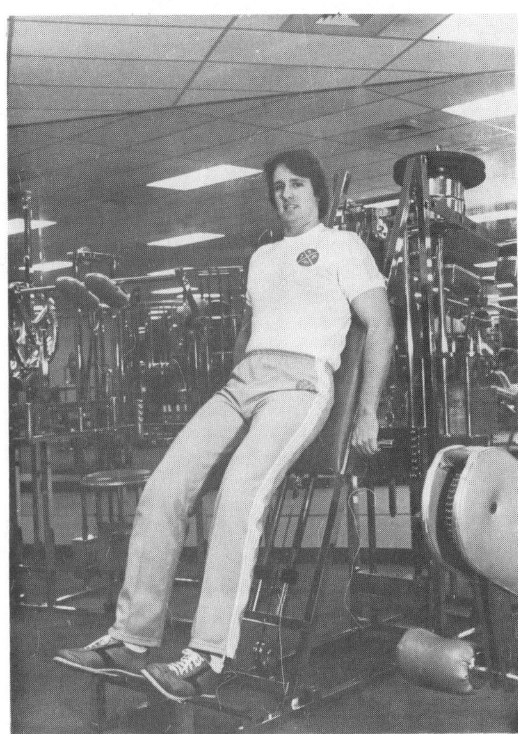

Step 2

HACK SQUAT

Actually, the hack squat is a variation of the "sissy squat," a form of knee bend pioneered and popularized by the West Coast bodybuilding guru Vince Gironda. According to Vince, the sissy squat is superior to the regular squat because it puts less strain on the lower back and also makes the leg appear longer through the development of the upper thigh muscles. In the sissy squat, you should hold the bar across the back as in the regular squats, but when you lower your body toward the floor you should keep the upper body in a line perpendicular to the floor. Your buttocks should be slightly tucked in, and your heels should be raised by a block. This exercise intensifies the leg workout from the knee all the way to the front of the hip. If you have short legs and want to make them look longer, then Vince's sissy squat will probably do the trick.

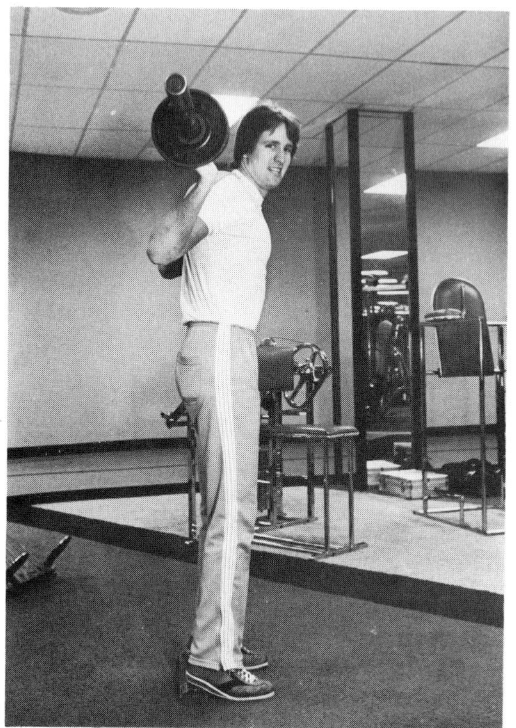

Step 1

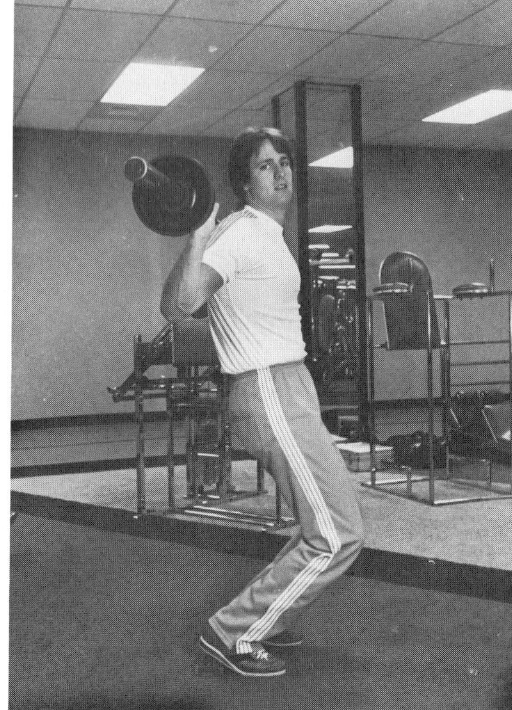

Step 2

SISSY SQUAT

LEG EXTENSIONS

Now that we have learned how to do the basic leg exercise, we need to describe supplemental exercises that will give you the kind of completely rounded development that is a must for any bodyshaping program. The leg extension is an important exercise, and can be used in conjunction with the regular squat and sissy squats in supersets. The most popular way to do the leg extension is on a leg extension machine, but remember: the movement was done for forty years before the machine was invented. Here's how to do it at home.

Pick up a set of ankle weights at the local sporting goods store. They cost anywhere from $5 to $15, depending on how fancy you want to get. Better yet, look around for a pair of "iron shoes," which are cast-iron sandals with leather or cloth straps. The iron shoes will accommodate a dumbbell handle and are thus far more versatile than the strap-on ankle weights. You can add weight to the iron shoes all the way to your limit.

If you do the exercise with ankle weights or iron shoes, sit down in a chair or on the edge of any sturdy piece of furniture (or on the edge of a porch, etc.). You might want to put a cushion under your knees to keep your legs from chafing against the porch, table, sofa, chair, or whatever you are sitting on. The movement begins with the knees bent at right angles and the feet hanging down. Raise both legs slowly until they are parallel to the floor. Hold for a count of two at the top of the movement. Then slowly drop the legs until they are in the starting position. Repeat for the requisite number of reps. This exercise concentrates on the muscle that locks the knee at the top of the movement, and on the front thigh during the first two-thirds of the movement. It is a great knee strengthener and will also help you get rid of any fat that might have collected around the tops of the kneecaps.

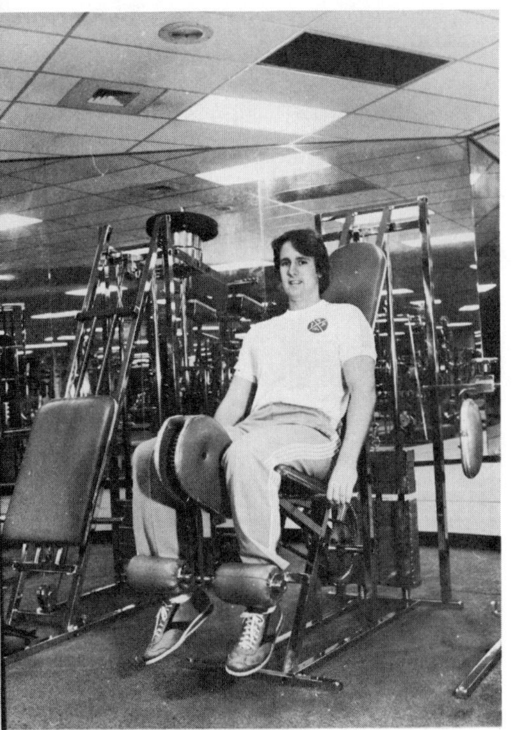

Step 1

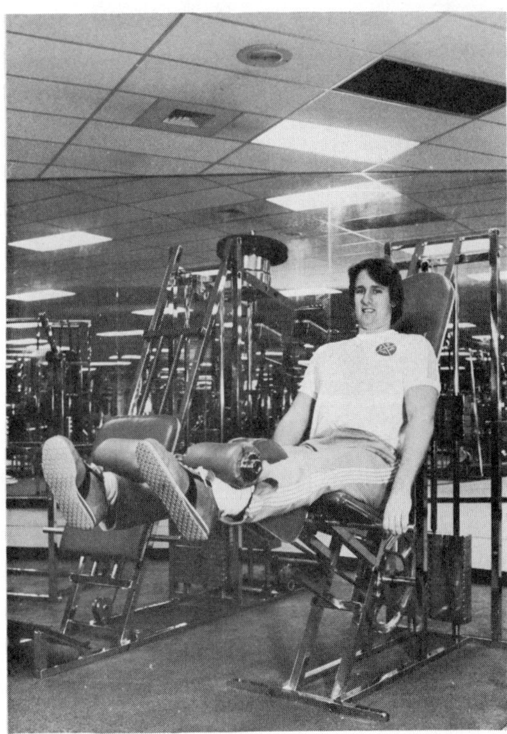

Step 2

LEG EXTENSION

LEG CURLS

Next on the list of upper leg exercises is the leg curl, which parallels the curls done for the arm biceps. The leg curl isolates the leg biceps or back of the thigh, and supplements the workout given to the back of the leg during the full squat. No leg is symmetrical without leg biceps development, and the leg curl will give you that fullness in the back of the leg that you want. The exercise is done with ankle weights or iron shoes, or on a machine. The movement begins with the leg extended, and ends with the foot pulled back until the heel touches the buttocks. If you are working with the iron shoes or with ankle weights, the greatest intensity can be achieved by doing the movement in a standing position. This way, the tension on the leg bicep is constant and doesn't diminish at the top of the movement. Do the exercise slowly and mechanically. Don't jerk the leg up in an effort to use more weight than you can handle in strict form. Hold at the top of the movement for a count of one, and then slowly let the foot back down to the floor.

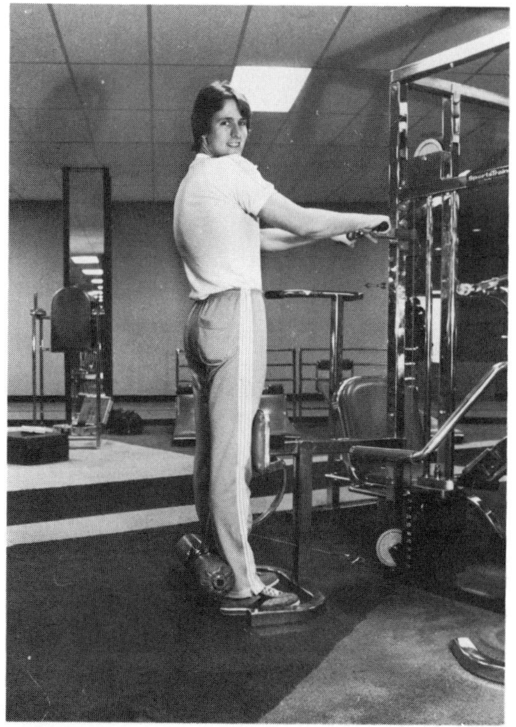

Step 1

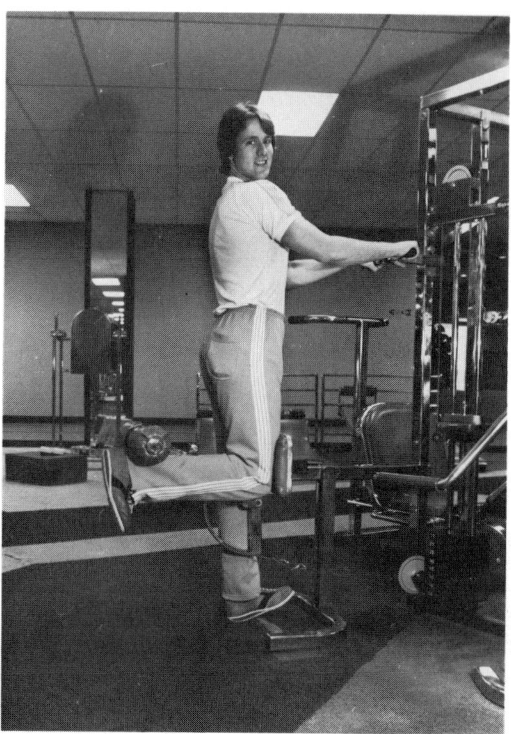

Step 2

LEG CURL

LEG PRESSES

This is a popular leg exercise which does not work the hips as does the full squat, but concentrates on the front and side of the thigh. If done properly, it can also work the backs of the legs when you bring the knees all the way down to the chest. The safest way to do leg presses is with a machine. The danger of not using a machine lies in dropping the weight on your neck. In the old days, bodybuilders actually balanced a heavy barbell on the soles of their feet as they lay on their back and pushed the weight up. We woudn't recommend this at all unless you have a person spotting you in the lift with his hands firmly grasping the barbell. It ain't worth it, guys, so don't risk injury. If you don't belong to a health club, get someone to help you with this one. If you do belong to a health club, don't do what Bill Grant did last year. He was bouncing the weights at the bottom of the lift, bounced off a twenty-five-pound plate, and caught it right in the face. It can ruin your whole workout! Whether you do the lift with a little help from your friends or at a club, you should start it on your back (or in the seat of a Universal, Dynacam, or Nautilus machine), with your knees against your chest. This is important if you want to get the full benefit of the lift. Otherwise, you are doing only a partial movement. Straighten your legs out almost all the way, but don't lock your knees or you might suffer an injury. Always keep tension on the thigh muscles, and bring the legs back as slowly as you straightened them. This is a heavy-duty exercise, and you should use as much weight as you can handle for ten to twelve reps at the beginning.

CALF EXERCISES

The calves are the most neglected of all leg muscles. They don't respond to exercise as quickly as the arms or the thighs, and they also achieve a burning sensation more quickly than any other muscle in the body. The calves are extremely dense, and are accustomed to the high-repetition movements that are naturally found in walking, jogging, and running. Moreover, since the calves are used as much as or more than any other muscle in these low-weight high-rep endurance movements, they are usually lacking in the explosive strength that we associate with the arms. It takes a while for them to loosen up and start developing, but persistence will win you a good set of calves. There are many ways to do calf "raises" but they all have one thing in common: you start with the heel slightly below the toe (stand on a plank or a book) and end with the calf flexed as tightly as it will go. The two basic ways to do the calf raise are either standing or seated. The standing calf raise develops the upper calf muscle (the gastrocnemius), while the seated raise concentrates on the lower calf muscle (the soleus). The difference comes from the fact that the knee is bent in the seated raise while it is straight in the standing raise.

Whether you do calf raises in a seated or a standing position, certain things remain true of the exercise. (1) To develop the outer portion of the calf, you should do the movement with your toes together and your heels apart. (2) To concentrate on the inner portion of the calf, you should do the movement with your toes pointed outwards. (3) To make sure that you develop the entire calf, you should do raises with the feet straight, or parallel. A good method is to perform six sets of calf raises: two with the toes apart, two with the toes together, and two with the feet parallel.

Further, you should do calf raises with the fullest movement possible. You should place the toes on a block at least three inches high, so that the heel can drop well below the level of the toe at the bottom of the movement.

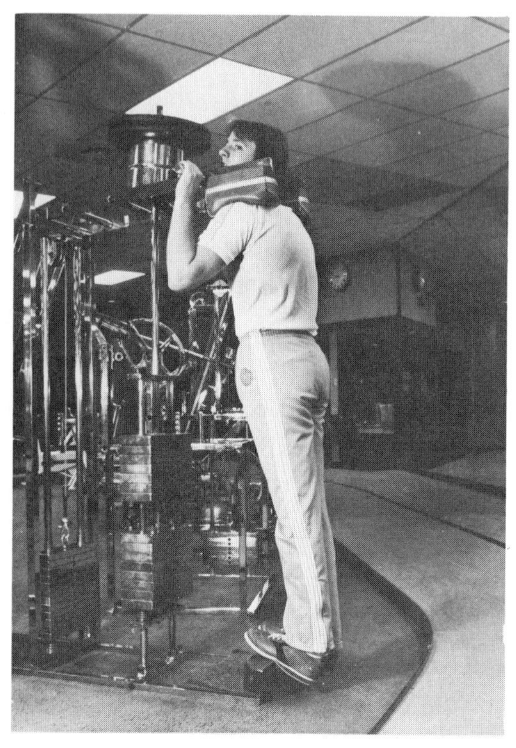

Step 1

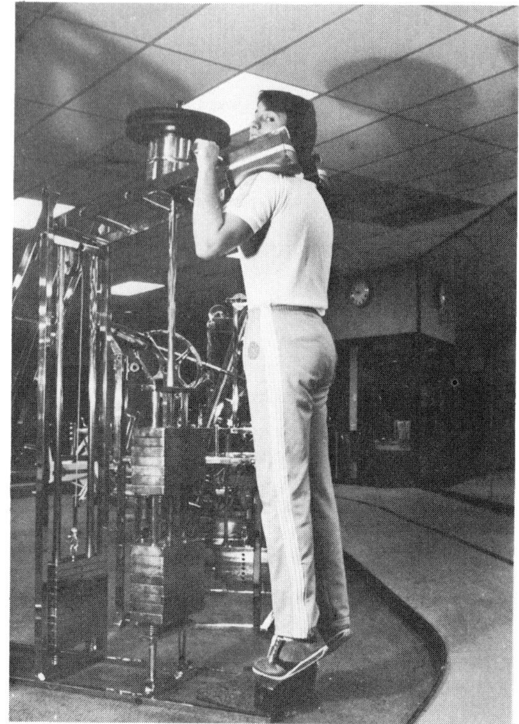

Step 2

CALF EXERCISE

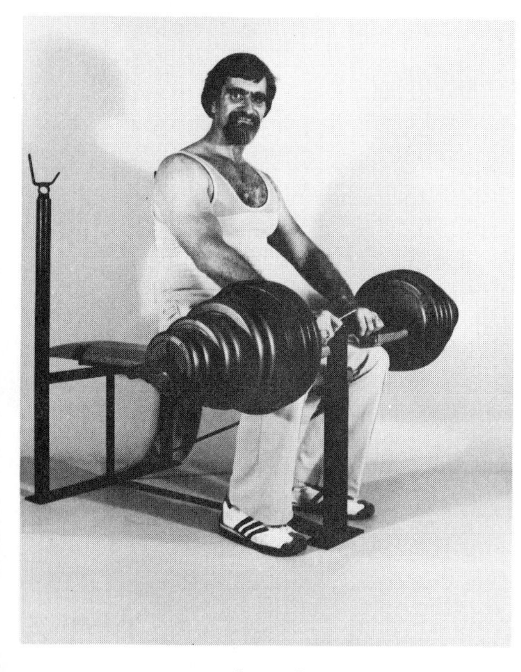

Step 1

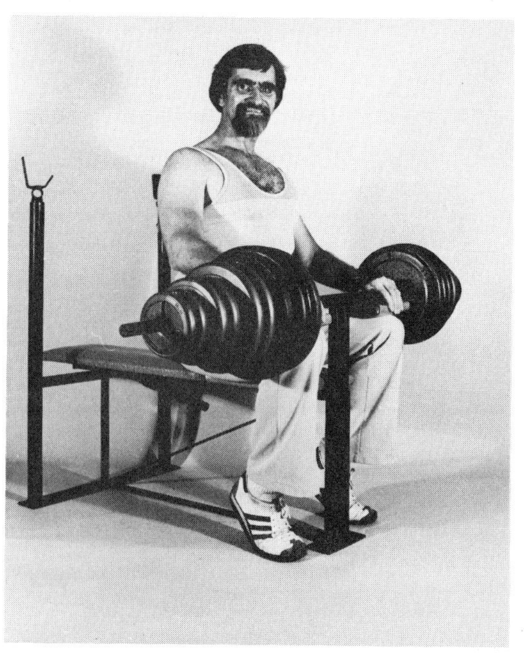

Step 2

SEATED CALF RAISE

This gives the calf a good stretch, and gives you a much longer contracting movement. Also, when you flex the calf muscles and rise on your toes to the top of the movement, you should go all the way to the top—as far as you can possibly go—so that the muscles flex to their maximum.

All the movements should be done fairly slowly, so that you don't cheat by bouncing out of the bottom of the movement. The calf muscles are hard to develop; they take more work than any other muscle group except the muscles of the forearms. Keep after them with a persistent, systematic workout each exercise period and they will respond.

EXERCISES FOR THE HIPS

Men do not usually collect fat in the bottom of the hips, but they do collect it at the top. Some men have large hip muscles, and some have very small hip development. If your buttocks are large and you are not particularly fat, you probably have naturally large buttocks muscles. If this is the case, you will want to avoid doing heavy squats because they will make the muscles even larger, with the result that your bottom will stick out all the more. Further, if you are one of those who collect fat around the hips, heavy squats will not make the hips less fat, but will merely push the fat farther out. If you have a fat bottom, do high-repetition hip exercises and get yourself on a strict low-calorie, low-carbohydrate diet. When it comes to fat around both the hips and the waist, diet is 80 percent of the fight.

Nevertheless, the best all-around exercise for the hips is the squat. There are also a number of other exercises that will help you to trim the hips without adding muscular bulk. Here are the best ones.

STANDING BACK LEG RAISE

Put on ankle weights or a set of iron shoes. Stand erect, supporting yourself by a chair, door frame, or some sturdy object. Swing the leg in an arc slowly to the rear. You won't have a very wide range of movement, so it's best to do the swing slowly in order to get the maximum benefit from it. Bring the leg slowly back to a point where the feet are side by side, then repeat the movement. At the beginning, you should use enough weight to make the twelfth or fifteenth rep the last one you are able to do in strict form.

STANDING SIDE LEG RAISE

Here you will begin as you did in the back leg raise, but the movement will be directly out to the side. It may help to keep the foot parallel to the floor throughout the movement (this is good practice for the karate side-thrust kick) in order to keep your body from turning in the direction of

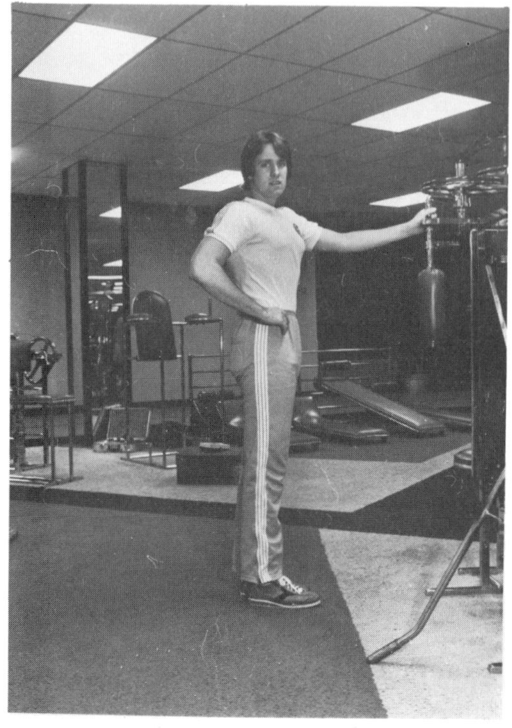

Step 1

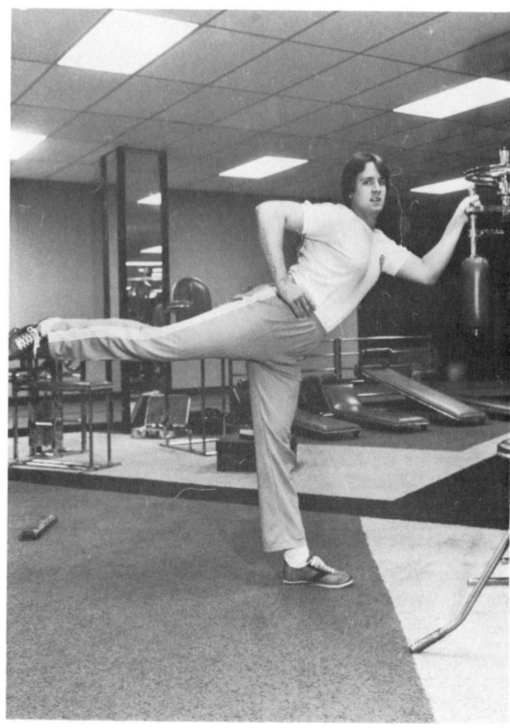

Step 2

STANDING BACK LEG RAISE

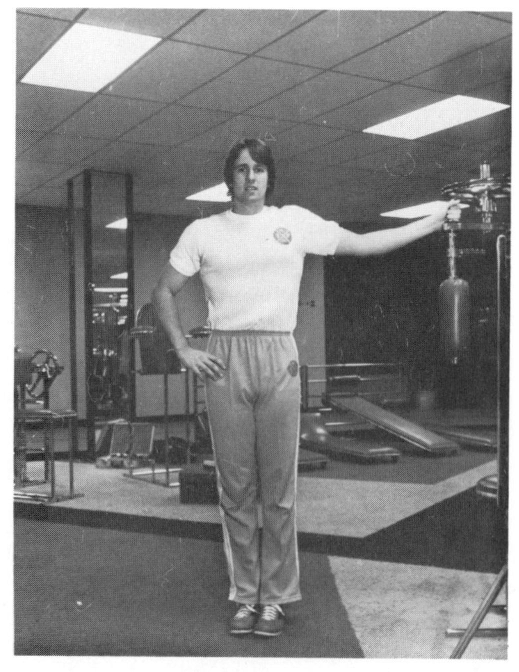

Step 1

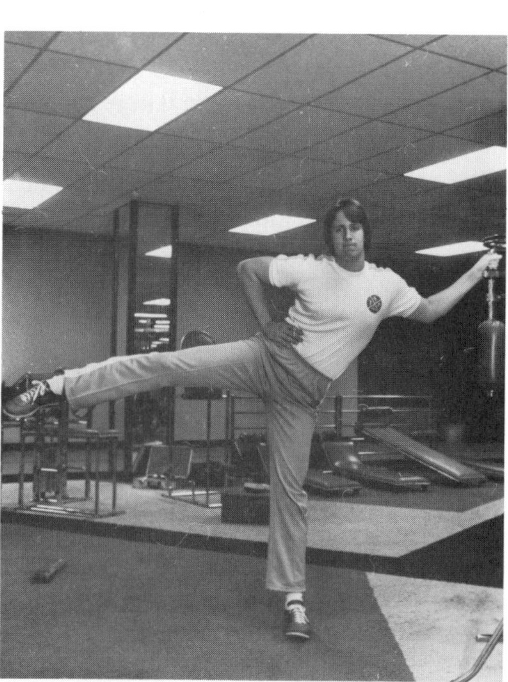

Step 2

STANDING SIDE LEG RAISE

the swing. This is also a high-repetition exercise, and you should not use very heavy weights. Try to bring the leg up the side until it is parallel to the floor, then slowly bring it back down to the starting position. This will work the sides of the hips.

STANDING FRONT LEG RAISE

Again, use the iron shoes or ankle weights. This time you should bend your knee as you bring your leg up, and try to touch your chest with the knee. Do the movement slowly, and after you have brought the leg all the way up, slowly return to the starting position. This will work the front of the pelvis where the leg muscles tie in to the abdomen. You will find that it works the abdominals too, and is a good supplementary exercise for the waist.

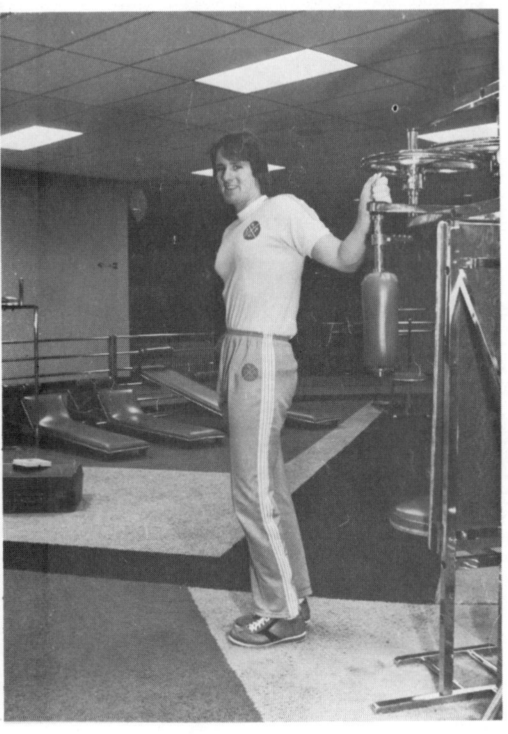

Step 1

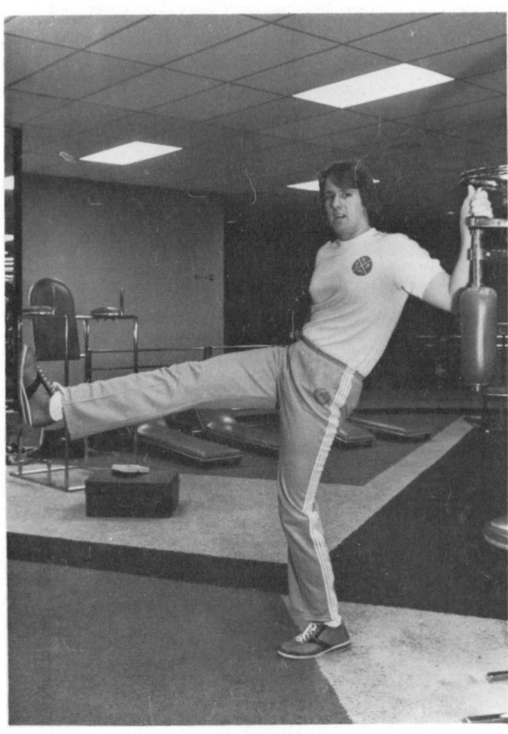

Step 2

STANDING FRONT LEG RAISE

RECLINING LEG RAISES

All of the leg raises can be done from a lying position. This way the muscles are worked from a slightly different angle. In the *back leg raise,* you should lie on your stomach and do the raise with as little hip movement as possible in order to isolate the muscles. In the *side leg raise,* you should lie on your side and raise the leg until it is about forty-five degrees from the floor. If you go higher, you will release the tension on the muscles and will lose some of the effectiveness of the exercise. Also, you should take care not to roll your torso toward the back (a natural inclination), so that the movement will remain essentially a movement to the side. The *front leg raise* is chiefly an abdominal movement; we'll describe it in detail in the next section on the waist.

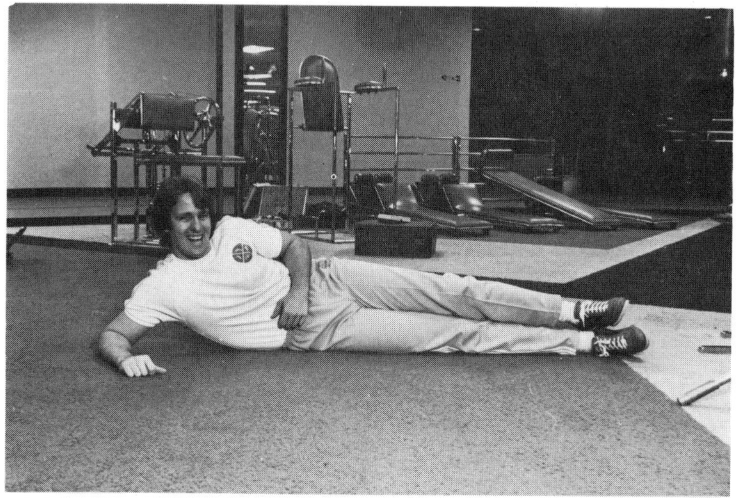

Step 1

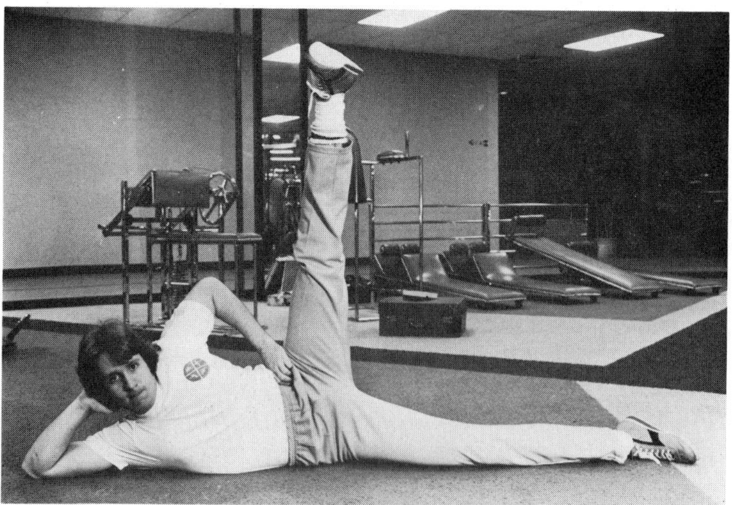

Step 2

RECLINING LEG RAISE

THE HIP THRUSTER

The purpose of this exercise is to strengthen the muscles and trim the area in the back of the hips. Lie on the floor on your back and bend your knees, bringing your feet to a position where the heels are almost touching your bottom. Place your arms at your sides. Now raise up on your shoulders, pushing your pelvis toward the ceiling as far as you can. You will feel your buttocks clench at the top of the movement. Hold still at the top for a count of three, then slowly return to the starting position. Your feet should remain stationary throughout the movement, and you should be supported by your feet and your shoulders at the top of the movement. If you have a tendency to collect fat in the back of your hips, this will help you to trim it off. If you want to strengthen the hip muscles, place a barbell plate on your abdomen before you start the movement. Be sure that the plate doesn't slip at the top of the movement. You don't want to make an emergency trip to the dentist.

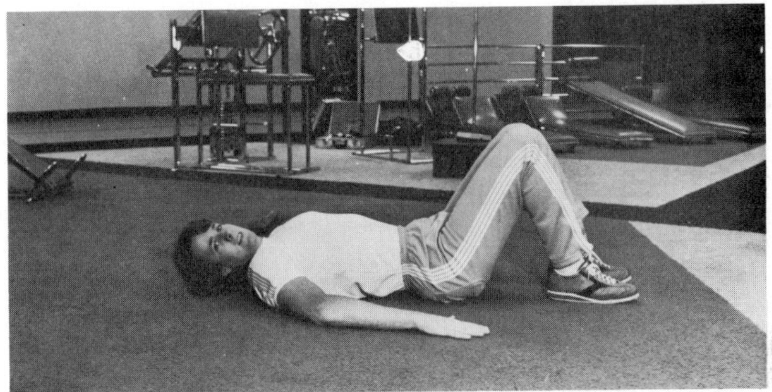

Step 1

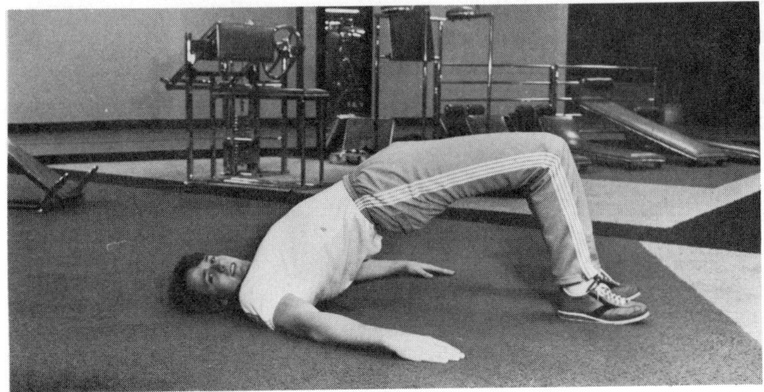

Step 2

THE HIP THRUSTER

EXERCISES FOR THE WAIST

The one place where all men collect fat is around the waist. Even tall, skinny guys sometimes have a pot in front, which is a dead giveaway that although they are lean they are not in shape. The average man collects fat in front, from the sternum all the way to the pubis, and on the sides and to the back in the form of the infamous "love handles" or "kidney pads." The fat in front will diminish relatively quickly with effort and diet. The fat on the back and to the sides is the hardest fat to get rid of for men. Ralph has the problem himself, and has fought it all his adult life.

There have been many times over the last twenty years when Ralph has dieted heavily without exercising. Even when his weight got down to 160 pounds, the fat on the sides held on as if he had never been on a diet. His father had "handles." All his uncles on his mother's side of the family have them. He has them. When he tried the old-fashioned side leans with a dumbbell to get rid of them, he merely developed the external oblique muscles and pushed the fat farther out.

John Grimek and Arnold Schwarzenegger both prescribe bentover twisting movements for "handles." Franco Columbu maintains that running is the only known cure. Frank Zane does twists and also runs. All the top bodybuilders use one kind of twist or another. Almost nobody does side leans anymore as a waist-trimming exercise. We should point out, however, that if you do not have a fat problem in this area, and if your abdominal development is lacking on the sides, you should perform some side leans on a regular basis to build the area up. Be warned, though, that the external obliques develop very rapidly, and you can lose the trim waist you're after before you know it. Take a look at some of the muscle magazines and you'll see what we mean. Paul Grant of Wales appears slightly overdeveloped in this area, as does Ron Teufel. Frank Zane's obliques are more developed than most, but he is saved by his magnificent symmetry and polish. We talked to Frank when he visited Houston in 1979, and chatted for a few minutes about waist training. He verified that at one time he did a lot of side leans, and he quickly overdeveloped the obliques in relation to the rest of his body. One look at Mr. Olympia now and you can see that whatever unbalance he suffered, he more than corrected it in the ensuing years.

Side leans aren't the only controversial waist exercises. There are differences of opinion among most bodybuilders about how the waist should be trained. West Coast bodybuilding guru Vince Gironda says that you should work the abdominals the same way that you work any other muscles: moderate repetitions, and under no circumstances every day. Ed Gugliani, another West Coast gym owner and title holder, advises high repetitions, daily workouts, and fast movement. Frank Zane has been quoted as saying that he does forty-five minutes of situps a day. Gironda says that situps work the psoas muscles that tie in to the back instead of the abdominals. Rick

Wayne, former editor of *Muscle Builder* and himself possessor of one of the most incredible midsections in bodybuilding, has recommended crunches over situps for etching definition into the "abs." What should you do?

The common thread that runs through all these versions of the ideal waist workout is that the abdomen needs to be worked out and should not be neglected for the more glamorous arms, lats, and pecs. The abdominals give the bodybuilder that polished look necessary to win contests. Abdominal work will give the average person the kind of trim waist that is associated with youth, vitality, and strength. The truth is that the abdominals seem to respond differently to exercise from person to person, and you will have to experiment until you find the ab exercise that works for you.

If you take a look at all the bodybuilders mentioned above—Zane, Grimek, Gironda, Columbu, Guliani, and Schwarzenegger—you will find that they all have fabulous abdominal muscles. Also they all have very strong opinions about how you should work your abdomen. But they differ widely, and in Gironda's case, vehemently, about how you should go about it. Here are some tips on how to make your waist workout work for you, regardless of which exercise you do.

1. Concentrate on every movement, whether it is a twist, a crunch, or a situp. Make each movement count. Keep the concentration up the same way that you would if you were trying for your record bench press.
2. Vary the movements. Do them slowly with continuous contraction of the muscles one day and try rapid movements the next. Don't allow your abdominals to adjust to the exercise that you are doing.
3. Shake up your waist by adding weight to situps on occasion. Arnold Schwarzenegger says that hardly anybody uses weight in abdominal movements anymore, but every gym we've ever visited will have a couple of guys with fantastic abs doing slow situps on the slant board with a twenty-five-pound plate held against their chest.
4. Some bodybuilders say that if you work the abs every day you will smooth out. Others say that if you don't work the abs every day you will smooth out. Try it both ways, starting with three times a week, and see which method works best for you. Go for at least three weeks before you make a judgment about changing the routine.
5. When you first begin working out with weights, you shouldn't spend a lot of time on the abdominals. You will find that heavy leg work in the form of squats and leg presses will do wonders for the abdominals indirectly. Since the legs have the largest muscles in the body, they use a lot of fuel. If you are on a good diet, then solid leg work will help you to peel the fat off your abdomen quickly.
6. Whatever you do, don't get into the trap of thinking that situps and

twists will trim the waist if you do more of them than any other exercise. Situps and twists don't use up much fuel. We've seen hundreds of fat men over the years wasting their time doing thousands of situps while neglecting heavy leg work. They always get discouraged and quit working out. They usually become critics of weight training because for them it didn't work. If they had concentrated on *weight training* instead of situps and twists, they would have succeeded.

These are the basic rules. Now let's get on with the exercises.

SITUPS

Situps are the oldest, most popular form of abdominal training. They are a good exercise, despite their detractors, but they should be done in a specific way for maximum benefit. Slant boards are often used in order to put more pressure on the abdominals, hence increasing the intensity of the exercise. Most slant boards, however, are not well designed, and you will find that your legs will tire before your abdominals as you try to hang on with your toes to a padded foothold at the top of the board. Further, most boards are built in such a way as to make it difficult to keep the knees wide apart, which is essential if you are to isolate the abdominals and keep the psoas muscles from doing most of the work.

The advantage of a slant board is that it enables you to keep the tension on the abs throughout the range of the movement. If you buy a slant board, or if you make one out of an old board and some padding as we did, be sure that there is a strap to hold your feet. That way you can concentrate on working the abs without the distraction of worrying about keeping your feet under the foothold.

The movement begins with the body flat and (if you are on a slant board) the head at the lower end of the board. The knees should be wide apart, and should remain apart throughout the movement. The arms can be folded across the chest (if you are a beginner), or the hands can be placed either behind the head or at the temples. If you put your hands behind your head, be sure that you don't help yourself up by pulling on the back of the neck with your hands. This defeats the purpose of the exercise.

Bring yourself up slowly, consciously tensing the abdominal muscles as you rise. Come all the way up until your chin would touch your knees if they weren't pointed outward. Then slowly return to the starting position. Don't be discouraged if you can't do many situps. They'll become easy before you know it. After months of them, Ralph once did 2,001 just to be able to say that he did it. It took him almost forty-five minutes. But when he first started working out again on his fortieth birthday (eight years ago), he could barely do seven.

Use this basic situp technique, whether you are on a slant board or the floor or on a bed. If you have a back problem, you may have trouble doing

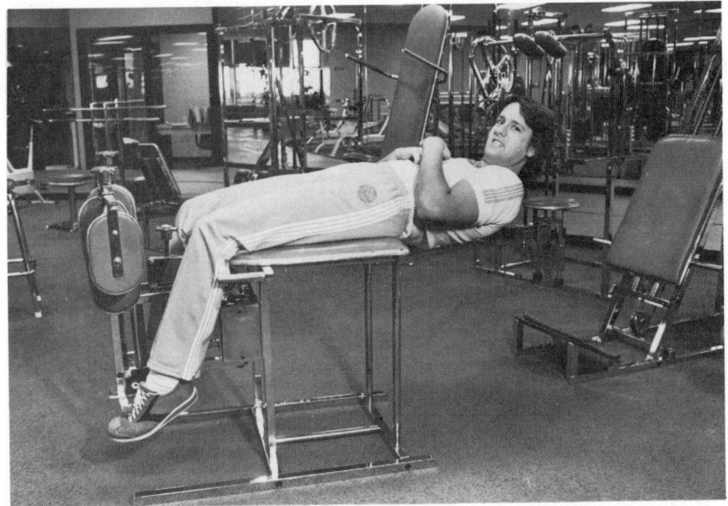

Step 1

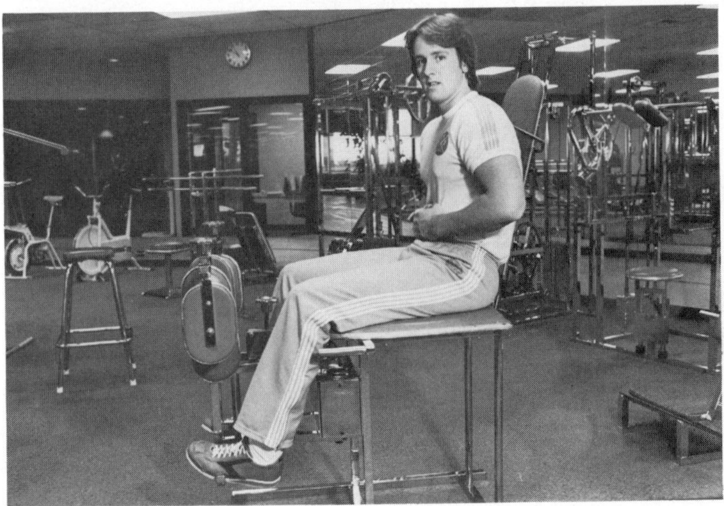

Step 2

SITUPS

situps, since they put a lot of pressure on the lower back. If the slant board hurts your back (it does Ralph's), try doing situps on a mattress or other soft surface. If you concentrate on what you're doing, you can get the full range of movement, and it'll be a lot easier on your aching back. If you do situps on the side of a bed, don't cheat by pulling yourself up with your legs, but keep the knees wide apart and bring yourself up slowly. Don't use the bounce of the innerspring mattress to help you up!

CRUNCHES

This is a variation of the basic situp, and is cited by many bodybuilders and coaches as being superior to the situp in isolating the abdominal muscles. It's also a lot less painful if you have an old back injury like Ralph or like Rick Wayne. There are several ways to do the exercise.

The Basic Crunch

Lie on your back, hands at the temples, and bring your shoulders off the floor as if you were doing a regular situp. However, raise up only until the shoulders clear the floor. Keep the small of the back on the floor and contract the abdominal muscles as tightly as you can. Hold for a count of three, then slowly let yourself back down.

Crunch with the Knees Together

In this variation, bend the knees and bring them up until the thighs are almost pointing at the ceiling. Raise up until the small of the back is just off the floor and your chin is almost touching your knees. Hold for a count of three and slowly let yourself back down.

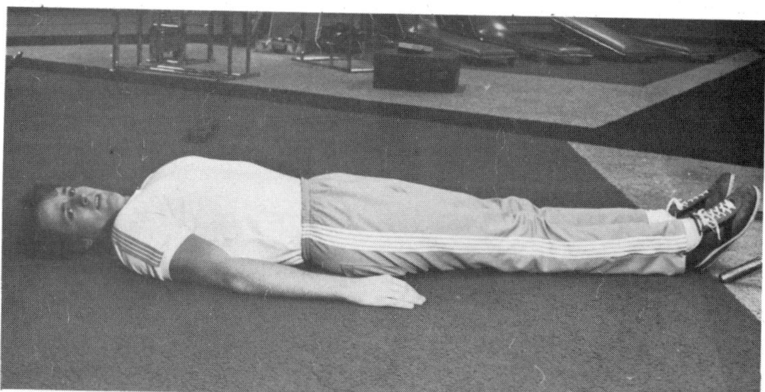

Step 1

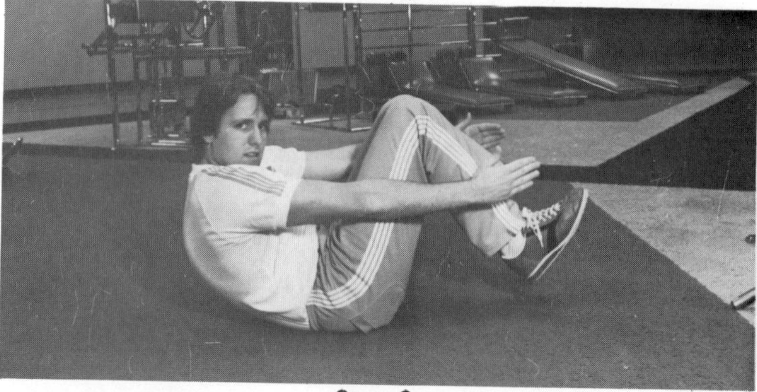

Step 2

CRUNCH WITH THE KNEES TOGETHER

Crunch with the Knees Apart

This time keep the knees wide apart and bring yourself up so that your back is just off the floor. Hold for a count of three and let yourself back down.

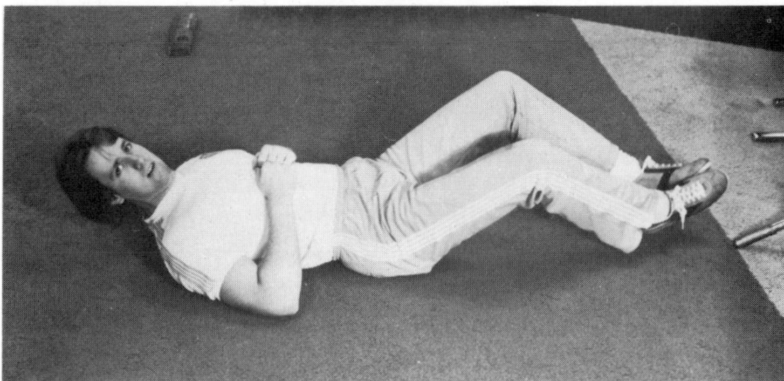

Step 1

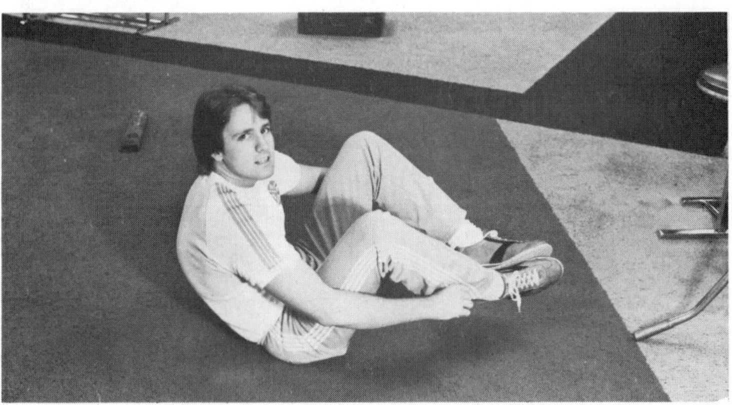

Step 2

CRUNCH WITH THE KNEES APART

Crunch on a Slant Board

You can do crunches on a slant board, just as you can do situps. The tension is dramatically increased, and you should concentrate on flexing the abdominal muscles as you do the movement. You can do the exercise with the knees apart or together. Knees apart will still give you the best concentration on the abs themselves.

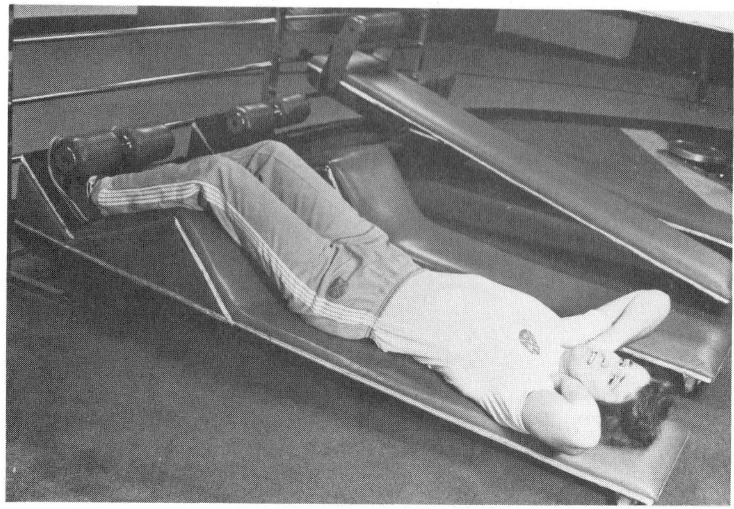

Step 1

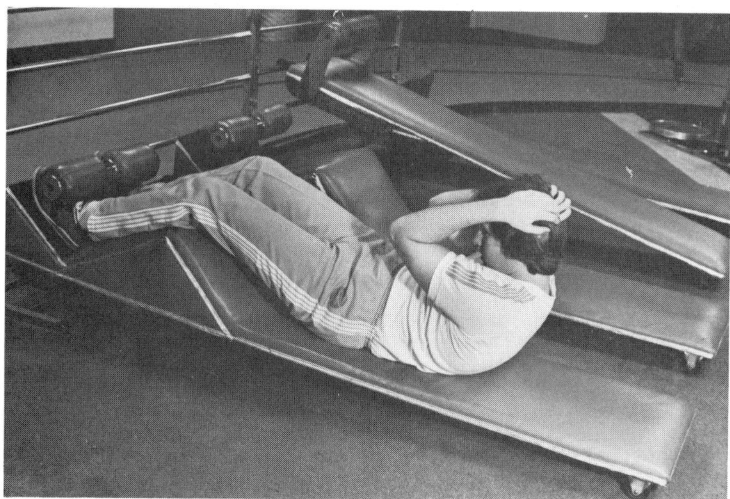

Step 2

CRUNCH ON SLANT BOARD

Crunch with a Lotus

This time put your legs into the traditional yoga lotus position. If you can't do a full lotus, place the knees wide apart and keep the legs crossed at the ankles. As you do the crunch, this time keeping the small of the back against the floor, at the top of the movement while you are holding the position for a count of three, bring the legs slowly off the floor and pull your pelvis toward your sternum. This will intensify the pressure on the entire abdominal region.

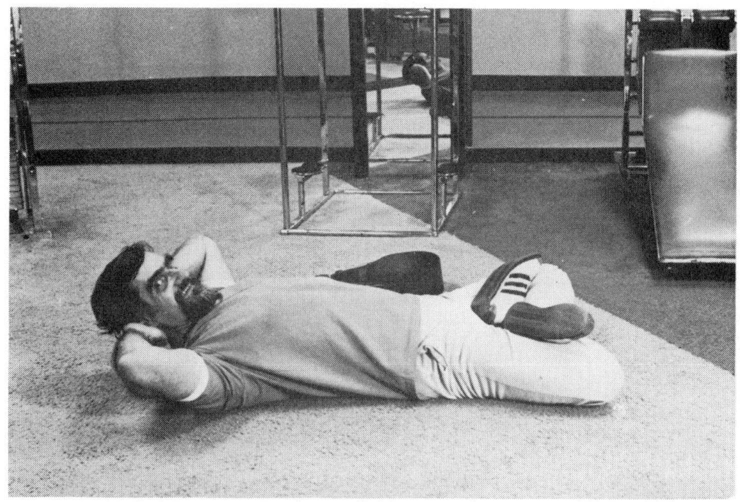

Step 1

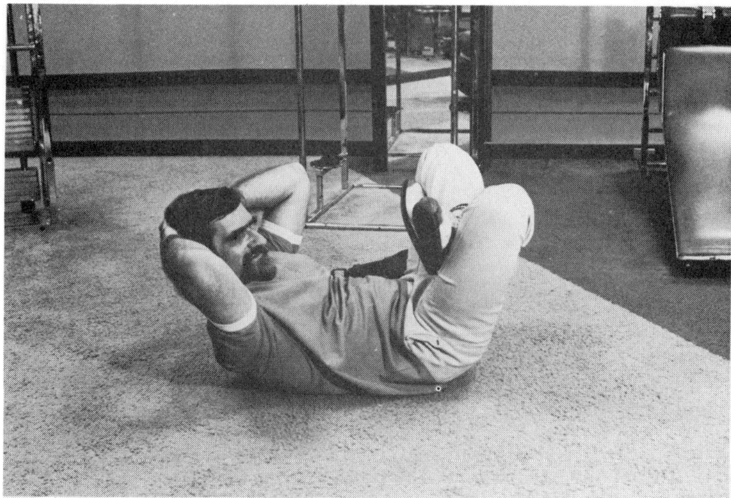

Step 2

CRUNCH WITH LOTUS

Crunch with the Feet on a Bench

Lie on the floor with your knees bent and your feet on top of a bench. Let them rest lightly. Do your crunch, and when you are at the top of the movement push your legs up slightly by pushing against the bench top with your toes. The purpose of this movement is to bring the lower abdominals into play at the top of the crunch. Although it would seem that you are merely pushing with the legs, a little concentration will show you that you are actually isolating the lower abdominal region along with the upper abs, and the burning sensation you get will be greater than if you had lifted your feet off the bench without pushing up with your toes. Don't take your heels off the bench top; hold for a count of three, then slowly let yourself back down. If you do it right, you will feel a burning sensation after only three or four reps.

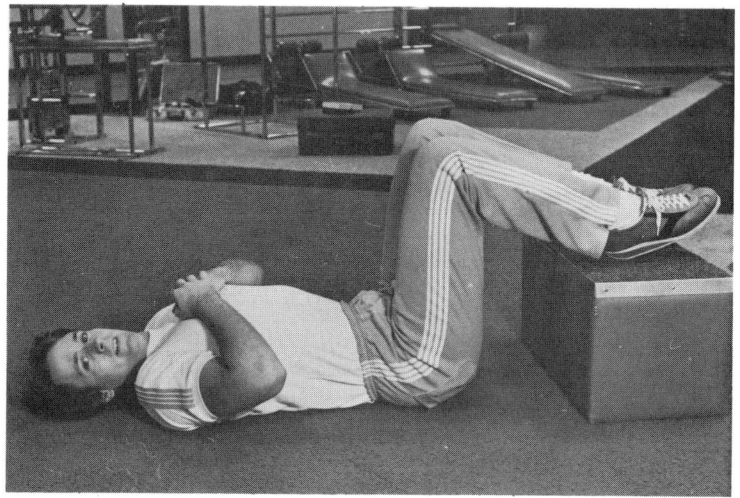

Step 1

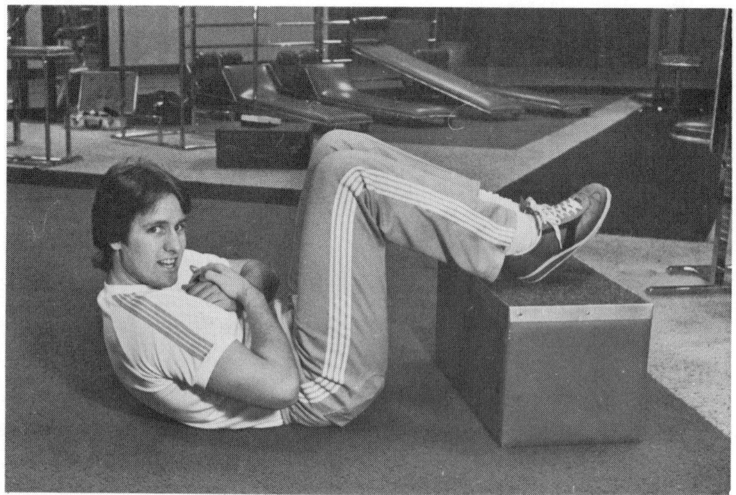

Step 2

CRUNCH WITH THE FEET ON A BENCH

Side Crunches

This time lie on your side as if you were going to do the reclining side leg raises described on page 97. Flex the external obliques, or side muscles, while pulling your legs off the floor. If you are already in good shape, you may be able to bring your upper body off the floor without using your arms as a prop. Arch your body to the side (which will be in the direction of the ceiling) and hold for a count of three at the top of the movement. Then slowly let yourself back down to the starting position. Do one side for a set of ten to twelve reps and then try the other side.

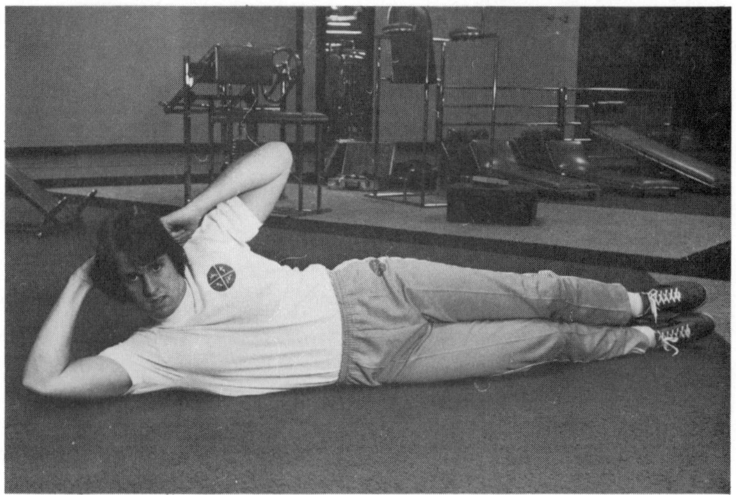

Step 1

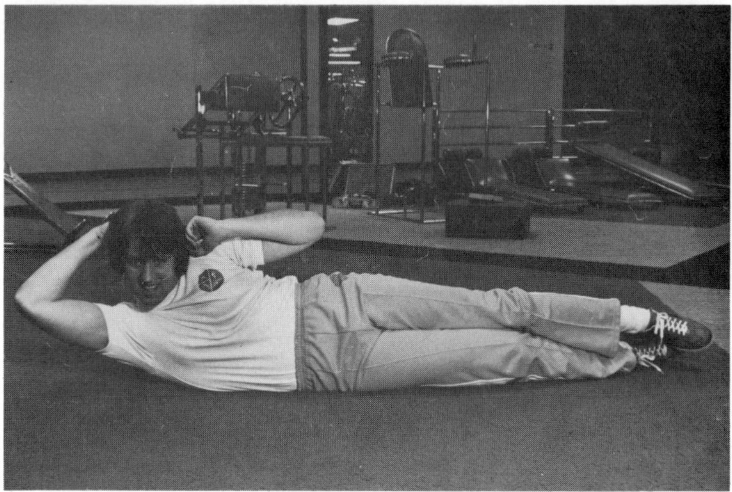

Step 2

SIDE CRUNCH

Back Crunches, or Spinal Hyperextensions

The back crunch is a variation of the spinal hyperextension, and is a good back strengthener. Lie on your stomach, extend your arms out in a position that would bring them overhead if you were standing, keep your hands and your feet together, and arch your back as far as you can. Hold for a count of three. If you hold for a count at the top of the exercise, it's a crunch. If you don't hold for a count, but let yourself back down immediately for another rep, then it becomes a hyperextension. The crunch comes when you hold the muscles in a completely contracted position.

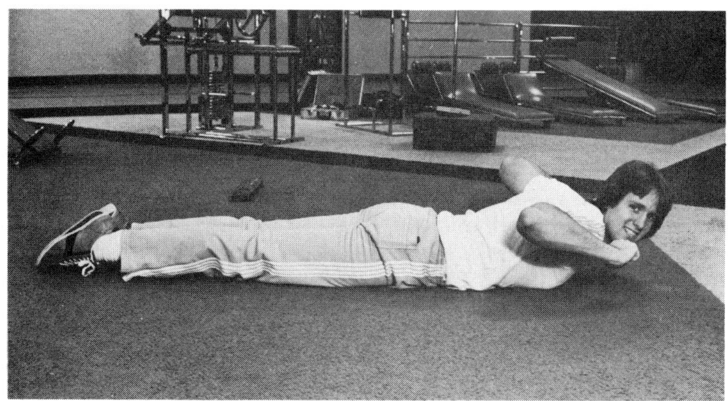

Step 1

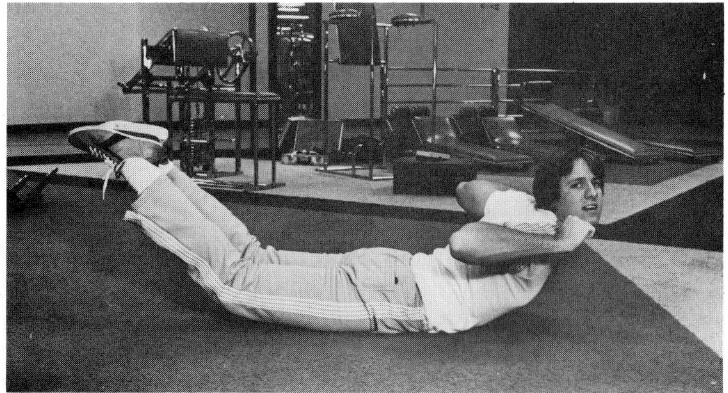

Step 2

BACK CRUNCH

TWISTS

There are basically two kinds of twists: with the back straight and with the back bent. The straight-back twists work the intercostal area under the arms and down the sides, and the bent-back twists work the sides to the back—in short, the place where the "handles" sprout.

Straight-Back Twists

These twists are best done in a seated position in order to immobilize the hips. If you do them standing, you will twist the hips inadvertently and lose most of the effectiveness of the exercise. Sit cross-legged on the floor or on the edge of a bench. Place an unweighted bar or a broomstick on your shoulders behind your head (don't hold it too high, or you will "saw" your neck), extend your arms out toward the ends of the bar, and twist from side to side. Do the movement as fast as you can. This exercise is primarily a stretcher and a massager, and it will give your waist that final polish it needs to be extra trim.

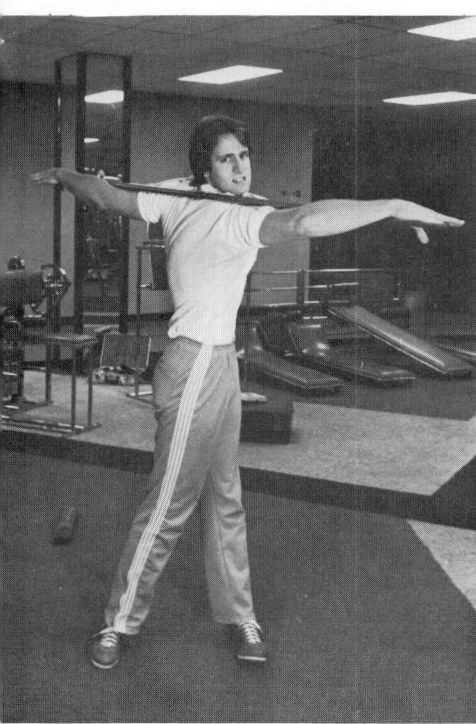

Step 1

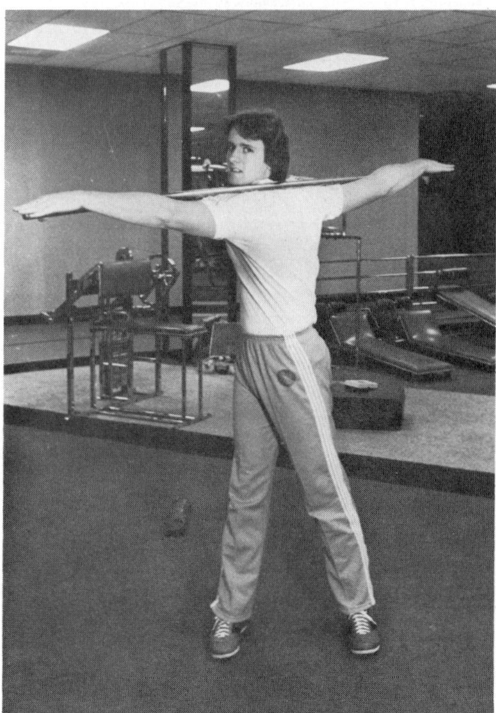

Step 2

STRAIGHT-BACK TWIST

Bentover Twists

These twists can be done standing or seated. They work best standing. Keep your knees straight, and bend from the waist until your upper body is parallel to the floor. Holding the bar or broomstick the same way that you do in the seated twist, rotate the body rapidly as far as you can go in either direction. If you do this one correctly, you will feel the sides begin to burn. The great advantage of the bentover twist is that it will help you trim the fat off your sides without making the external oblique muscles grow.

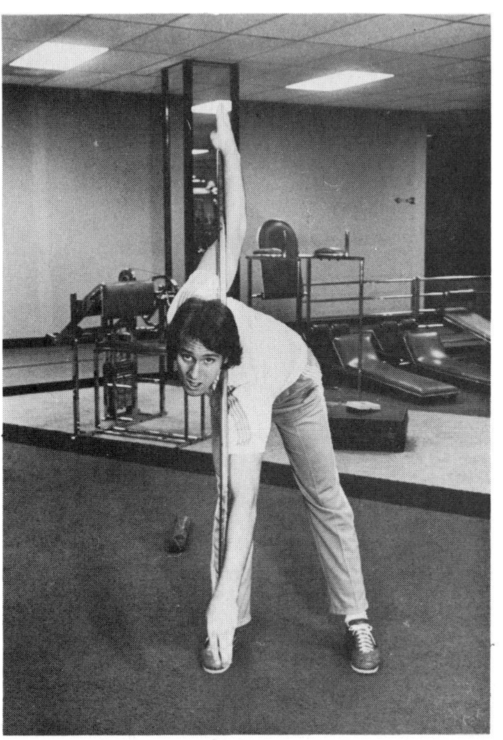

Step 1

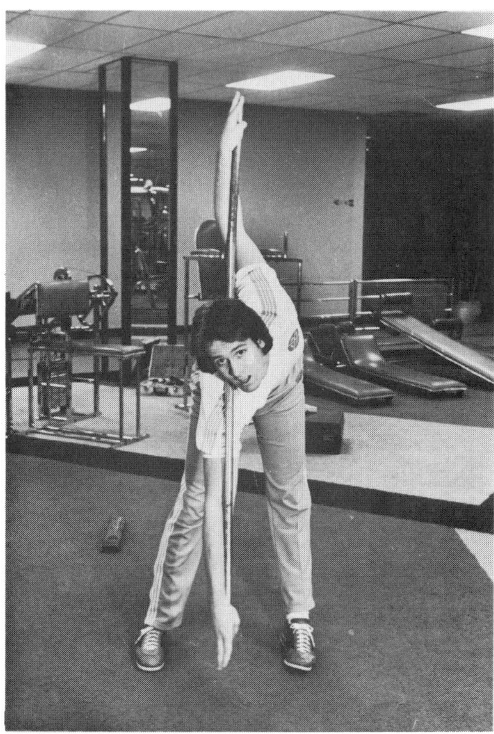

Step 2

BENTOVER TWIST

LEG RAISES

We've already talked about various leg raises as hip exercises. Leg raises can also be used to trim and tone the abdomen. Again, there are several variations.

Regular Leg Raises

When most people talk about leg raises, they mean this one. Lie on your back, bend your knees slightly, and raise both feet off the floor until your legs are a little past the forty-five-degree mark. Hold for a count of three, and then slowly lower the legs until they are almost touching the floor. Repeat the movement, keeping tension on the abdominal muscles at all times.

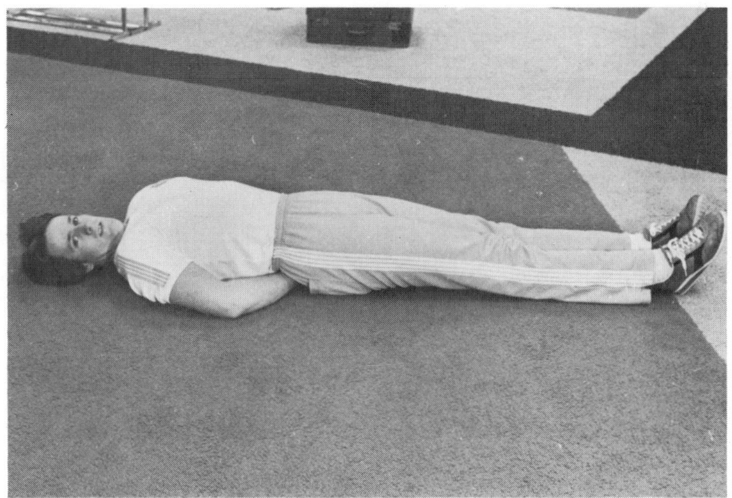

Step 1

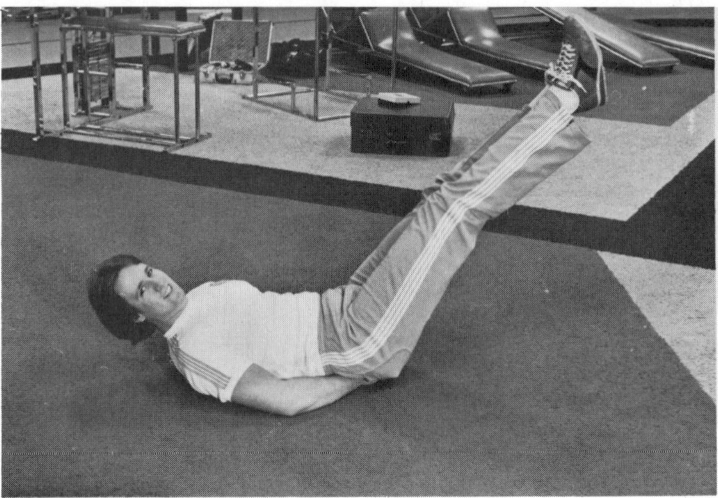

Step 2

REGULAR LEG RAISE

Vertical Leg Raises

These can be done on a chinning bar or on a set of parallel bars. The idea is to be vertical to the floor, and to bring your legs up in front of you. Bend your knees slightly to avoid back injuries, and hold for a count of three at the top of the movement. Your feet will eventually be above the level of your head, but don't overdo it at first or you will pull a kink in your back. A variation is to bend the knees and bring them up under the chin, holding for a count of three.

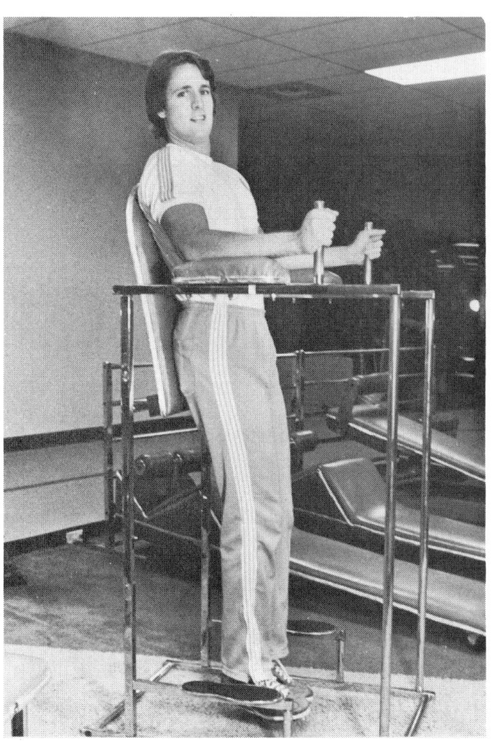

Step 1

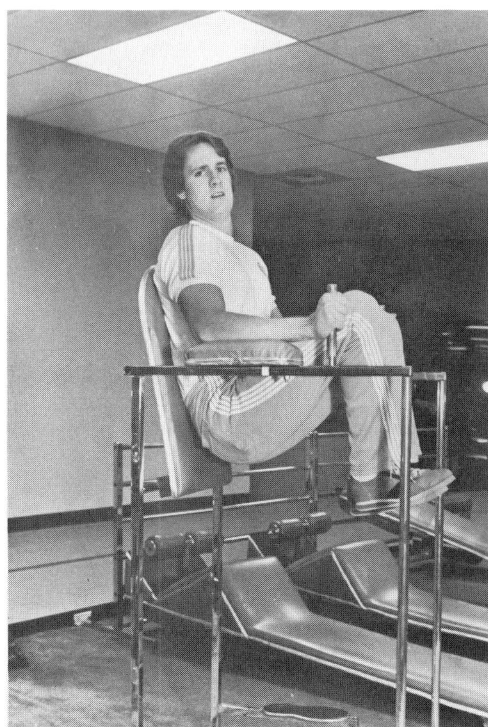

Step 2

VERTICAL LEG RAISE

Leg Raises on a Slant Board

Further intensification can be gained by lying on your back on a slant board with your head at the upper end of the board where your feet would normally be. Grasp the foothold with your hands and raise your legs, keeping the knees slightly bent, as you would if you were on the floor.

Alternating Leg Raises

This time, whether on a slant board, the floor, or hanging vertically, bring your legs up one at a time, so that they cross when they are about forty-five degrees from the plane of the body. This will work the lower abdominals from a slightly different angle and will round out your development.

Whatever way you do the leg raises, they concentrate on the lower abdominals, while crunches and situps work the upper abdominals. You need to do both leg raises and crunches or situps to work the entire abdominal area.

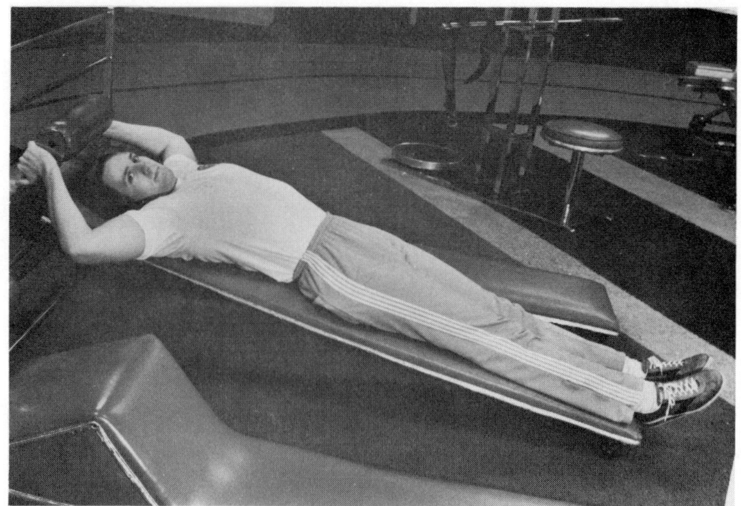

Step 1

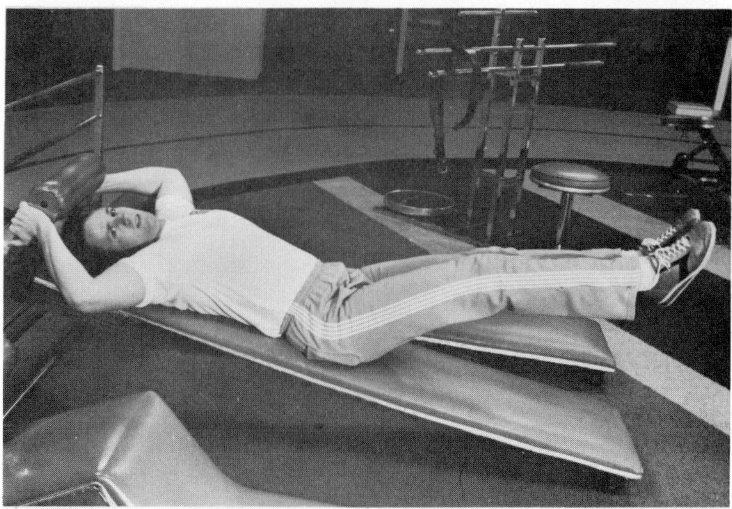

Step 2

LEG RAISE ON A SLANT BOARD

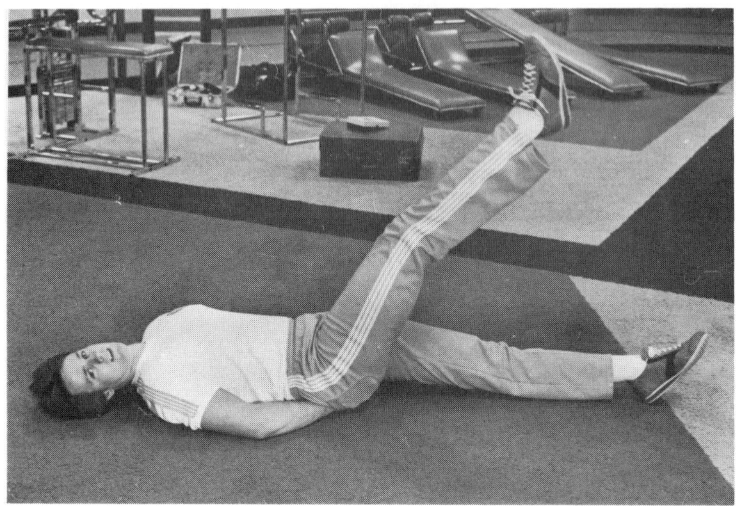

ALTERNATING LEG RAISE

EXERCISES FOR THE LOWER BACK

Since the lower back is the back part of the waist, let's make the transition to the back exercises with some exercises for that area.

SPINAL EXTENSIONS ON THE FLOOR

For a partial movement, you can do this one while lying on the floor as you would do the back crunch. Arch the back slowly, relax, and repeat for ten to twelve reps.

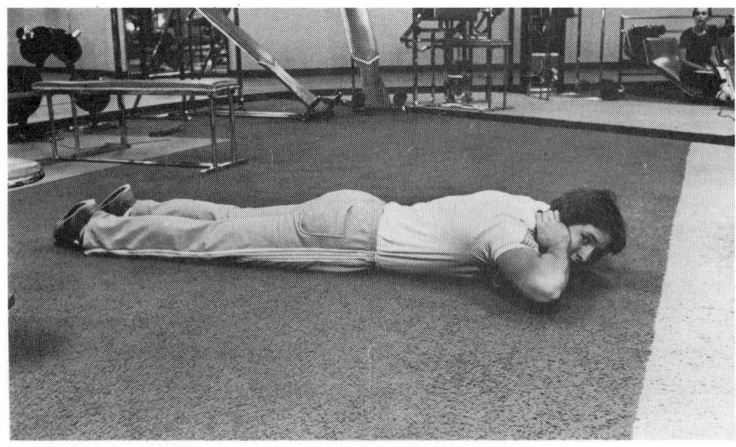

Step 1

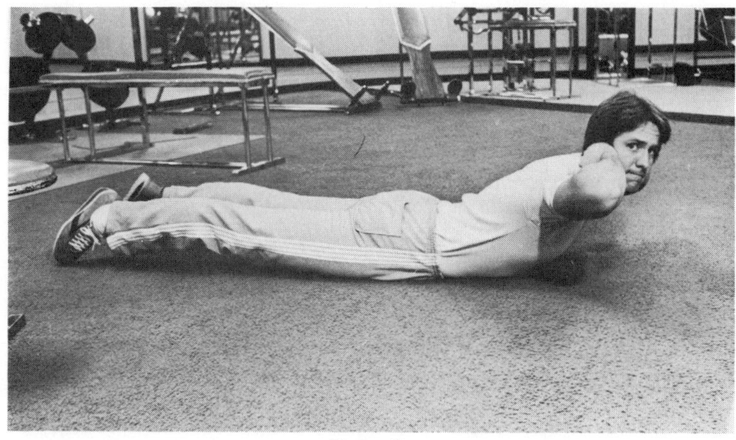

Step 2

SPINAL EXTENSION ON THE FLOOR

SPINAL EXTENSIONS ON A ROMAN CHAIR

A Roman chair is a bench with a foothold that allows you to bend at the waist while resting on a padded seat. If you sit on the seat, you can loop your feet under the foothold and do situps. If you lie on your stomach across the seat, you can do spinal extensions with a full range of movement. To do this, catch the backs of your legs at the Achilles tendon under the foothold while resting your pelvis across the seat. Place your hands behind your head and bend at the waist until your body is perpendicular to the floor. Then slowly rise until your body is parallel to the floor. Repeat slowly for ten to twelve reps.

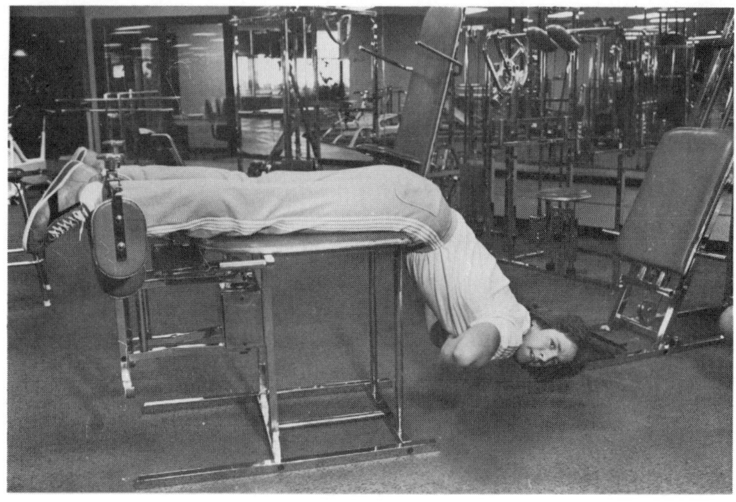

Step 1

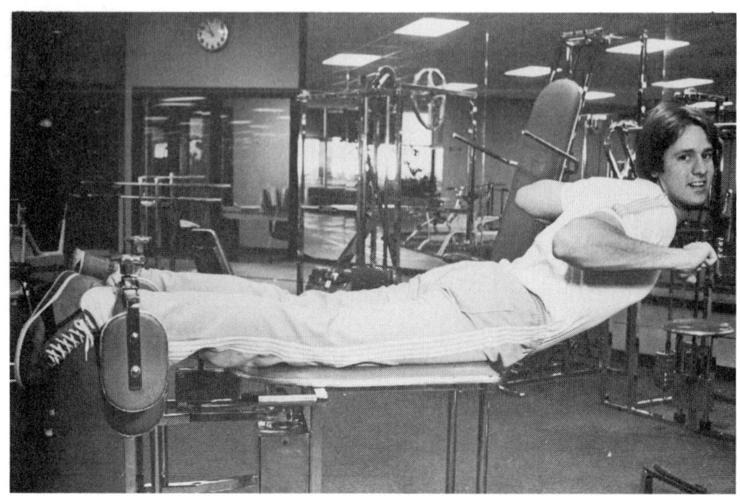

Step 2

SPINAL EXTENSION ON A ROMAN CHAIR

STIFF-LEGGED DEADWEIGHT LIFT

This exercise isolates the lower back muscles, and is both a strengthener and a trimmer. It should be done with a very light weight at the beginning, in order not to injure the back. Stand erect and bend at the waist while keeping your knees locked. Grasp a barbell with both hands and slowly return to an erect position, bringing the barbell up against the front of the thighs. Slowly let yourself down to the starting position and repeat. Don't bend your knees, and don't bounce at the bottom of the movement. Do the movement slowly and deliberately, with no jerks. Use a weight that will give you a flushed sensation in the lower back with twelve to fifteen reps. Breathe out as you go down and in as you come up.

REGULAR DEADWEIGHT LIFT

This one is used by powerlifters as training for one of their three competitive lifts. Stand erect, then bend at the waist while also bending your knees. Grasp the bar with your hands while keeping your knees bent and your back parallel to the floor. Slowly rise to an erect position while straightening your knees. You will be able to use considerably more weight in this lift than in the stiff-legged deadweight lift, but don't go overboard. It's a strenuous lift, and if you have any back injuries you should be extremely careful with it. After reaching an erect position, slowly bend at the waist and at the knees and return to the starting position. Breathe out on the way down and in on the way back up. Do ten to twelve reps.

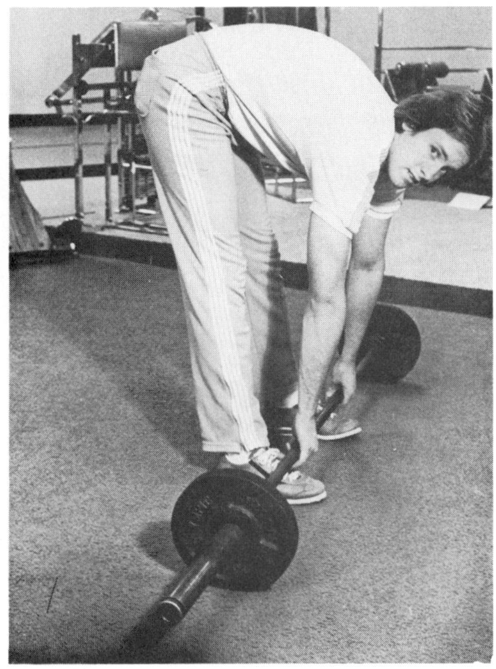

Step 1

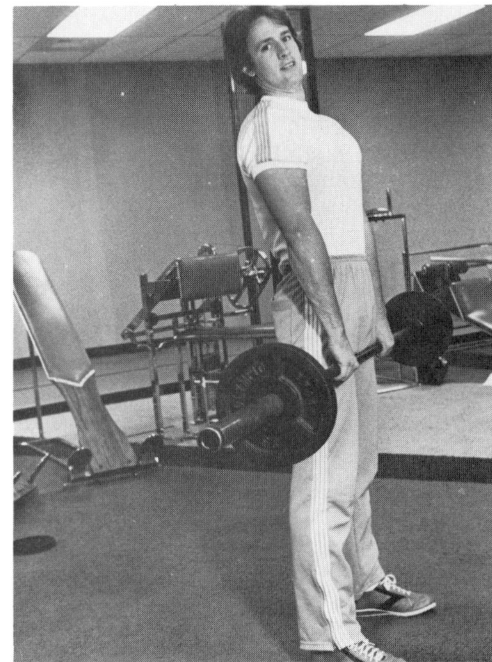

Step 2

STIFF-LEGGED DEADWEIGHT LIFT

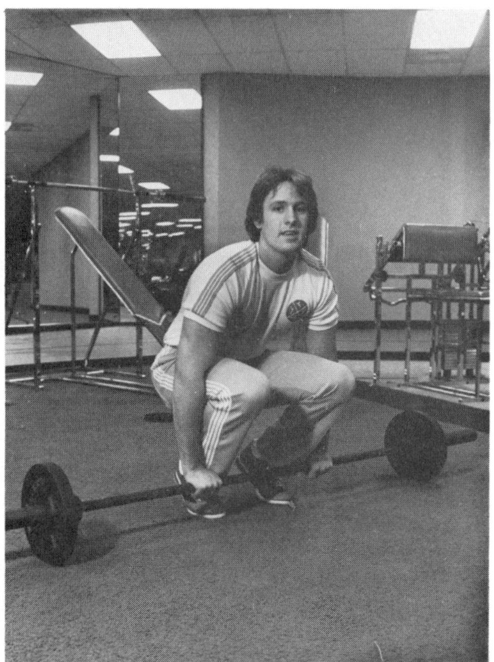

Step 1

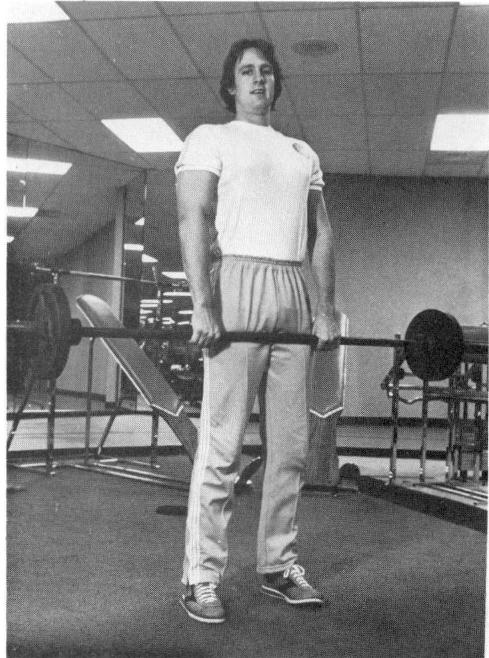

Step 2

REGULAR DEADWEIGHT LIFT

JEFFERSON LIFT

This is an oldie but a goodie. It's a combination back and leg exercise. Stand over a barbell, bend over while bending your knees, grasp the bar, and return to a standing position while bringing the bar up between your legs. You should grasp the bar with the palms facing each other as you would grasp a baseball bat. Hand spacing will depend on the structure of your body, but the hands are usually a little farther than shoulder width apart. Bend your knees, bend at the waist, and return to the starting position. Breathe in on the way up and out on the way down.

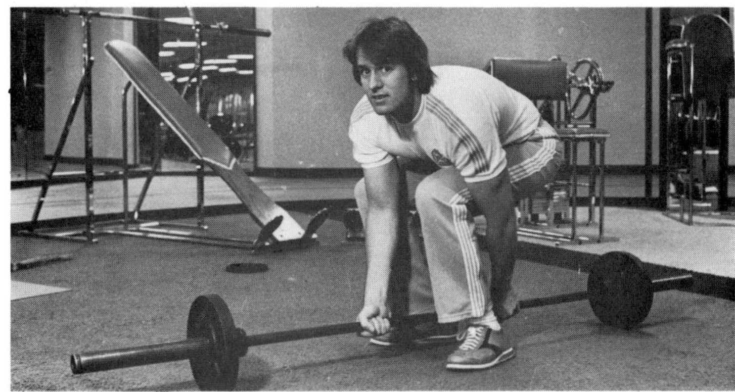

Step 1

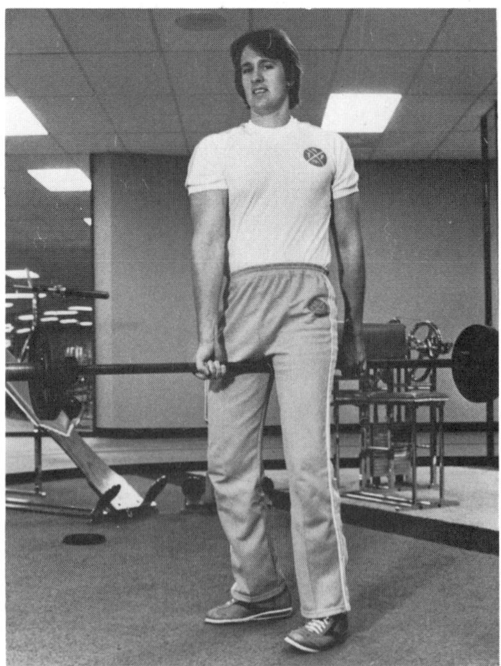

Step 2

JEFFERSON LIFT

EXERCISES FOR THE MIDDLE AND UPPER BACK

The upper and middle back is made up of two major muscle groups, the latissimus dorsi and the trapezius. The "lats" swing down underneath the arms and give you that "V" taper everyone wants. The "traps" insert at the neck and cover the upper back roughly in the shape of a manta ray, spreading out to the shoulder blades and tapering down the center of the back between the lats. The lats make you look wide and the traps give your shoulders and neck that muscular thickness that is always associated with strength and youth. You can't have an overall good build without developing these two important muscle groups. Superior traps and lat development combined with a trim waist will do more than almost any other components of your body to give you that special look that comes from weight training.

Let's do the lats first, and then work our way up the back to the traps.

LATISSIMUS EXERCISES

Wide-Grip Chins (Palms Facing away from You)

This is an old and familiar exercise, done by practically everybody who ever wanted to show off to the rest of the high school gang. The difference here is that you do the chin with a wide grip in order to isolate the lats.

Reach up and grasp a chinning bar so that your hands are placed farther apart than shoulder width; your palms are facing away from you. Pull yourself up slowly until your chin is on a level with the bar. Hold for a count of two. Then slowly let yourself back down. Be sure to get a full stretch at the bottom of the movement, but don't let the tension off the lats. Also, concentrate on making the lats do the movement instead of the arms. The temptation will be to use all the strength of the arms to pull yourself up to the bar. Try to make the lats do the work instead. The arms will always play a role in the movement, but you can minimize their role and maximize the lat work by concentrating on the back instead of the arms.

Wide-Grip Chins Behind the Neck (Palms Facing away from You)

We realize that this exercise is strangely named, but that's what they call it! It's a variation of the chin described above. This time, when you pull yourself up, pull yourself forward so that the bar will be behind your neck at the top of the lift. This will work the lats in a slightly different way, and will assure you of fully rounded development.

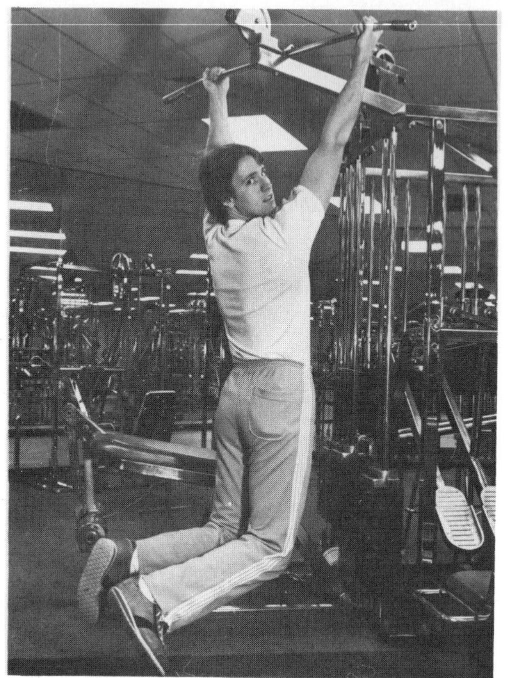

Step 1

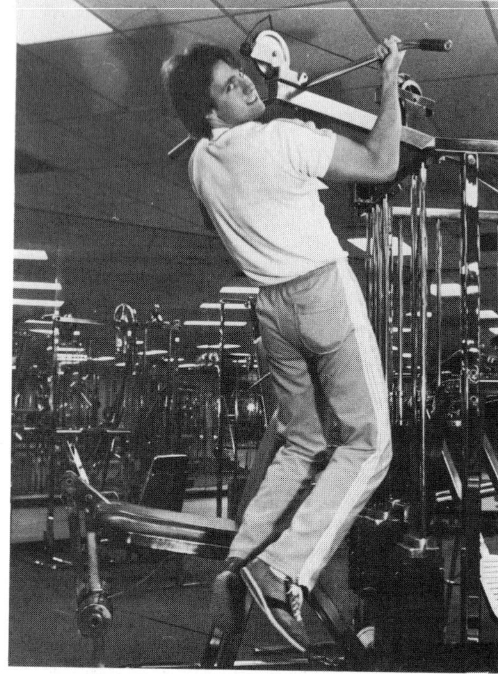

Step 2

WIDE GRIP CHIN

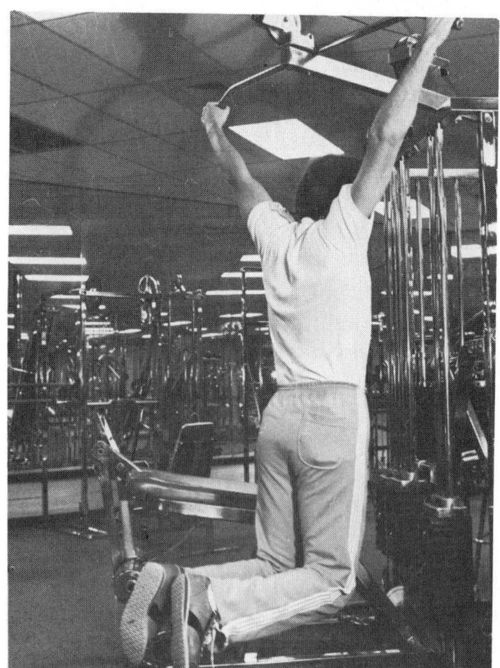
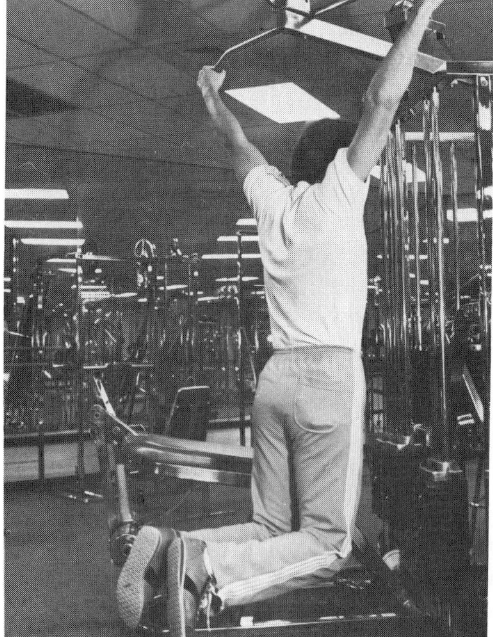

Step 1

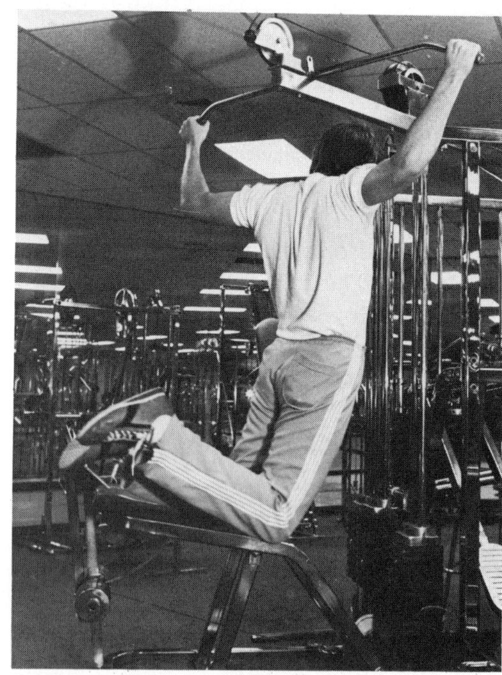

Step 2

WIDE GRIP "CHIN" BEHIND THE NECK

Close-Grip Chins (Palms Facing You)

Grasp the bar with your hands about eight inches apart; pull yourself up so that the bar is in front of your chest at the top of the movement. Keep your elbows close to your sides and concentrate on making the lats work. This exercise affects the lats in still another way and will help to build up the area immediately under your arms.

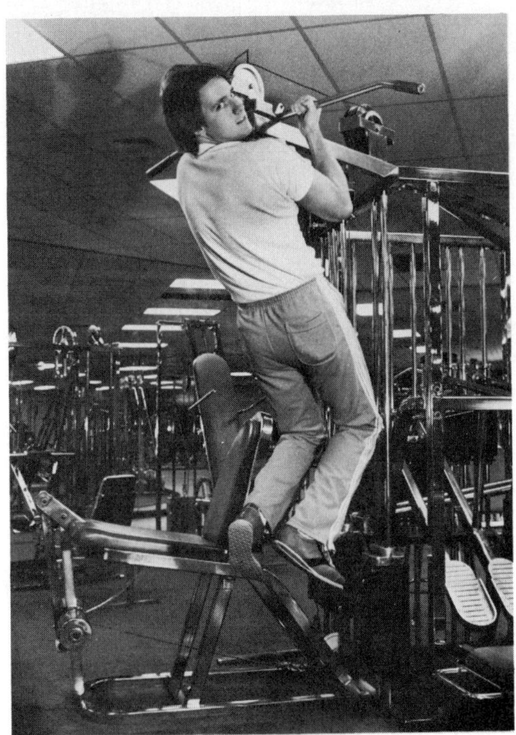

CLOSE GRIP CHIN

Reminders

A final note on chins: do all the movements slowly and deliberately. Don't bounce at the bottom of a movement. Minimize the effort of the arms and maximize the use of the lats. When you first grasp the bar, try to spread your lats as soon as you put tension on them. That way the entire range of the movement will be more effective. When you do the wide-grip chins behind the neck, arch your back and look to the front. This will intensify the movement. When you do the close-grip chins, do them with the palms facing you, and look up at the ceiling. When you get to the point where you can do more than fifteen, add weight by wearing strap-on ankle weights, iron shoes, or some barbell plates suspended by a strap from the waist.

Pulley Exercises

Another method of working the lats is by various pulley machines, common in most gyms and health clubs. When Ralph first started working out again, he realized that he would need either a pulley machine or a chinning bar. Since there was no place in our high-rise apartment to mount a chinning bar, he built a pulley attachment for the bench press/leg press bench we had bought at a local sporting goods store. It consisted of a metal bar about three feet long, a pulley with a hook that would fit over a barbell bar he had slid through the posts of the bench, about six feet of vinyl-covered one-quarter-inch cable, and a long-shank eyebolt with appropriate washer and nut. The whole thing cost about $11, and he's used it ever since. He simply threads the eyebolt through the center hole on some twenty-five-pound plates, pops on the washer and nut, and he's ready to go.

If you're not particularly enthusiastic about building your own, there are several pulley machines on the market, with prices ranging from a little over a hundred dollars all the way up to a couple of thousand. Whatever you get or build, be sure that you have both a high pulley and a low pulley. We'll explain why below.

In all pulley exercises, you will grasp a bar that is attached to a cable, which goes through a pulley and ends with weights, in the form either of barbell plates or of professionally machined rectangular plates in a rack. If you use a more primitive setup, you vary the weight by adding or subtracting barbell plates.

You should do all pulley exercises slowly and deliberately, just as you would do the chins for which many of them substitute. Don't yank on the bar, and don't bounce through the movements in an attempt to cheat on the effort. Be sure that each movement is done to the fullest extent possible, with a good stretch at the bottom of the movement and a full contraction at the top. Start with a weight that will tire you at eight to ten reps, and work your way up to sixteen to twenty reps.

When you get to the point where you are lifting a weight close to your own body weight, you may have to hold yourself down by wrapping your legs around a heavy dumbbell or barbell. A friend can help by placing his or her hands on your shoulders and applying downward pressure throughout the movement. If you're lucky enough to have access to a Nautilus machine you won't have to worry, because it includes belts to strap you in and hold you down.

Some pulley bars are straight, some are bent, and some are fashioned so that your palms face each other while doing the lift. Each pulley machine company will tout its own design as the best, so don't get upset if you read and hear a lot of claims and counterclaims. All of the machines have their merits, and different machines work the muscles in slightly different ways. Try them all if you have the chance, and you will eventually settle on the one that suits your particular skeletal and muscular structure best. Remember, the best way to assure total development is by working the muscles from every angle possible.

Here are the exercises. Have a good workout!

Pulldown Behind the Neck

This is the pulley version of the chin-behind-the-neck movement. The best way to do it is to sit on the floor, grasp the bar with a wide grip (palms facing away from you) lean your head forward, and pull the bar down until it is touching the top of the trapezius muscles at the base of your neck. It's better to sit with your legs stretched out in front of you than to have them doubled up under you, because if you do the latter the tendency is to lean forward too much. If this happens, the exercise becomes a mediocre pectoral exercise instead of a super lat exercise.

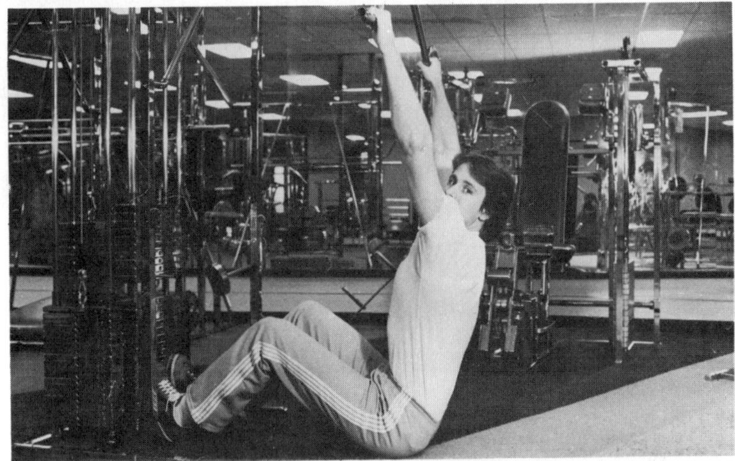

Step 1

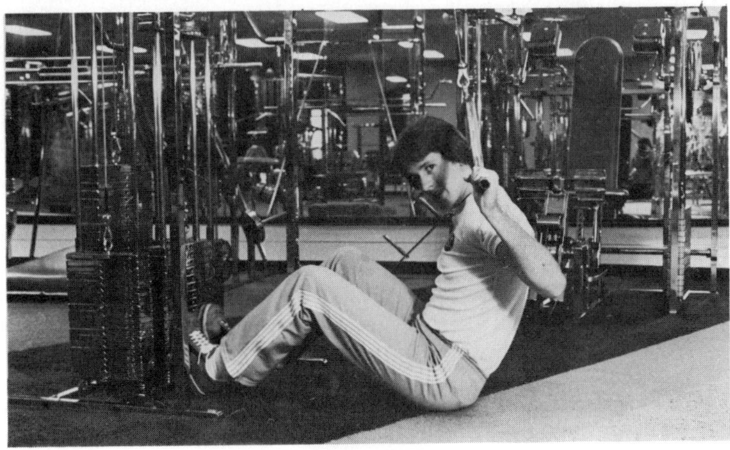

Step 2

PULLDOWN BEHIND THE NECK

Pulldown to the Chest (Palms Facing You)

Again, put your legs in front of you, and this time look up toward the ceiling or at the head of the pulley apparatus as you do the movement. Grasp the bar with the palms facing toward you, hands about eight inches apart. Pull the bar down slowly and return it slowly to the starting position. Some machines have double grips instead of a bar, so that you can keep your elbows close to the body and isolate the lats more easily.

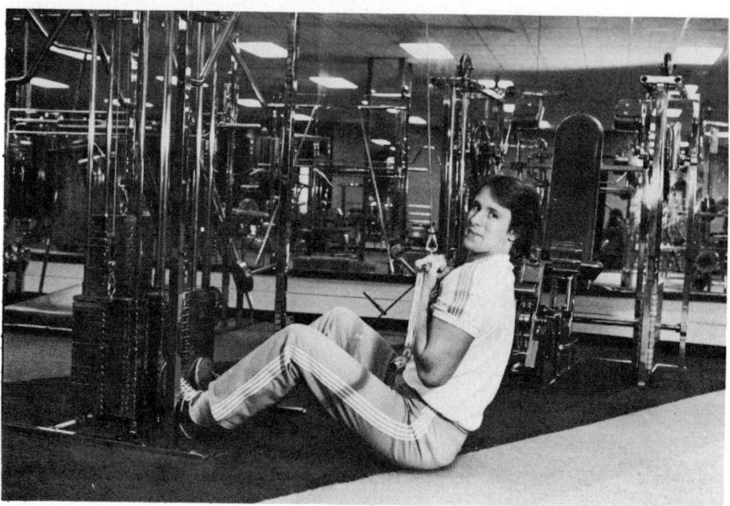

Step 1

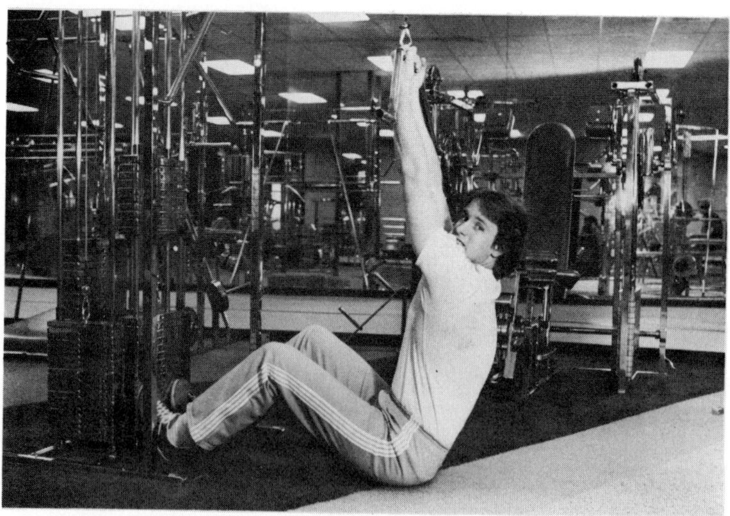

Step 2

PULLDOWN TO THE CHEST (palms facing you)

Pulldown to the Chest (Palms Facing away from You)

If you don't have access to a low-pulley machine, you can simulate the low-pulley movement by grasping the bar with the hands about six inches apart, elbows to the sides, and lying on your back on the floor before you begin the lift. You should place your feet against the machine frame about three or four feet off the floor, so that you can push yourself down and hold yourself down. Then pull the bar toward you until it is touching your chest right under the pectorals. This also is a variation of the bentover rowing movement, but it does not put the strain on the back that bentover rowing does.

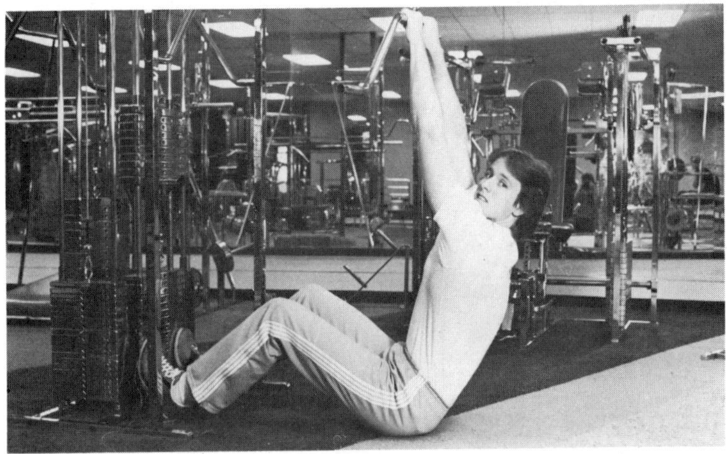

Step 1

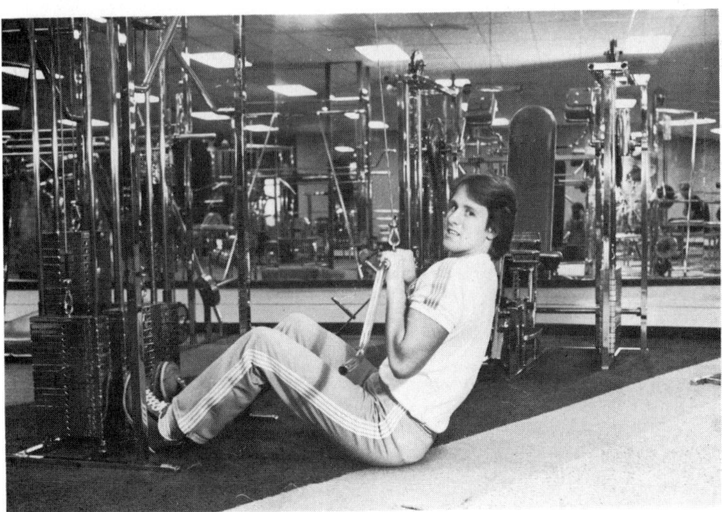

Step 2

PULLDOWN TO THE CHEST (palms facing away from you)

Low-Pulley Work

In this exercise, brace your feet against the machine frame or the footrests (if the machine has them); your legs are straight and your body is bent at the waist toward the machine. Grasp the bar or handgrips (separate handgrips are superior to a bar in this lift), keep your elbows close to your waist, and pull the grips until they are touching your chest just below the pectorals. Do the movement slowly, don't jerk or bounce, and concentrate on the lats. While the pulldowns behind the neck and to the chest work the upper area of the lats, this exercise tends to develop the lower portion of the lats for a fully rounded sweep from arms to waist. This exercise is also a good indirect way to help you get rid of those "handles" at the back and sides of the waist.

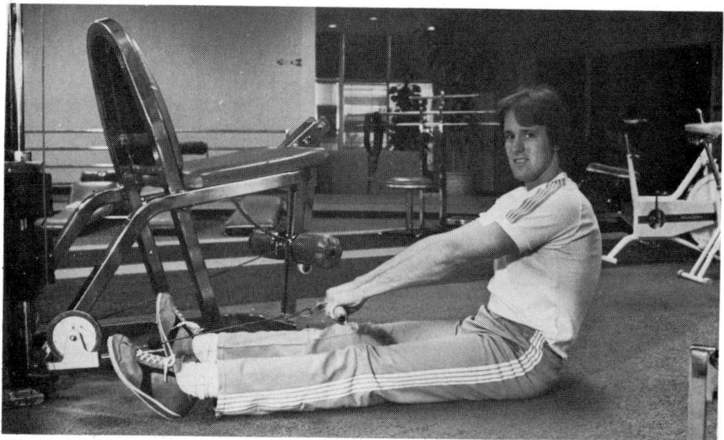

Step 1

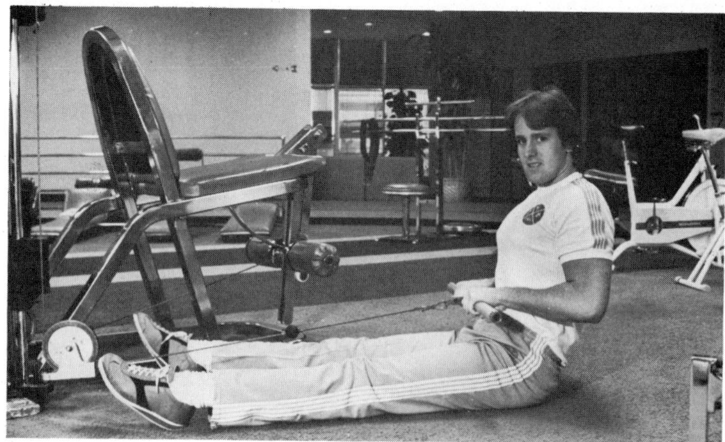

Step 2

LOW PULLEY WORK

Bentover Rowing

This is a controversial exercise which, if done properly, can give you terrific gains without danger of back injury. If done improperly—that is, with too much weight and with jerking movements—it can pop a strain in the lower back more quickly than any other exercise. It's done with (1) a barbell that has plates on both ends or (2) a barbell that has plates on the one end and the other end jammed against a stop or corner to keep it from sliding or (3) a simple lever machine. The last is nothing more than a bar that is attached to a metal or wood base on one end, leaving the other free for plate loading. Some rowing "machines" have a crossbar welded onto the main shaft so that your hands are placed with the palms facing the floor.

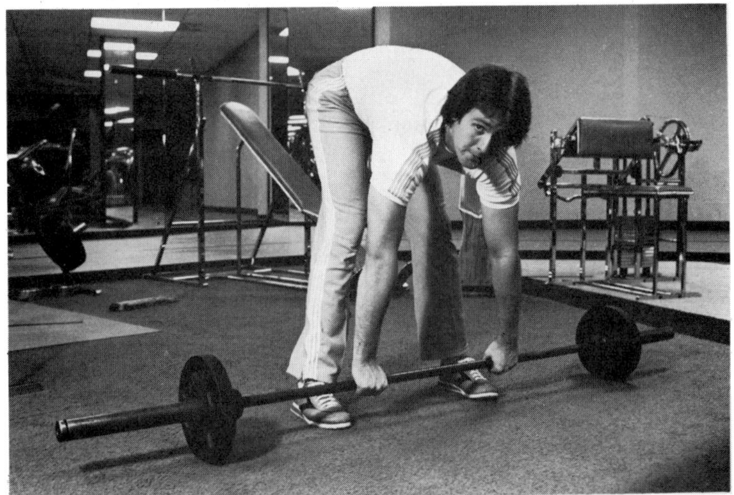

BENTOVER ROWING

Bentover rowing is done while standing with your body bent at the waist at about a forty-five-degree angle. Your elbows should be kept close to the body for lat work. The weight should be pulled up slowly until your knuckles are touching your chest just under the pectorals, then slowly lowered to the starting position. This movement works the latissimus muscles in the middle and lower areas of the back.

If you want to shift the load to your upper back, bring the weight up to a point higher on your chest while at the same time letting your elbows go wide so that the upper back contracts. Try pulling the weight up so that your knuckles come right under your chin. Place your arms so that at the end of the movement they are at right angles to your body, and your elbows are higher than the plane of your upper back. In bentover rowing, arms and hand position are the variables that determine the area of the back to be worked.

You should not lock your knees completely, but let them be slightly bent so that you will not put a strain on the joints. Further, since you will find that you increase weight rather quickly in this exercise, guard against using weight that is too heavy for your present lower back strength. If you have trouble or pain in doing this lift, substitute pulley work and take the strain off the lower back.

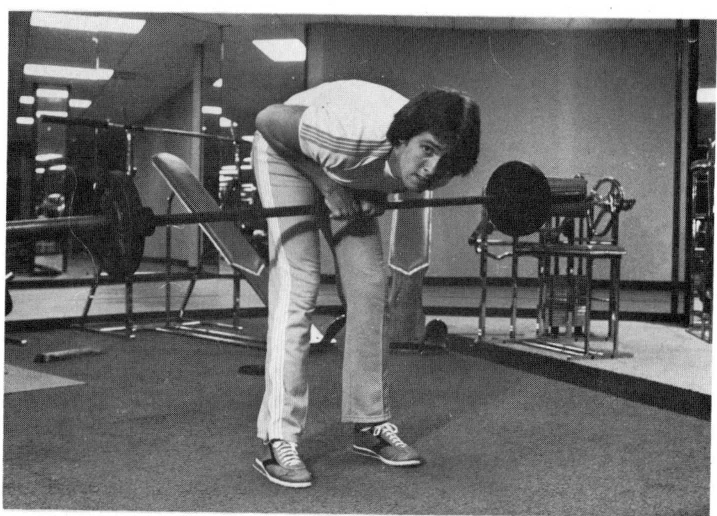

BENTOVER ROWING (close grip for middle back)

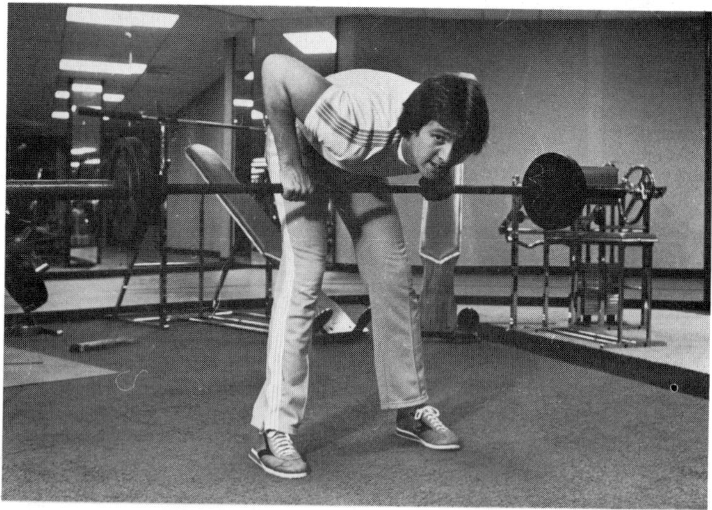

BENTOVER ROWING—ALTERNATE
(wide grip for middle and upper back)

One-Arm Bentover Rowing

In this exercise, you will use a dumbbell instead of a barbell. Place your feet about shoulder width apart and lean at the waist toward the floor until your upper body is almost parallel to the floor. Rest one hand on a bench for balance, and grasp a dumbbell with the other hand. Keep your elbows close to your sides, and bring the dumbbell up until it is even with the side of your waist. Then slowly return it to the starting position. Practice this lift until you feel a good stretch at the bottom of the movement and a good contraction at the top. Because of variations in individual structure, you will have to find the right "groove" that does the most for you. This is an excellent exercise for the lower lats, but you must concentrate on letting the lats do the movement instead of the arms. Think of your hands as merely hooks, and your arms as merely inanimate pieces of wood that connect the hooks to the lats.

TRAPEZIUS EXERCISES

Now let's move on up the back to the top. The last pose in the obligatory sequence of poses in any IFBB (International Federation of Bodybuilders) physique contest is the "most muscular" pose. It's the one where the bodybuilder will clench his fists in front of him, arch toward the front, flex the abdominals and the pectorals, and throw his trapezius muscles into full contraction by pulling his shoulders downward. That's when you see the maximum display of these muscles. It's also the most ungainly of all the obligatory poses. Unfortunately for bodybuilding's image, it's the one that photojournalists love the most for its very grotesqueness, and many people mistakenly think that bodybuilders look like that all the time.

It's a shame that this sort of thing happens, because many people base their evaluation of what weight trained muscles look like on what, unknown to them, is a formalized, obligatory requirement for contests. Consequently, when you talk about traps exercises, some people shy away because they don't want to look like a constipated version of Hercules.

Don't worry. The traps don't grow all that easily, and besides, when they are relaxed they add the depth and fullness to the neck and shoulder area that makes the difference between a symmetrical body and a lopsided one. Also, it's good to have both strength and size in the traps, since they are used in almost any lift that you make with the arms. You can't pick up a dumbbell off the rack without bringing the traps into play. Don't neglect them, and they will announce to the world around you that you are a force to be reckoned with!

Shoulder Shrugs with Dumbbells

Grasp a dumbbell in each hand; stand erect, with your eyes front, back straight, shoulders slumped toward the front. Hold the dumbbells to the front, with their handles making a triangle in front of you. Pull your shoulders up and back, arching your upper back between the shoulders, lifting the shoulders as far as they will go toward touching your ears. Rotate the shoulders all the way back while throwing your chest out to the front, and while bringing the dumbbells around to the sides of your body. Then let the shoulders continue to rotate downward until they have reached the starting position. Keep your elbows straight at all times, and resist the impulse to bend your arms and pull the dumbbells higher by contracting the biceps.

The object of this exercise is to work the traps, not the arms. The shoulders will move in a circle so that the entire bulk of the traps is worked. You should do ten to twelve reps at the start, with enough weight so that the final rep is a real effort. If you do it right, you should feel a nice burning sensation on about the ninth or tenth rep.

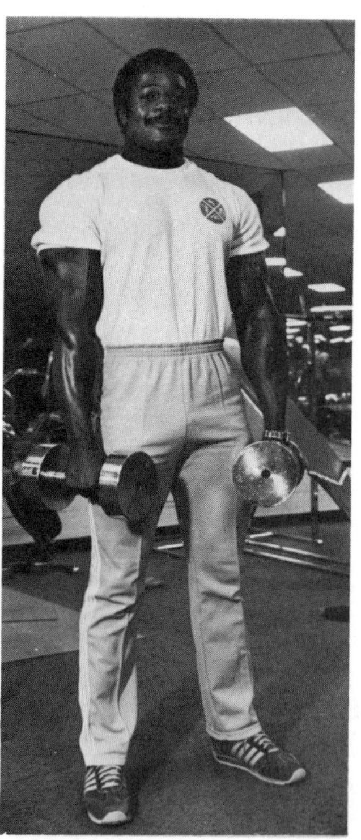

Step 1

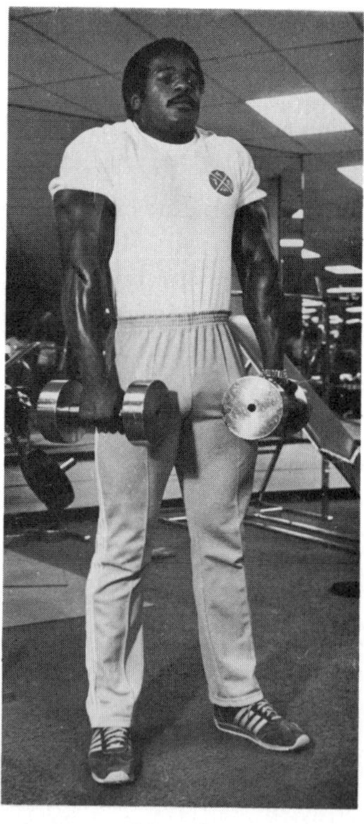

Step 2

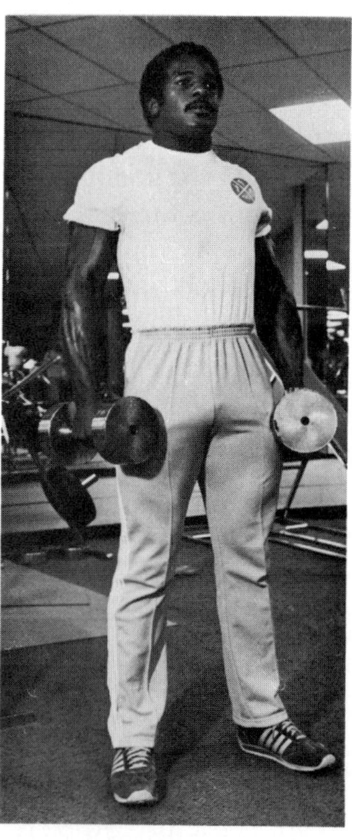

Step 3

SHOULDER SHRUG WITH DUMBBELLS

Shoulder Shrugs with a Barbell

This exercise is done essentially the same way as the dumbbell shrug, but this time you will use a barbell. Grasp the bar with your hands about eight inches apart: keep your arms straight, palms facing you; and rotate your shoulders through the movement.

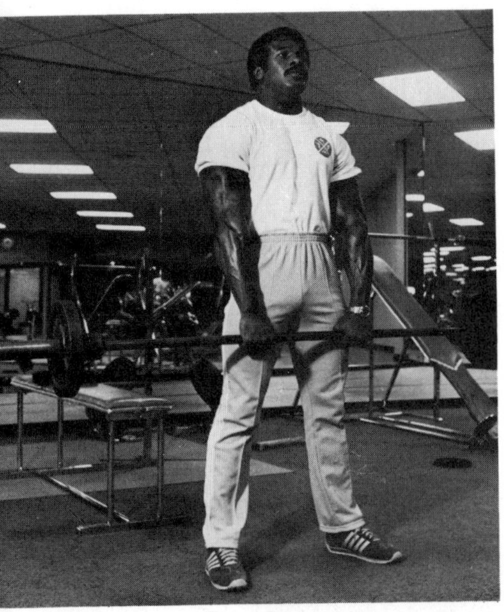

Step 1

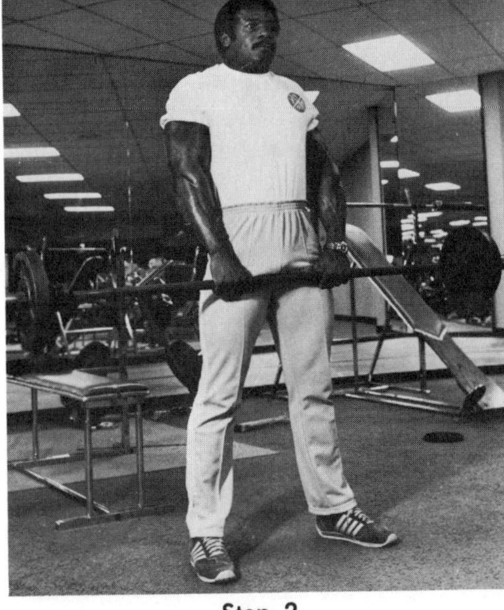

Step 2

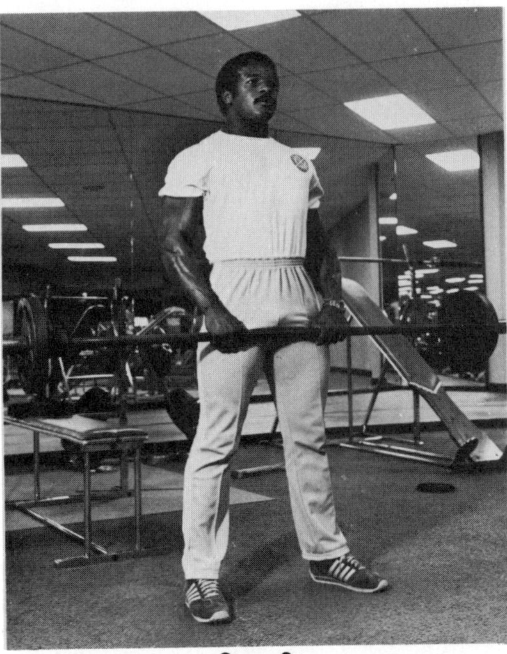

Step 3

SHOULDER SHRUG WITH BARBELL

Upright Rowing Motion

This exercise works the traps as well as the shoulders. Grasp a barbell with your hands about four inches apart, the palms facing you. Stand erect, back straight or slightly arched, and lift the barbell in straight line from in front of your thighs to a point in front of your face. At the top of the movement, lift the bar a little past the level of your chin, and you will feel the traps come into play in an effort to continue the movement overhead. If you start the movement with the shoulders slumped forward and contract the traps throughout the movement, you will receive the maximum effect on the traps. Keep your elbows high throughout the movement, and think of your hands as hooks. Concentrate on letting the traps and the deltoids do all the work.

A cautionary note: one of the most painful injuries Ralph ever suffered occurred while doing upright rows with only seventy pounds. When you get the bar about even with the top of your chest, there is a tendency to let the arms take over the lift. Perhaps this is a holdover from prior conditioning in doing "snatching" movements, which aim to bring the weight from the floor to an overhead position. Whatever the cause, if you allow your arms to pull too high, you will place undue strain on the

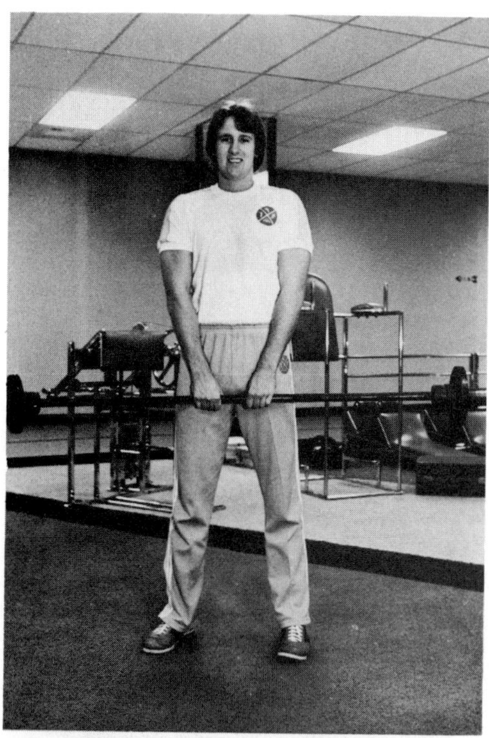

UPRIGHT ROWING MOTION

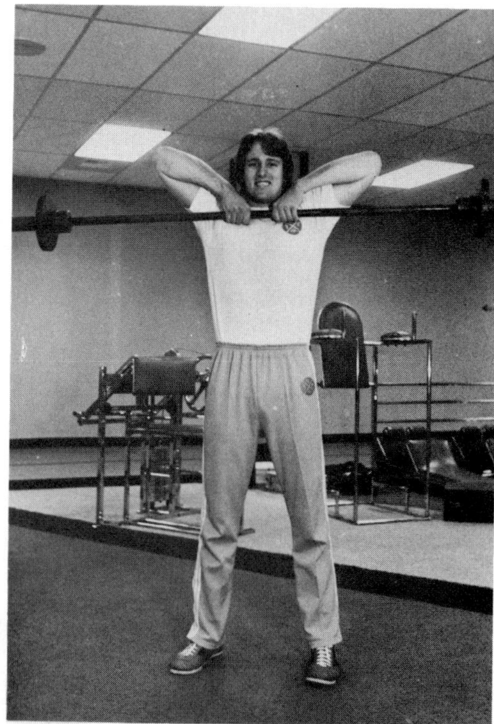

UPRIGHT ROWING MOTION WITH BARBELL

forearms, especially the ropelike muscle that runs from the elbow across the top of the forearm. Once that muscle is pulled, it takes a long time for it to heal. Ralph was injured on the last of twelve reps. He felt the muscle give, felt a twinge, but really didn't pay much attention to it. Within an hour, the arm was all but immobilized.

So, remember: in this exercise, concentrate on letting the traps and the shoulders do the work. Keep the bar as close to your body as you can, and don't jerk it up. Let the movement be slow and smooth, with a hold at the top for a count of two.

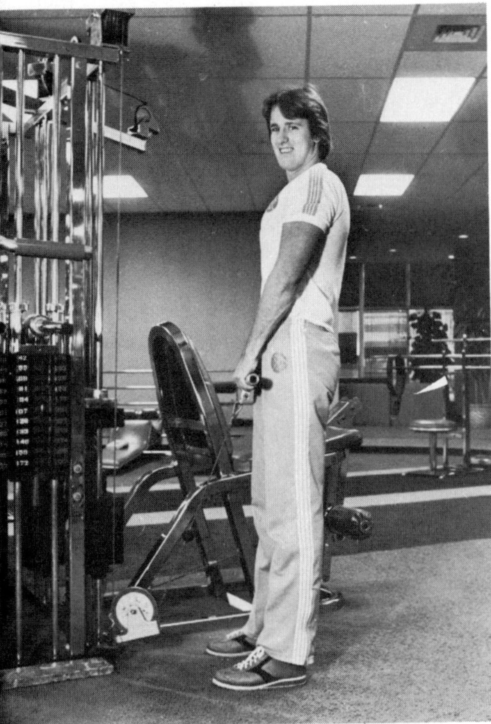

Step 1

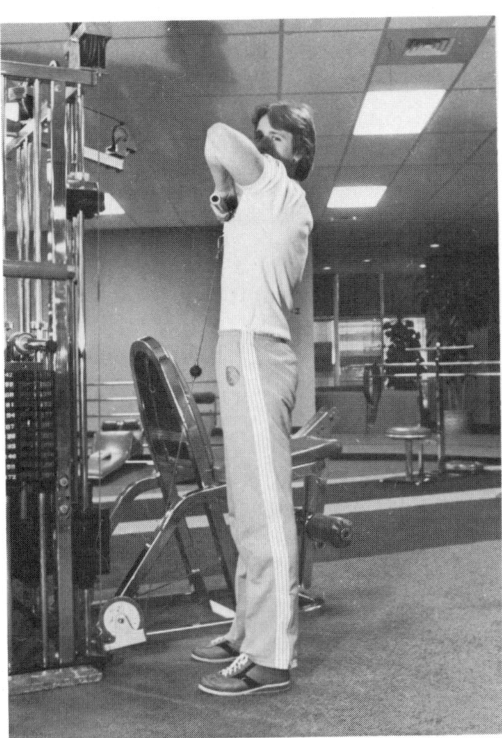

Step 2

UPRIGHT ROWING MOTION WITH MACHINE

EXERCISES FOR THE CHEST

We'll leave the back now and go on to the other side of the body: the chest area. The chest is made up of the pectoral muscles, the large slablike muscles that cover the area from the collarbones to the sternum. There should be a sharp separation between one side and the other, and the line at the bottom of the pecs should be clean and free of fat. The collarbones should not be prominent, but should be covered at the top by the upper pectoral. There should also be strong tie-ins between the pecs and the deltoid, or shoulder, muscles.

In addition to building up muscular mass, you should also do exercises that expand your chest and limber up your rib cage. These exercises don't involve much weight, and are primarily breathing exercises. Among them, the most popular is the two-arm pullover, which is described in detail on page 149.

In seeking a symmetrical body, you should never neglect pectoral development. You don't have to build huge slabs of meat like the pros do, but there's nothing that attracts attention more quickly than a person with a small waist and a large chest. If you strive to improve your posture as well, walking always with the chest out instead of hidden away as if you were ashamed of it, you will find that some of your back problems and chronic shoulder and neck aches will disappear. The only time you should slump your shoulders is when you are getting ready to do shoulder shrugs!

Let's begin with the heavyweight of all chest exercises.

THE BENCH PRESS

This is by far the most popular weight training lift. It's the glamour lift, and if your gym or health club has a bench press rack, that's where you'll find most of the heavy-metal types. It's not unusual to see otherwise sane, normal men grinding out rep after rep, set after set, on the bench, until they can hardly lift their arms to wipe the sweat from their foreheads.

Maybe it's because they can lie down to do the lift. More than likely, it's because it's possible to run up some pretty impressive poundages in a relatively short time. The bench press is a compound exercise—it works the arms and the anterior deltoids as well as the pectorals—and it will add inches to your upper body faster than any other single exercise.

We offer several words of warning about the bench press, and implore you to take them seriously. Along with the leg press with a free barbell, the bench press is one of the few weight training exercises that can be truly dangerous if you're not careful. You may remember the young man who played the male lead in Antonioni's movie *Zabriskie Point.* After the movie, his luck changed; he got into trouble and wound up in a state prison doing three to five years for robbery. While in prison he got interested in weight training, and tried doing heavy bench presses without a spotter. One day it finally caught up with him, and they found him dead with the bar lying across his neck. Last year another amateur weight trainer died of the same cause, with his helpless four-year-old son standing beside him.

If it sounds like we're trying to scare you, it's because we are. We would really be shirking our duty if we failed to tell you when to be careful. Nobody wants to get hurt in any sport, especially if the purpose of that sport is essentially constructive. So whatever you do, don't do the bench press with heavy weight unless you have a spotter handy who has the strength to lift the weight on up if you are unable to complete that last rep. It's just good sense.

This is especially true if you're never done any weight training before. In order to make the maximum gains in the bench press, you should handle poundages heavy enough to put sufficient stress on the muscle fibers to cause them to enlarge, to build. That means that the last few reps should really be squeezed out, almost past your limits. This is fine when you're doing stiff-legged deadweight lifts. If you can't make that last rep, you can always let the bar go. If you let the bar go when you're doing heavy bench presses, it'll go right down on your neck. If you're just a beginner in this fascinating form of exercise, you probably won't be able to tell just when you are reaching your limits. A missed last rep on the bench press is a hell of a way to find out.

There are many ways to get around this. One, of course, is to have a spotter. Another is to buy or build yourself a bench rack that has bolts or shelves to throw the weight onto if you can't make it all the way to the top. In fact, there are some bench press racks, such as the Safety Gym frequently advertised in *Iron Man* magazine, which have structural safeguards built into the design that enable you to do a wide range of exercises normally requiring a spotter, all with complete safety. Check them out if you're planning to build your own home gym. If you go to a gym or health club, take a look at the equipment and make sure that either it is safety equipment or that you have a spotter handy. Some clubs stock the regular bench rack but do not provide a spotter. In that case, either work out with a friend or get one of the attendants to spot.

Enough said. Time to get to work.

The exercise is done with a barbell. The longer the bar the better, since you will want to place your hands wide in order to throw most of the weight on the pecs. After doing a few warm-up movements for your shoulders, lie on your back on the bench; reach up and make sure that your hands are spaced so that they are equidistant from the respective ends of the bar. If you don't space your hands correctly, you may find out too late that you are off balance.

Lift the barbell off the rack, and bring it down slowly to a point toward the bottom of the pectorals. Everybody has a slightly different "power groove," and you'll have to experiment in order to find out where yours is. When you find the right groove, you'll see what we mean. You'll have more power in the groove, and you'll experience less strain on your wrists, elbows, and shoulders. The weight will move smoothly throughout the movement, and you'll feel a great surge of power every time you lock onto the right track.

For some people, the groove is higher, up around the top of the chest.

For us the groove is lower, almost down at the sternum. So try the lift a few times with light weights and find the right groove. It's as important as finding the right groove or line on an auto-racing track. It's where you get the maximum performance.

When you reach the bottom of the movement, slowly push the weight back up to the starting position. Whatever you do, don't bounce the bar off your chest! We work out in a local gym occasionally, and every day there is a young man there—let's call him Jerry—who gives us shudders whenever he gets on the bench. He places a folded towel on his chest to

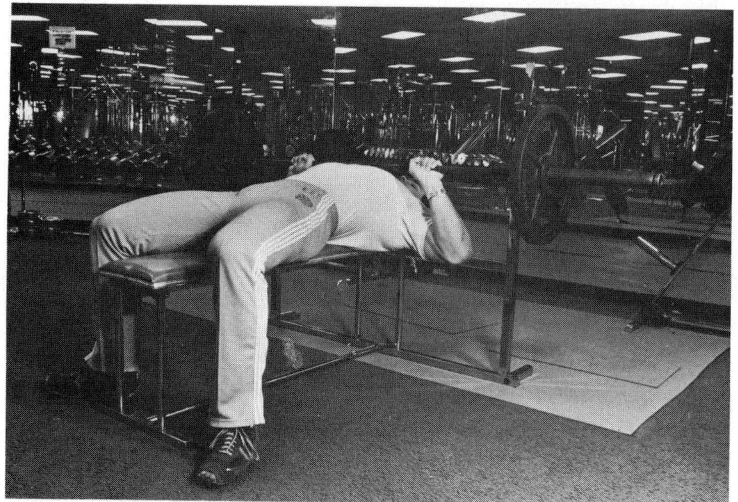

Step 1

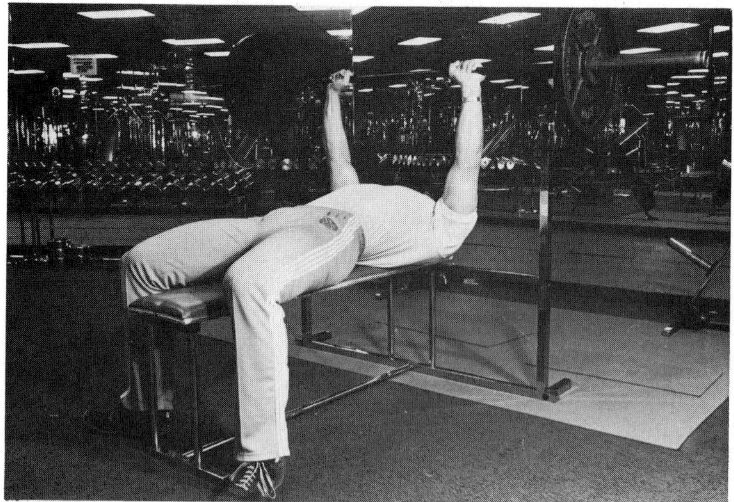

Step 2

BENCH PRESS

soften the blow, and then brings 195 to 215 pounds down on his chest with a *whomp!* and bounces it back up in the air.

Let's stop for a moment and talk about what Jerry's doing. In the first place, the bench press has three basic phases as the weight is pushed up to arms' length. At the bottom of the lift, and for the first few inches, the anterior deltoids do most of the work. Think about it for a moment. Your chest muscles are stretched to the side, the bar is touching your chest, and your pecs have no leverage. Your triceps have no leverage yet, because your arms are fully bent. It's the anterior, or front, deltoids that start the movement of the barbell back up. There is a sticking point about three inches off the chest when the pectorals begin to take over from the anterior deltoids. For the next few inches, the pectorals do more and more work until a second sticking point is reached about a foot off the chest, as the triceps begin to take over from the pecs. The last eight inches of the lift are done principally by the triceps, with assists from the pecs and the anterior deltoids. That's why it's called a compound lift.

Our young friend is lacking in anterior deltoid strength. He's making up for it by bouncing the barbell off of his chest at the bottom of the lift. That way he gets enough momentum from the bounce to get the bar up into pec territory, and if it's a vigorous bounce, he can skip right through the pec range into the triceps range for the end of the lift.

What is Jerry accomplishing? Well, for one thing, he's using a more impressive poundage than he would be if he weren't bouncing. To some people, this means a great deal. However, he is cheating himself out of whatever anterior deltoid and pec development the lift might give him, because the bounce is taking care of inertia at the bottom of the lift instead of shoulder and pec strength.

In turn, this means that he will reach a sticking point in the lift as far as poundages go, and he will not be able to go past that sticking point until he learns to do the lift correctly—slowly down, no bounce, and slowly back up.

Another young man at the gym, Joe, is 5′ 6½″ tall and weighs around 165 pounds. He does repetition bench presses with weights of 275, 280, and 300 pounds. Each time, the lift is done slowly and deliberately. When he started working out, he could barely lift 90 pounds. That was only two years ago!

Close-Grip Bench Presses

A variation on the regular wide-grip bench press is the close-grip press. For this, you place the hands about a foot to eighteen inches apart and keep the elbows closer to the sides. The exercise becomes more of a triceps movement and less of a pectoral movement. Later on, in the arm-exercises section, we'll describe another variation that is one of the favorite arm builders of the first Mr. Olympia, Larry Scott.

You might want to do two sets of wide-grip bench presses, and then follow them with close-grip presses. This will work the pectorals, the deltoids, and the triceps in at least two different ways, and the result will be a better rounded program. Try it and see how it works for you.

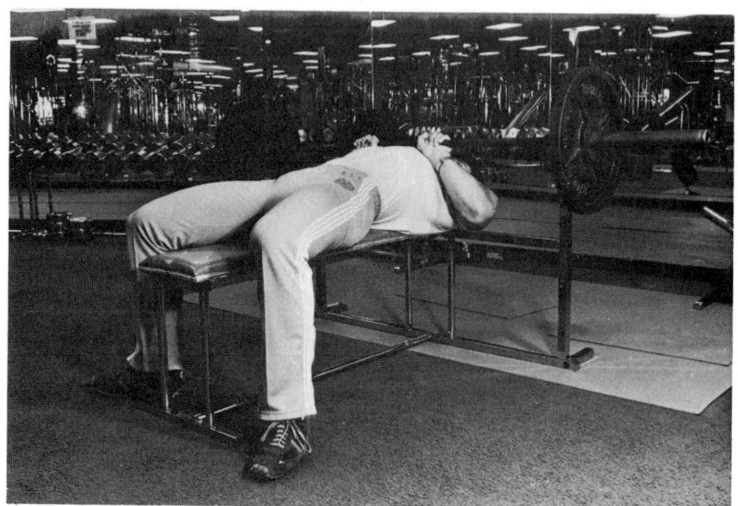

Step 1

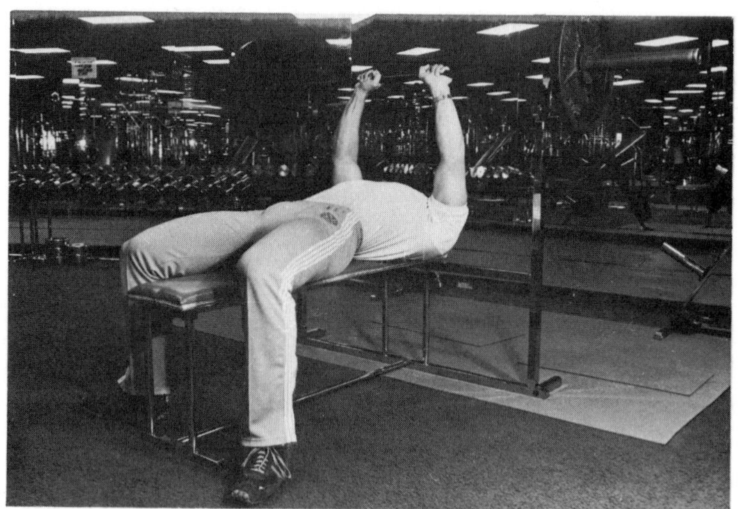

Step 2

CLOSE-GRIP BENCH PRESS

Incline Bench Presses

The most popular variation on the regular bench press is the incline bench press. This is done while you lie on a bench that is about forty-five degrees from the floor. Often you can use a squat rack to hold the barbell and can slide the incline under it. Care should be taken not to bite off more than you can chew when doing this one. The upper pecs are not usually that strong, and you can get into trouble in a hurry if you don't watch out. Also, you will not be able to handle as much weight as you do for the regular bench press, so don't try it with the same weight that you regularly use.

The incline bench press shifts the work load to the upper pecs, although the middle and lower pecs receive a thorough working out, too. If you want to balance your upper and lower pec development, this lift is a must. You can use either a barbell or dumbbells for this lift. The barbell will be easier to handle, because you won't be having to balance both dumbbells in the air. However, you should use both in the lift, because they work the pecs in different ways. The hand positions are the same for both dumbbells and barbell, and the movement will add poundages to your regular bench press.

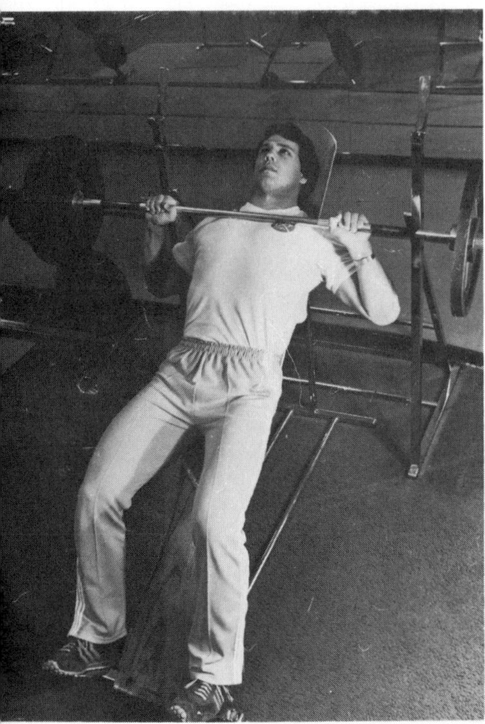

Step 1

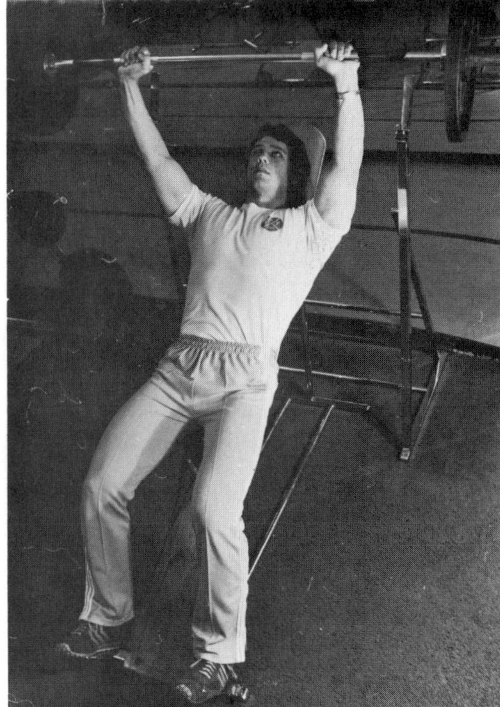

Step 2

INCLINE BENCH PRESS

Decline Bench Presses

Lie on an incline bench with your head at the bottom and press the barbell toward the ceiling. This works the lower pecs.

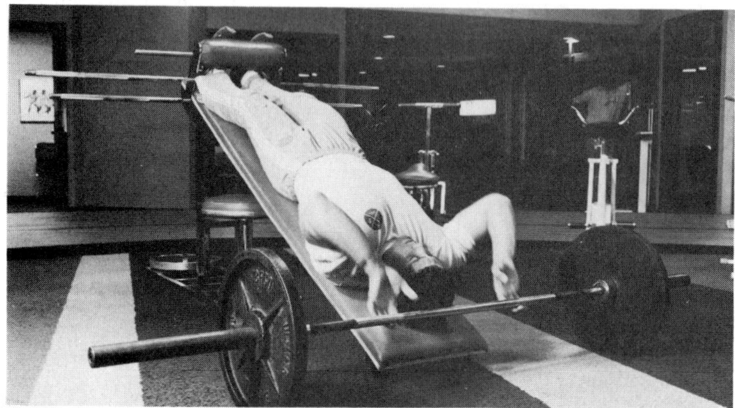

Step 1

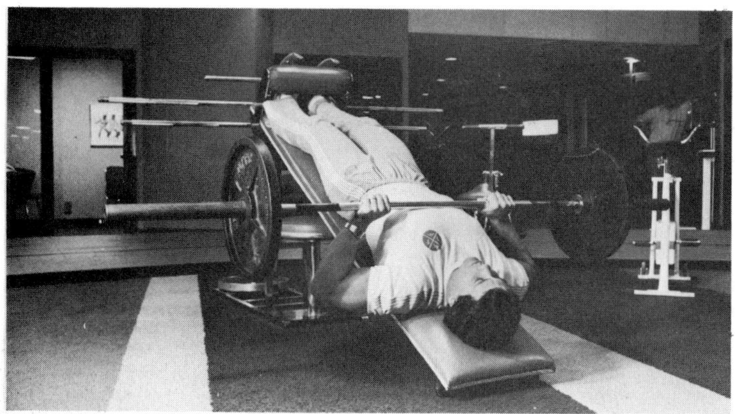

Step 2

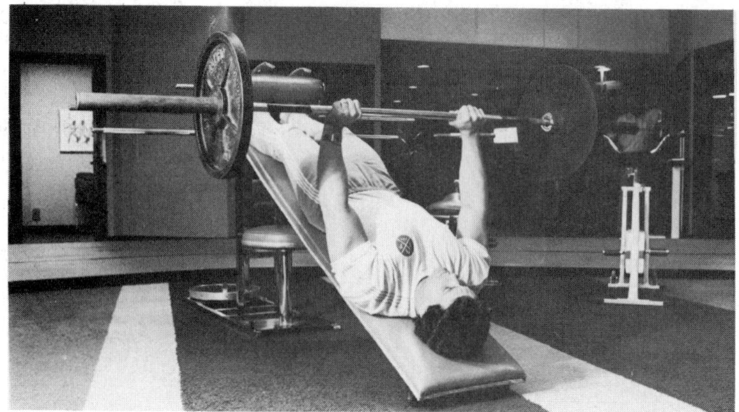

Step 3

DECLINE BENCH PRESS

Partial Bench Press Movements

When you do the regular wide-grip bench presses, try coming up only halfway before bringing the weight back down to the chest. This leaves the triceps out of the lift, for the most part, and gives the pectorals most of the work load. You may remember the scene in the movie *Pumping Iron* when Louie ("The Incredible Hulk") Ferrigno was doing bench presses under his father's supervision. He was doing partial movements, burning the pecs and concentrating on chest development.

When you are doing bench presses, resist the temptation to arch your back excessively. Many people try to force the weight up by arching their back (it makes it easier for the triceps to take over the lift), and often pull the lumbar muscles in the process. Certainly in competition you aren't allowed to arch your back, and except for the rare occasion when you might be in trouble with more weight than you and your spotter can handle, it's better to do the lift with the back flat on the bench.

Also, make sure your spotter knows how to spot. Gyms are always rife with stories about how inept spotters grabbed barbells by one end instead of the middle in a futile attempt to help out somebody who had pushed his muscles to the limit.

FLYES

The second most popular chest exercise is the "flye," a barbarous name taken from the old nomenclature, "flying exercises." There are several ways to do flyes, each working the pecs in a slightly different way. They also can be done either on a flat or an incline bench. The incline bench works the upper pecs, while the flat bench works the entire pectoral area.

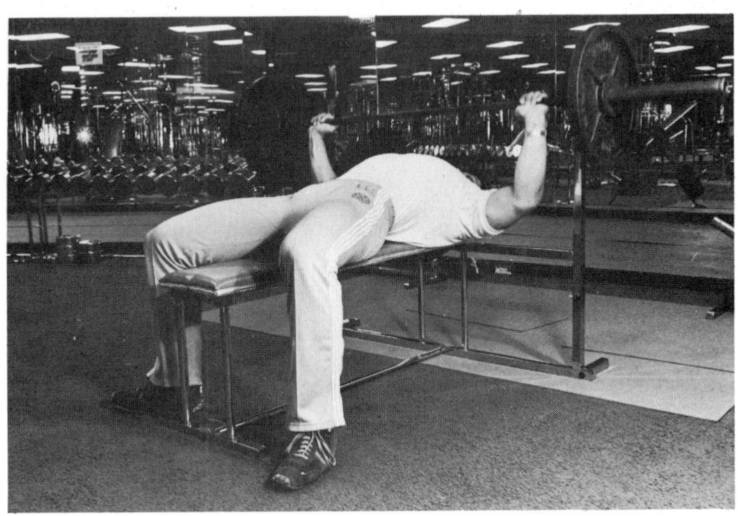

PARTIAL BENCH PRESS MOVEMENT

The Straight-Arm Flye

In this form of the flye, dumbbells are hoisted to a position over your chest while you are lying on your back. Bring the dumbbells down to your sides in an arc that is perpendicular to your body, stopping when your arms are almost parallel to the floor. Then bring the arms slowly back to the starting position. You won't be able to handle much weight on this one; if you do try to handle too much, you run the risk of elbow injury. Go easy.

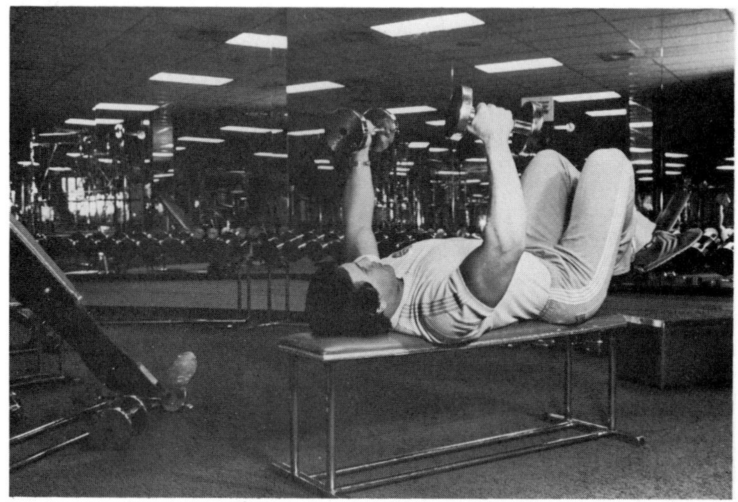

Step 1

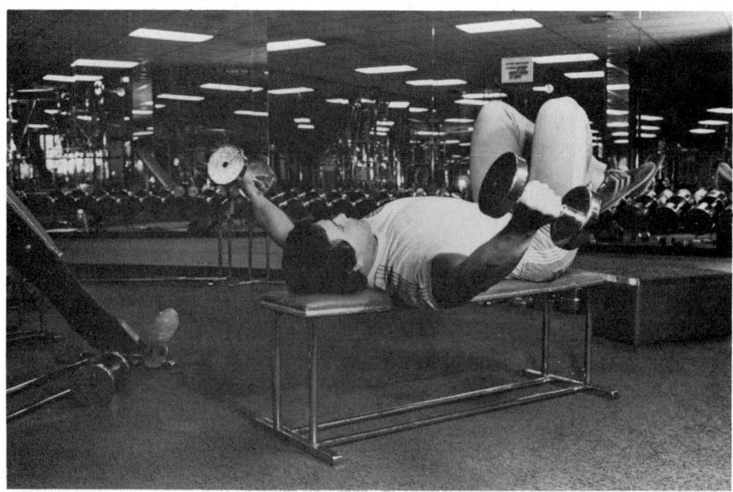

Step 2

THE STRAIGHT-ARM FLYE

The Bent-Arm Flye

Begin the same as above, but bend the elbows as you bring the arms down. Since the elbows are bent, you can bring the upper arms down past the plane of the body, and thus get a much better stretch of the pecs at the bottom of the movement. Bring the arms slowly back to the starting position.

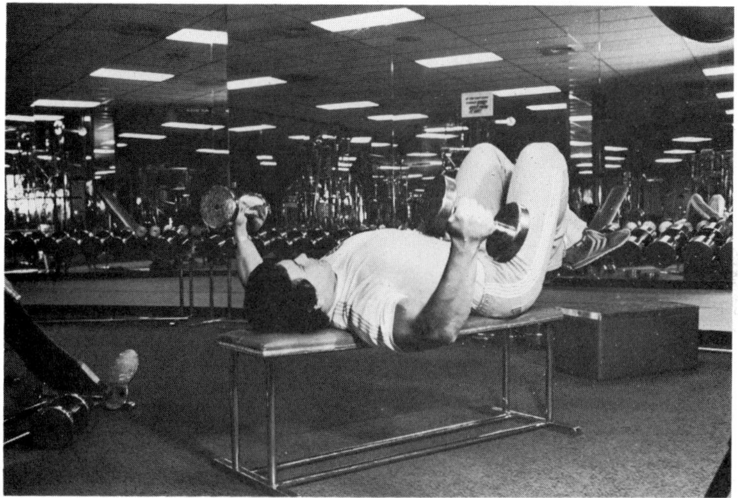

THE BENT-ARM FLYE

Hand Positions for the Flyes

Most people have the palms facing them at the top of the lift, and rotate the arms so that the palms are facing front at the bottom. Consequently, when the arms are down and extended out from the sides, the palms will be in the same position as they would be for the bench press. However, you may find that the pecs get a better stretch if you leave your hands in the position they started, and do not rotate the arms on the way down. Try it both ways and you'll see the difference.

When doing flyes, you should not allow yourself to rest at the top of the lift, but should immediately lower the dumbbells back down to the sides. When you do flyes on an incline bench, you should lower the dumbbells in an arc that is perpendicular to the floor. That places the greatest work load on the upper pecs.

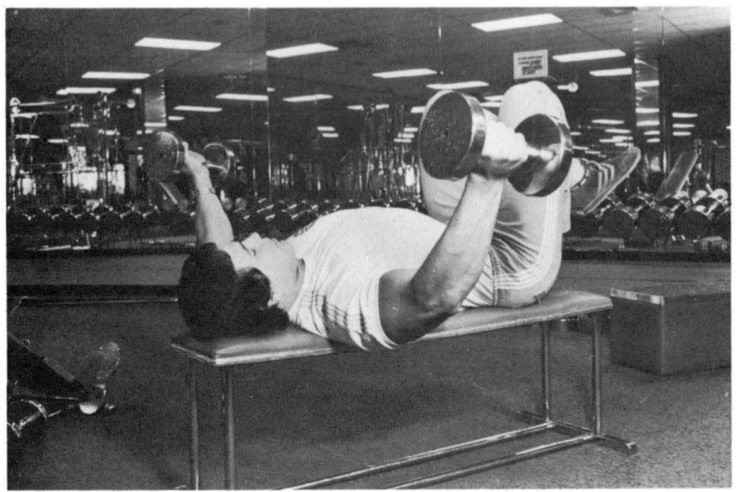

Step 1

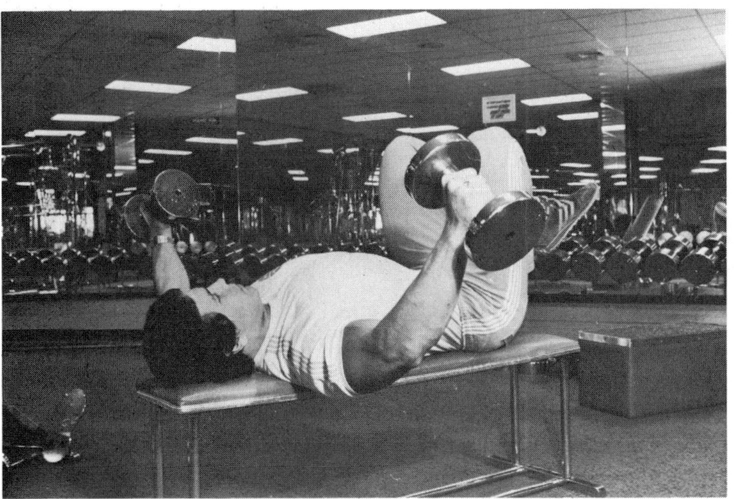

Step 2

HAND POSITIONS FOR FLYES

Parallel-Bar Dips

One of the finest lower and center pec exercises is the parallel-bar dip. This exercise can be done with no weight at the beginning, and with weight added in the form of ankle weights, iron boots, or barbell plates strapped around your waist. Grasp the parallel bars, lift yourself up into an arm-extended position, arch your back, and slowly drop all the way until the top of your chest is even with your hands. Keep your arms close to your body and you will feel the concentration on the triceps and the center of the chest. Let your elbows point outwards and you will feel the pecs take over. Find the right groove between the two elbow positions and do ten reps. When you get to the point that fifteen reps are easy, add weight.

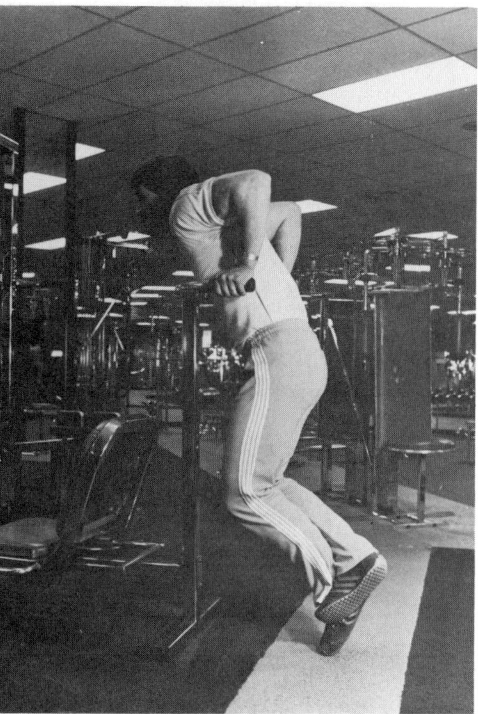

Step 1

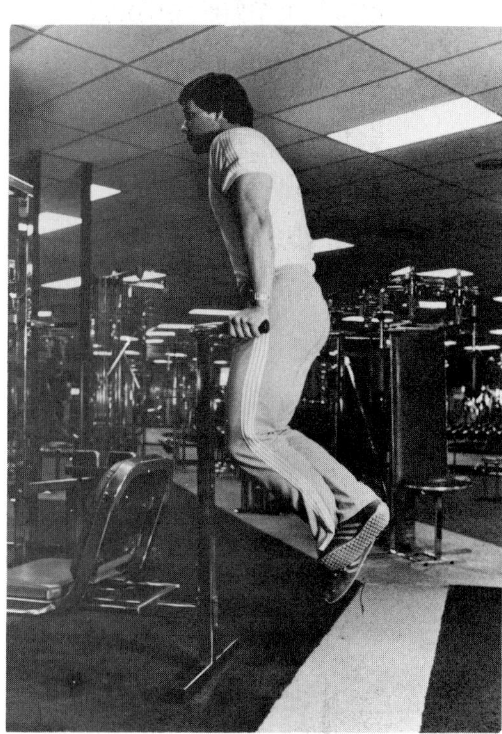

Step 2

PARALLEL-BAR DIP

Crossover Pulleys and Crossover Machines

Some of the better-equipped gyms and health clubs have pulleys that can be pulled across in front of the chest for maximum pectoral work. Machines are also now quite common for crossover work. You can do a lot of shaping and refining on the pecs with these devices, but the mass builders are still the bench press and weighted dips.

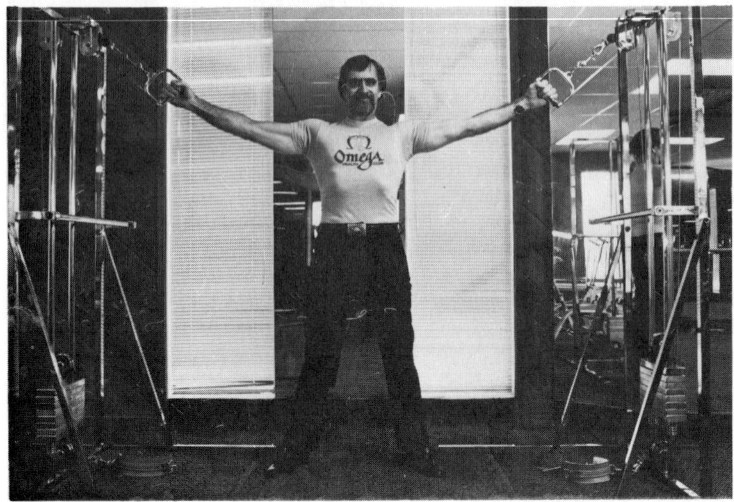

Step 1

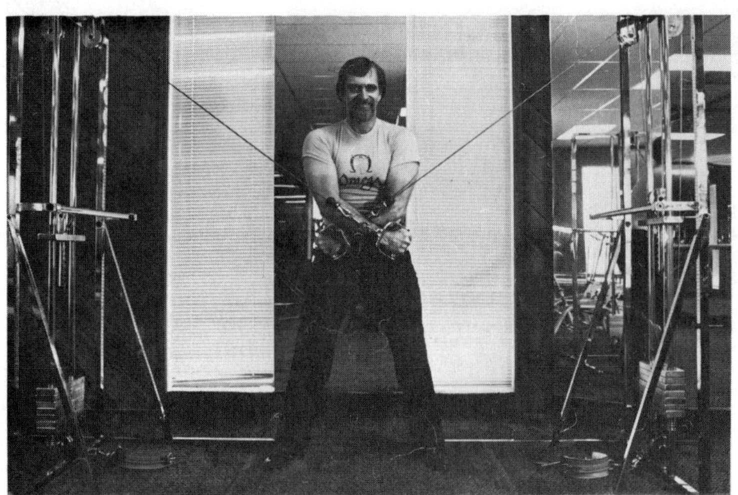

Step 2

CROSSOVER PULLEY PULLOVER

PULLOVERS

Another compound exercise that benefits the chest is the pullover. There are several ways to do it, and it works not only the pectorals but the latissimus and the serratus muscles under the arms as well. Pullovers are also a good chest expander if you breathe properly during the movements. Here we go.

Straight-Arm Pullovers

Lie on a bench crosswise, so that your shoulders are supported by the bench but your back is arched and your hips are off and below the level of the bench. Your head should not be supported by the bench. Grasp a dumbbell not by the handle but under the plates on one end. (Make sure the plates are securely fastened—you don't want them coming off on your face!) Extend your arms toward the ceiling until the elbows are straight. Now you are ready for the movement. Take as deep a breath as you can and slowly lower the dumbbell to a point slightly below the level of the bench and at the top of your head. At the bottom of the lift, you should bend the elbows slightly in order to maximize the pressure on the lats and on the serratus muscles to the front and under the arms. Then slowly raise the dumbbell until it is almost overhead. Don't let the pressure off the lats, pecs, and serratus, but immediately go into another cycle. When you bring the weight up, keep your arms straight so that you will be putting the maximum tension on the muscles of the torso. Breathe in on the way down and breathe out on the way up. This is a high-rep exercise, so you should start with about ten to twelve reps. Don't use much weight. This version is as much a rib-cage expander as it is a muscle builder.

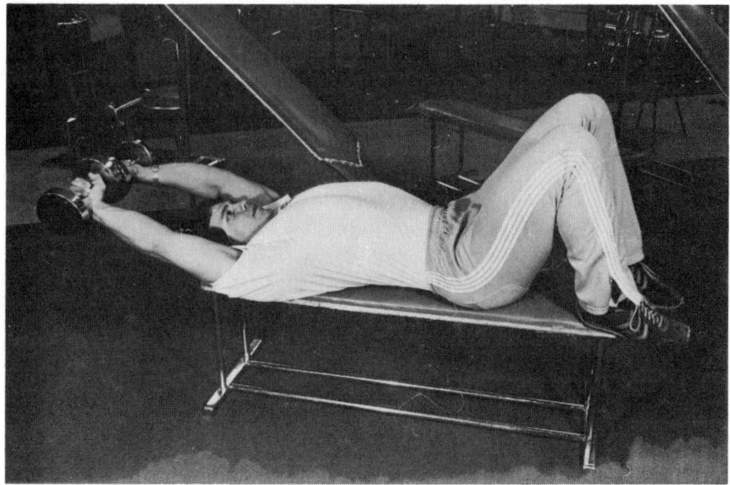

Step 1

STRAIGHT-ARM PULLOVER

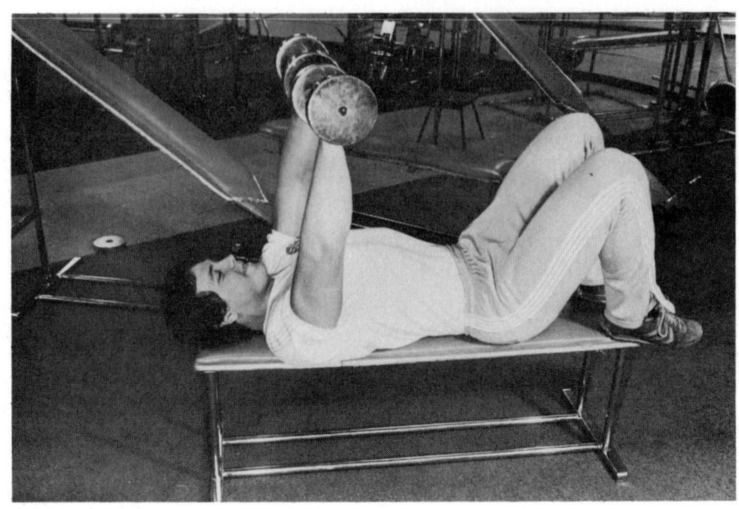

Step 2

STRAIGHT-ARM PULLOVER

Bent-Arm Pullovers

In this version, the breathing remains the same and the weight is held in the same way. However, here you should bend the arms at the elbows as you lower the weight so that the forearms will be about forty-five degrees from the floor at the bottom of the movement, with the upper arms parallel to the floor. You will be able to handle much more weight this way, but the movement will not be as good for chest expansion. The added weight will give the lats and the serratus muscles a good workout, as well as the lower portion of the pecs.

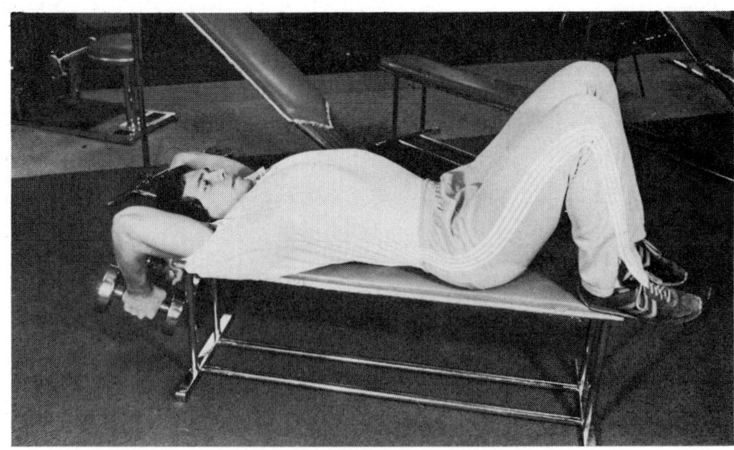

Step 1
BENT-ARM PULLOVER

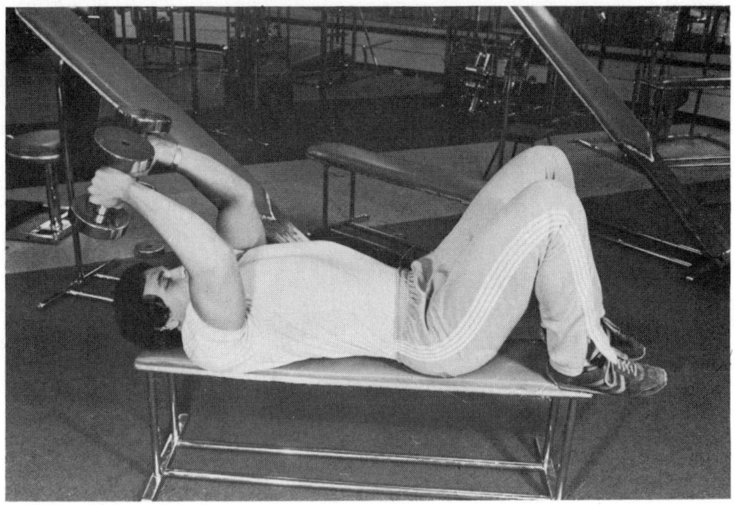

Step 2

BENT-ARM PULLOVER

Pulley Pullovers

You can use a pulley machine for pullovers if one is available. Most clubs have overhead lat pulleys, and they can be used for pullovers merely by changing the position of your body when you use them.

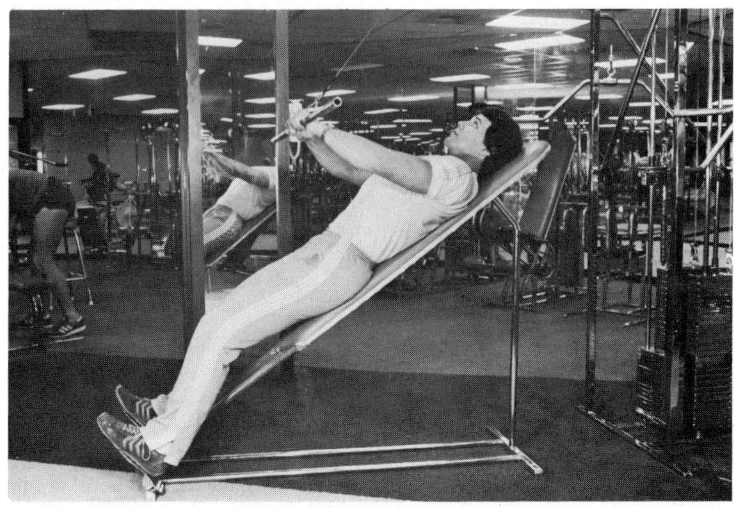

Step 1

PULLEY PULLOVER

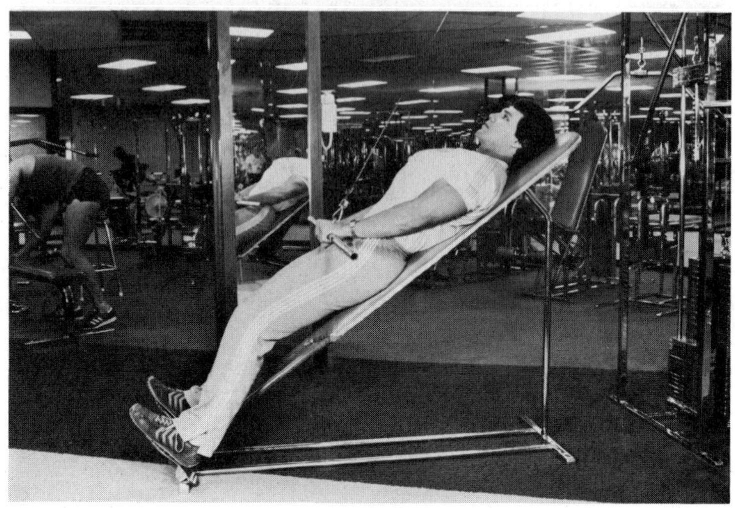

Step 2

PULLEY PULLOVER

Straight-Arm Pulley Pulldowns

This exercise duplicates the straight-arm pullover, but some people (including Ralph) find that it works the serratus area much more efficiently than the regular pullover. Here it is a pulldown. Stand erect, facing the pulley machine. Grasp the bar with both hands, palms facing downward. Keep your elbows straight, and pull the bar down to a position in front of your thighs. As you make the downward sweep, lift your shoulders slightly so that you will get a good stretch of the lats and serratus. You will feel the pecs flex at the bottom and sides. Do the movement slowly in strict form. You won't need much weight. This is not a mass builder, but a refining movement that will give you that extra bit of chiseling necessary to make the serratus and the lower pecs stand out in sharp relief. Do twelve to fifteen reps.

Bent-Arm Pulley Pulldowns

This is essentially the same exercise as above, but this time use more weight and bend your arms as you make the downward sweep. You'll find that the arms tend to take over the movement. Concentrate on the pecs, lats, and serratus so that it doesn't become merely a modified triceps pushdown (as described on page 178). For this one, do ten to twelve reps as a start.

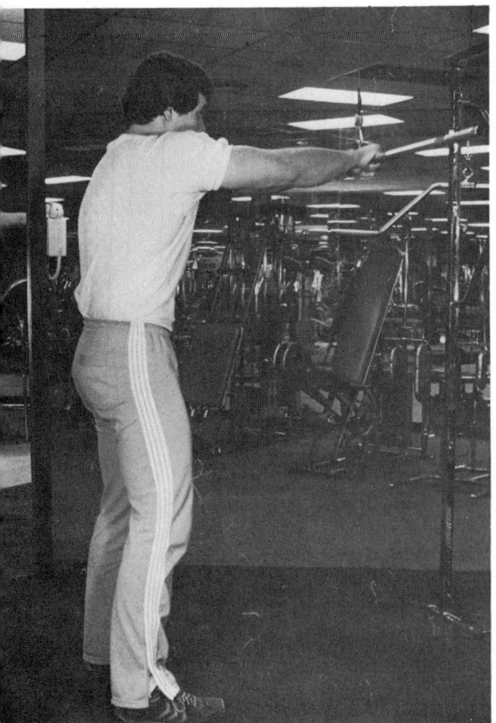

Step 1

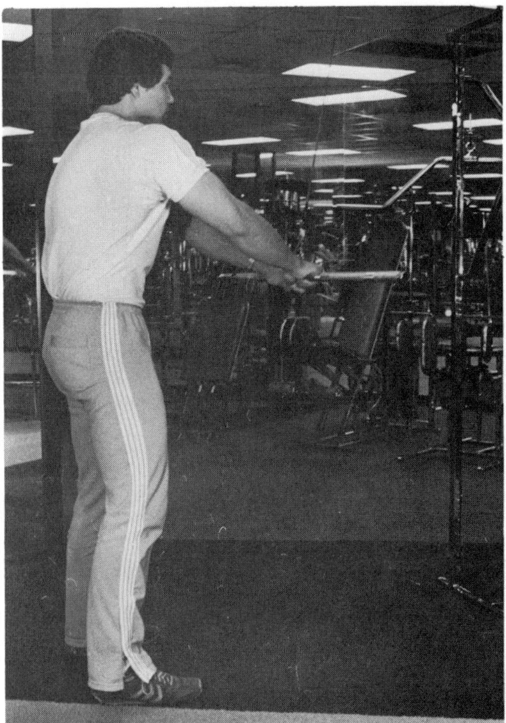

Step 2

STRAIGHT-ARM PULLEY PULLDOWN

Bent-Arm Pulley Pullovers

This one is a true pullover, since you will be pulling the bar over your head. Stand facing away from the pulley machine, reach back and grasp the bar, and with elbows slightly bent bring the bar over your head and downward to the front. Be careful not to crease the top of your head with the cable. Do ten to twelve reps at the beginning.

EXERCISES FOR THE SHOULDERS

Since we've already described an excellent anterior deltoid exercise in the section on the chest, let's go now to the shoulders and compile a list of deltoid movements. The deltoids are delta-shaped muscles (hence the name) that serve as capstones for the upper arms. They lift the arms up when we are standing, and to the front or back when we are lying on our backs or our stomachs.

Broad shoulders are always associated with masculinity, and a person with good shoulder development is usually given more respect than some-

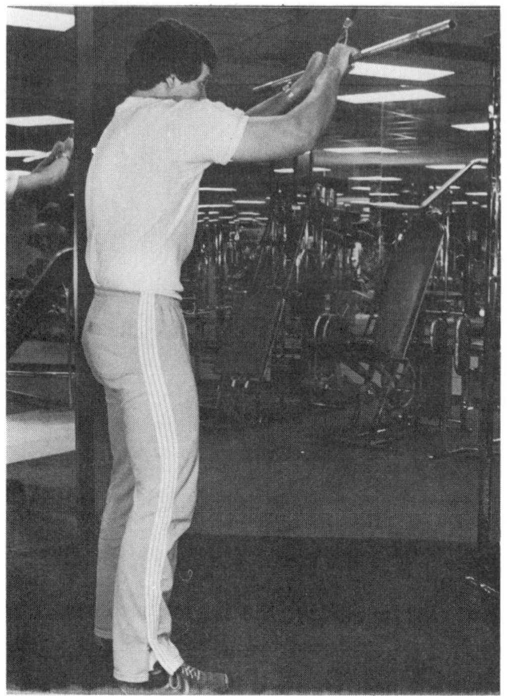

Step 1

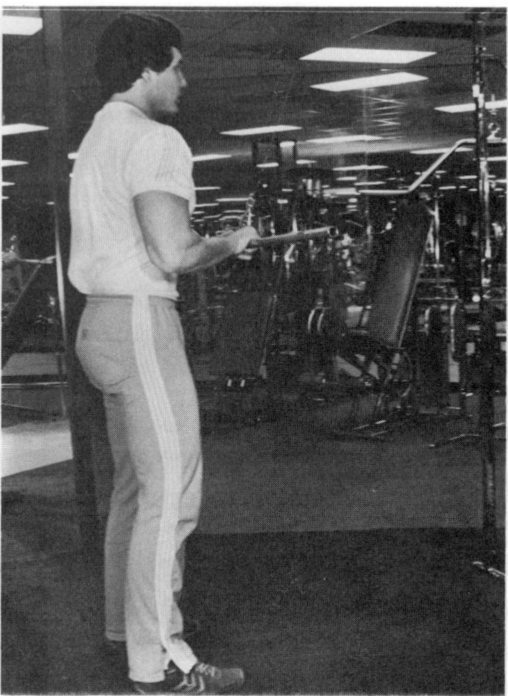

Step 2

BENT-ARM PULLEY PULLDOWN

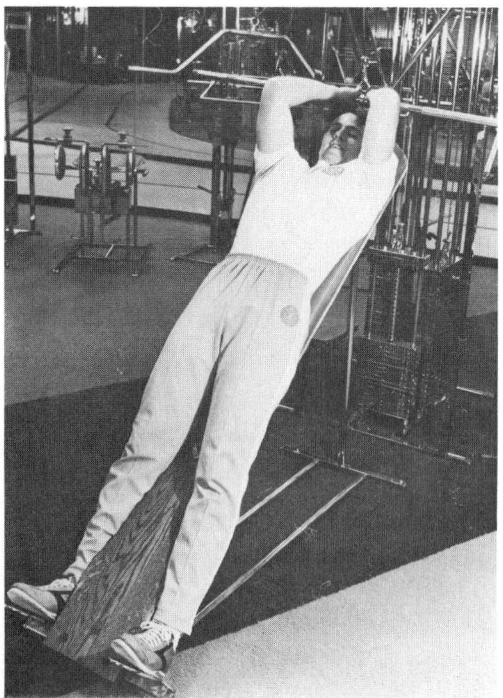

Step 1

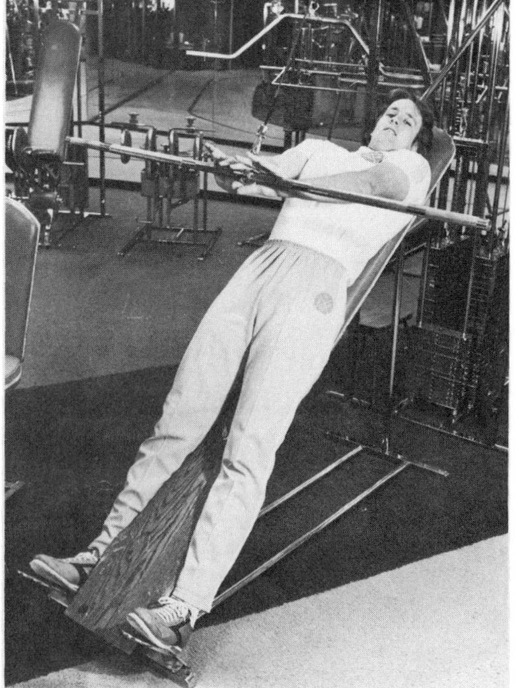

Step 2

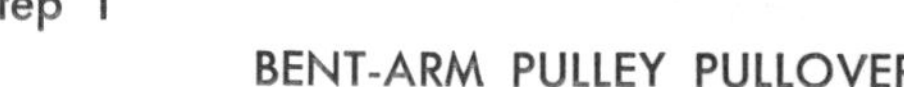

BENT-ARM PULLEY PULLOVER

body with narrow, sloping shoulders. Almost all suit jackets have padded shoulders in them, so the evidence is abundant that human beings give broad and strong-looking shoulders a special place in their evaluation of the male of the species.

To make your shoulders look their best, you should be sure to work all three heads of the muscle group. We've already talked about the bench press as a good anterior deltoid exercise. Here are some more shoulder exercises to make those pads unnecessary.

ANTERIOR RAISES

Stand erect, with either a barbell or two dumbbells held in your hands, palms facing you, arms straight, weight resting on the front of the thighs. Slowly raise the weight to the front until it is almost overhead. Don't carry the movement to the point where tension is taken off the deltoids. Don't swing the weight up, but lift it slowly. When you reach the top of the movement, lower the weight slowly down to the starting position. You should keep your arms straight, but don't lock your elbows. Use enough weight to really feel it on about the eighth or ninth rep, but not enough to force you to swing it up to complete the movement. This exercise works the anterior and lateral deltoids.

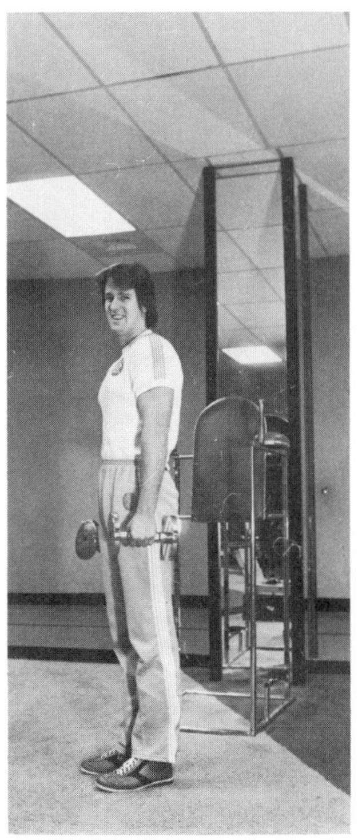

Step 1

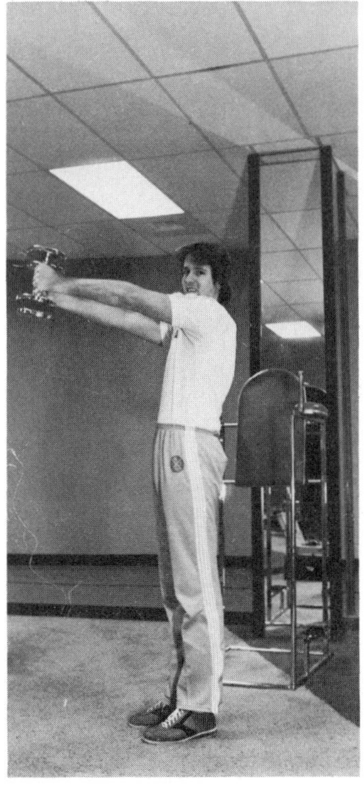

Step 2

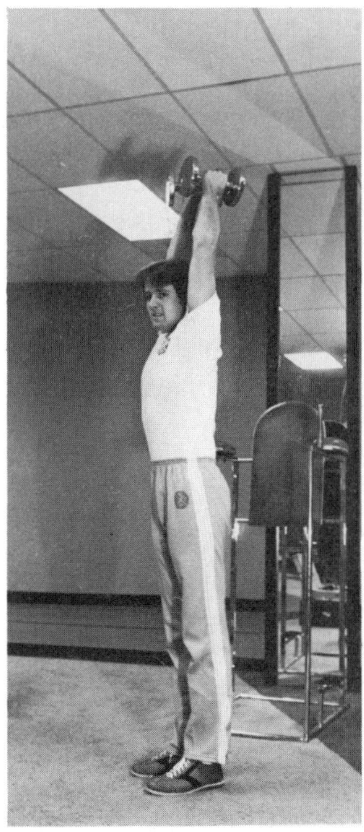

Step 3

ANTERIOR RAISE

LATERAL RAISES (STANDING)

This exercise isolates the lateral, or side, deltoid. Stand erect, with a pair of dumbbells at arms' length, palms facing each other, resting in front of your thighs. Bring the weights up in an arc that ends almost overhead, but not far up enough that the tension is taken off the deltoids. Return to the starting position. Again, don't swing the weight and don't use "body English" to get the dumbbells overhead. The key here is strict movement.

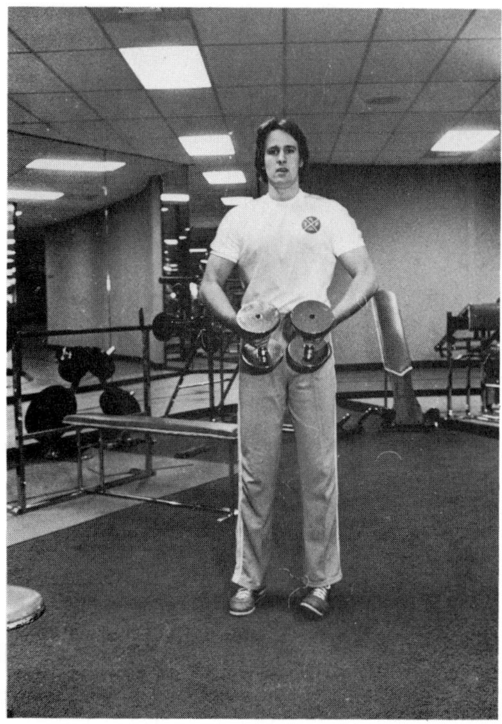

Step 1

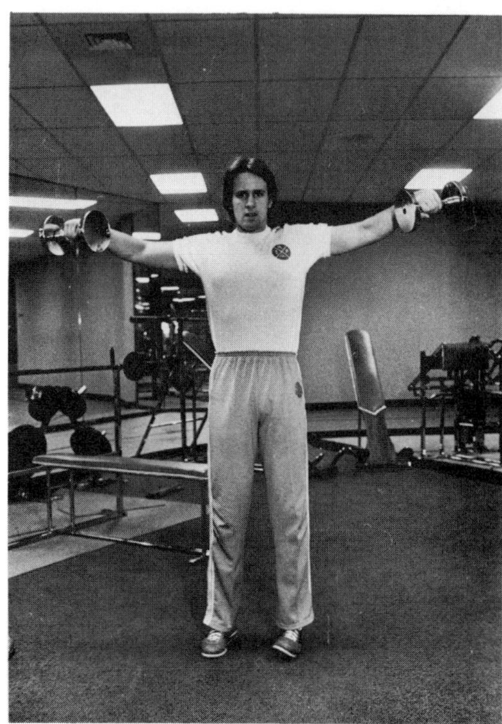

Step 2

LATERAL RAISE (standing)

LATERAL RAISES (SEATED)

Here's a good one, shown to us by Danny Tobol, the 1977 Mr. Teenage America. Sit on a bench, lean slightly forward, and hold two dumbbells in your hands, palms facing each other, with the ends of the dumbbells resting on the tops of your thighs. Bring the dumbbells up and to the back until they are higher than your head; your arms will be bent ninety degrees at the elbows. At the top of the movement, your forearms should be perpendicular to the floor and your upper arms should be back to the point that the lateral deltoids are fully contracted. Hold for a count of one, then *slowly* lower the arms in an arc to the starting position. When the dumbbells reach the tops of the thighs, don't let your deltoids rest, but immediately start the movement again. Do ten to twelve reps. Even the strong guys find that they have trouble using two 20-pound dumbbells for this one.

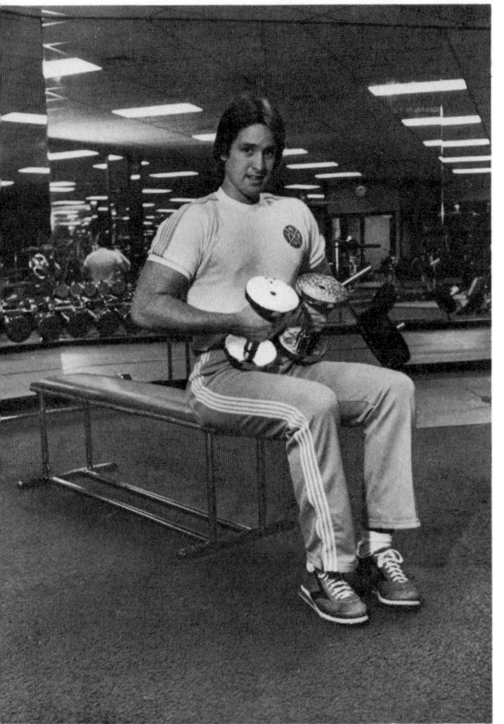

Step 1

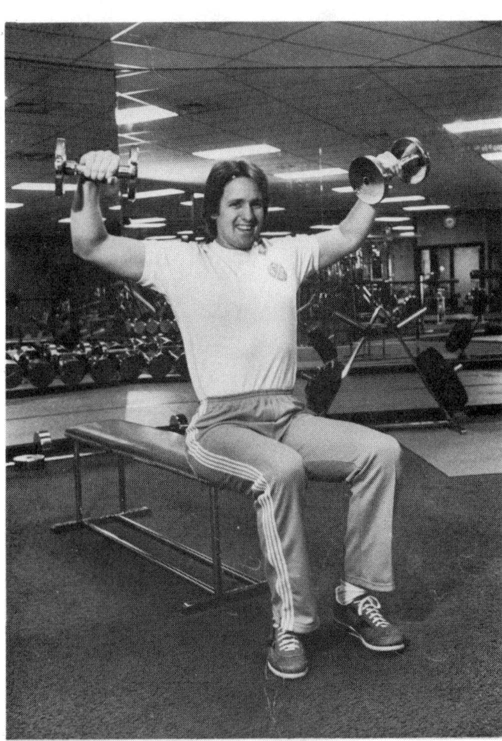

Step 2

LATERAL RAISE (seated)

POSTERIOR RAISES

Stand erect, then bend at the waist until your upper body is parallel to the floor. Grasp two dumbbells, palms facing, and bring your arms up in an arc from the floor to a position as high as you can get them while keeping them perpendicular to your body. Don't let them angle to the back if you can help it, but keep the tension on those posterior deltoids. When you reach the top, let the dumbbells slowly back down to the floor, and then repeat the movement. After ten to twelve reps you will feel this one like you never felt an exercise before.

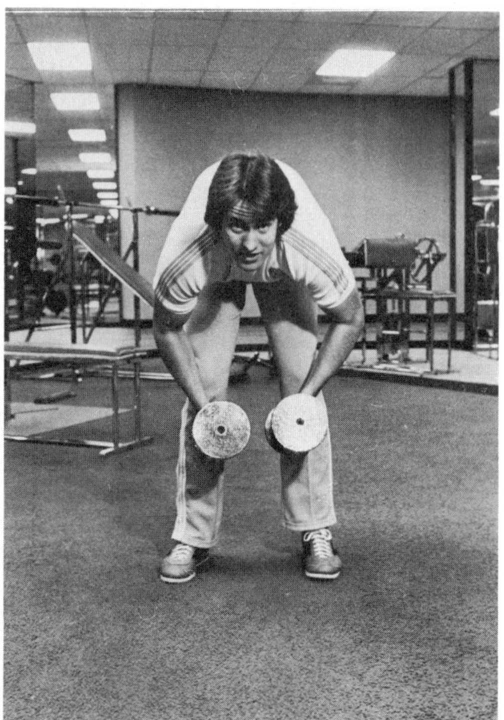

Step 1

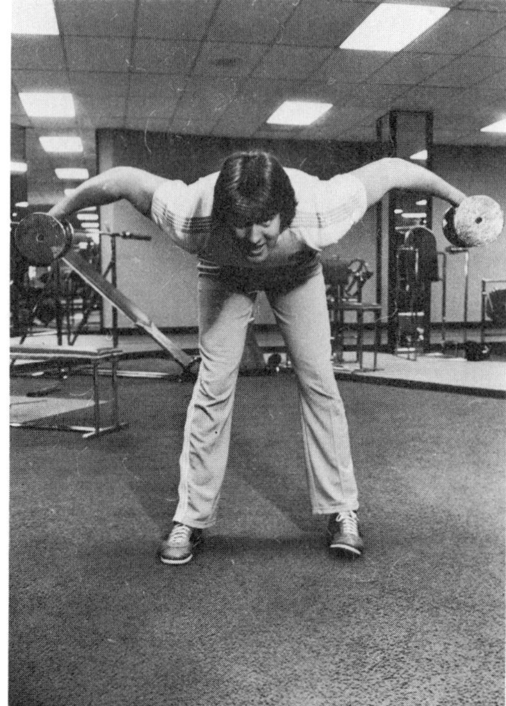

Step 2

POSTERIOR RAISE

THE MILITARY PRESS

One of the oldest standbys in weight training is the military press. It takes its name from the erect, "braced" posture of the body during the lift. While it is primarily thought to be a triceps exercise, it is also an excellent exercise for the deltoids, especially in the last few inches of the lift. Stand erect, with a barbell held in your hands, palms facing front, thumbs not opposing, resting at the top of your chest. Lift the barbell up and slightly back so that at the end of the lift it is in line with the back of your head. This is necessary both to maintain balance and to work the lateral deltoids.

The Seated Press Behind the Neck

This exercise is a variation of the military press, and intensifies the role of the lateral and anterior deltoids in making the lift. It is done in a seated position so that you can concentrate on the lift without the shifts in balance necessary in the standing press. Begin the lift with a barbell resting on your shoulders behind your neck, palms to the front, hands a little better than shoulder width apart. Lift the barbell up until your arms are fully extended over your head. Slowly lower the weight to the starting position. As in the military press, the anterior deltoids do most of the work at the beginning of the lift, the laterals take over after the initial few inches, and the triceps and the posterior deltoids complete the lift.

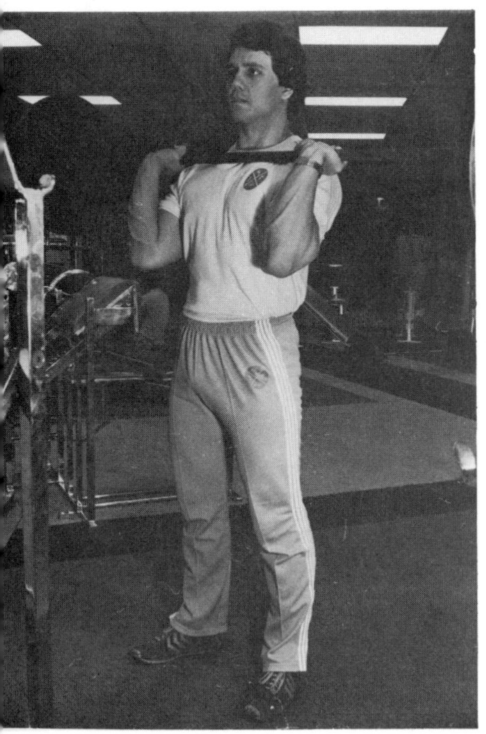

Step 1

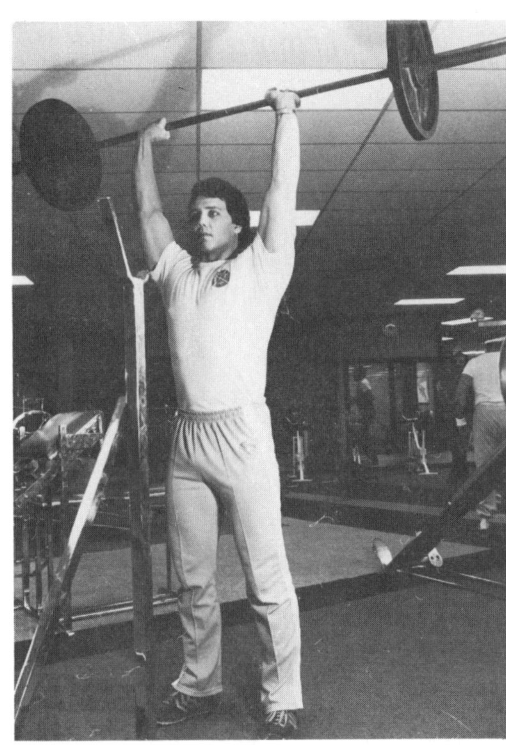

Step 2

MILITARY PRESS

EXERCISES FOR THE ARMS

Over the years there have been more ads in the muscle magazines on how to build big arms than ads for all the other body parts put together. We have padding for our shoulders, and suits that cover everything else. But eventually, you're going to have to take your coat off, and if it's summer you'll want to wear polo shirts. And there you'll stand with two toothpicks sticking out of your shoulders!

Another scenario: you're lying on the deck by the pool at your singles apartment complex and that jerk from B-961 comes over and starts talking to the chick you were about to offer a drink. One look at his arms immediately takes you back to high school when that other jerk, who was on the football team, did the same thing. You've always wanted big arms. You've never had them, and you've never really believed the Charles Atlas

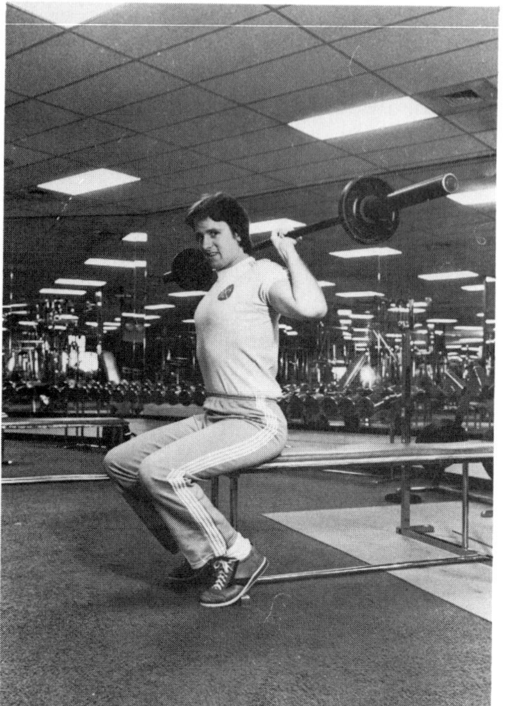

Step 1

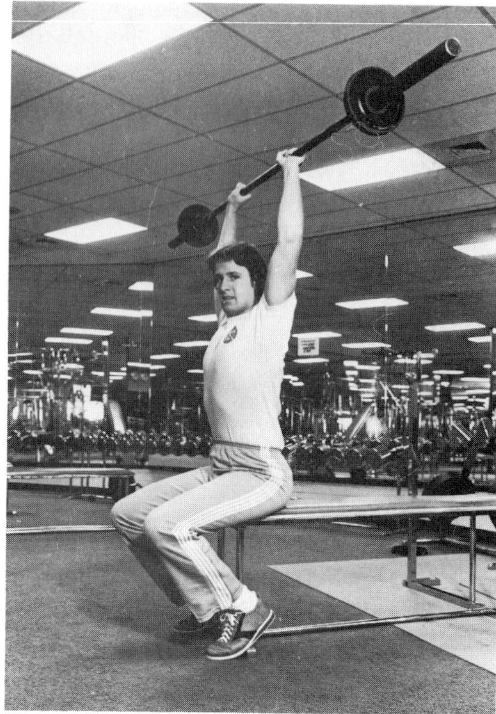

Step 2

SEATED PRESS BEHIND THE NECK

ads. And you've never taken weight training seriously either, because the muscle magazines have always been tucked away in *that* shelf with all the other fringe-group special-interest tabloids.

One of the reasons that bodybuilding has always had such a bad press in this country is the way in which it has been presented to the public by its own magazines. It's only been in the last half decade that bodybuilding magazines, especially Joe Weider's *Muscle Builder,* have come up to the standard of excellence enjoyed by other magazines.

As a consequence, muscle building has been less credible than it could have been. And you didn't have the chance to build the arms you wanted to build.

And now you're lying on the deck at the pool looking at that guy from B-961, wondering what he knows that you don't know. What he knows is that there are zillions of exercises that will build your arms. Do them consistently and with enough zeal and you can have the arms you want. And remember: the beauty of weight training is that the decision about how big you want to be is largely up to you. If you want monstrous, bulging biceps and you have the determination and the genes to build them, these exercises will do the trick. If you want to have muscular arms on a par with a champion swimmer, tennis player, or other top competitor, the same exercises will do the trick. How you want to look is strictly up to you.

THE BICEPS

The biceps are usually the showy muscles of the arm. They are what are seen most by people standing in front of you, and they denote great strength in pulling things toward you (such as girls, trees, motorcycles, assorted bars, and anything your interest might fasten on). They bulge out of your sleeve like baseballs if they're developed well, and they come in all shapes and sizes.

Sergio Oliva, Mr. Olympia before Arnold Schwarzenegger, had huge arms, probably larger than Arnold's. Sergio's biceps are long, however, and don't have a peak. Arnold's arms, on the other hand, have an incredible peak that slopes up suddenly like the last 500 yards up Mt. Everest. The two men represent the two extremes of biceps development. A lot of it has to do with the way they trained, but more has to do with genetics.

Whatever your inheritance, here are the exercises.

Two-Arm Curls with a Barbell

This one used to be called the military curl. Stand erect, holding a barbell at arms' length in front of you, palms to the front, resting across the tops of your thighs. Keep your elbows at your sides and slowly lift the barbell in an arc until it is at a position about nine to ten inches from your chin. Don't let it "fall into" your chest at the top of the movement, because that will release the tension on the biceps and lessen the effect of the exercise. Lower the barbell slowly back to the starting position. Don't swing it up and don't let it fall. Keep the tension constant on the biceps throughout the movement.

This exercise is the basic mass builder of all biceps movements. Although cambered curling bars became popular several years ago, a straight bar is best for the biceps. The theory behind the curling bar was that there would be less unproductive tightening of the forearm muscles if the hands were turned slightly so that the thumbs were pointed up. Bodybuilders soon realized, however, that one of the chief functions of the biceps was the "supination" of the hand—turning the hand to a palms-up position (as opposed to "pronation," which would turn the hand in the other direction). The curling bar prohibited that final supinating contraction, and thus prevented maximum growth of the biceps. So now it's back to the straight bar for curls.

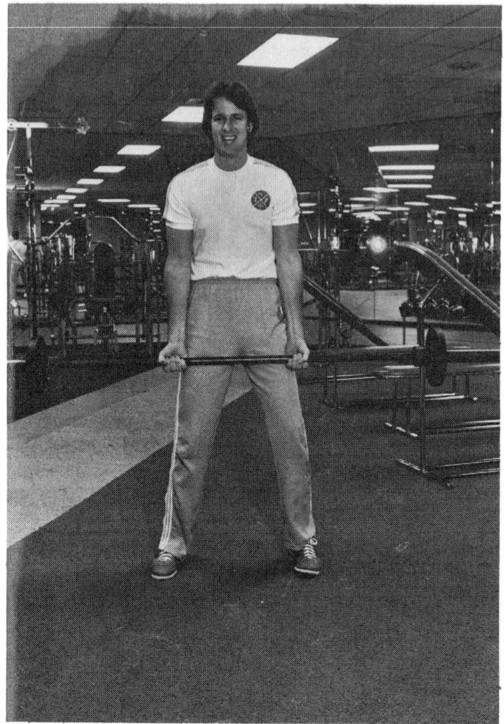

Step 1

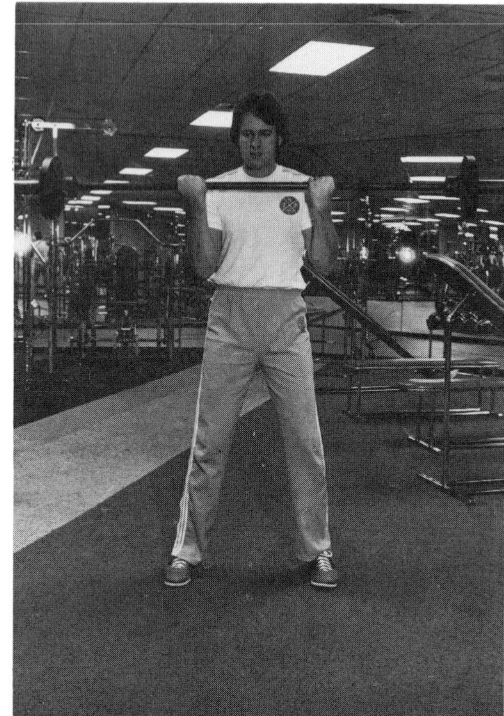

Step 2

TWO-ARM CURL WITH BARBELL

Barbell Curls with a Preacher Stand, or Scott Bench

The genesis of the preacher stand is shrouded in mystery. It's sometimes called a "Scott bench" after the first Mr. Olympia, Larry Scott. One magazine credits Vince Gironda with inventing it, another credits Scott himself. The device probably appeared in many places at about the same time, because it is a logical refinement of the technique used for the regular barbell curl. Whatever its origin, here's how it works.

The preacher stand is a flat surface, either on a slant or vertical, against which you can place the upper arms while doing dumbbell or barbell curls. It keeps you from cheating on the lift, and thus assures a strict, intensive pull throughout the movement. If used correctly, it concentrates the effort on the belly of the muscle, and hence develops it to its fullest potential.

The stand usually has an extension to sit on, but some are on pedestals so that you can stand while doing the lift. Grasp the barbell as you would for the regular curl, bring it to the top of your chest, and lean over the stand, placing your elbows against the padded board. Let the barbell down slowly

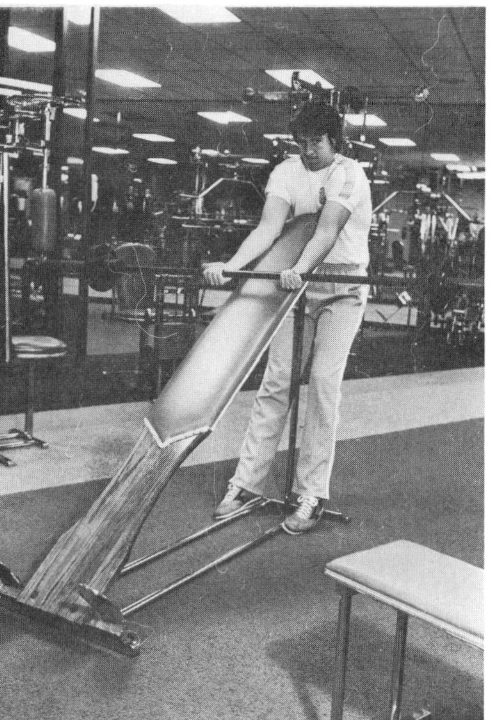

Step 1

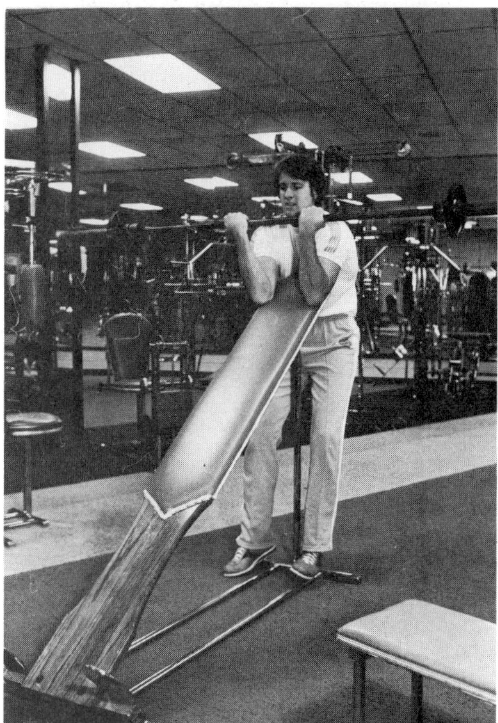

Step 2

BARBELL CURL WITH A PREACHER STAND, OR SCOTT BENCH

all the way, but not far enough to allow the elbows to lock in a straight position. If you do that, you will lose leverage completely, and the result could be a painful elbow injury. Conversely, don't stop halfway down, or you will miss the best part of the lift.

Return the barbell slowly to the top of your chest, and repeat the movement. If you want to develop the outer head of the biceps, keep your hands placed fairly close together and the elbows wide. If you want to peak the inner bicep, keep the hands placed wide and keep the elbows close together on the stand. Don't try to use your body to swing the weight up. Be sure to let it down as slowly as you bring it up.

Bentover Barbell Curls

Stand erect, with a barbell grasped palms away from you, resting at the tops of your thighs. Bend at the waist until your upper arms are perpendicular to the floor. Now curl the barbell with a slow, deliberate movement until it is as close to your chin as you can bring it. Don't swing it up. Now lower the weight and repeat. This movement isolates the biceps in much the same way as the Scott bench, and it will help you to peak the muscles.

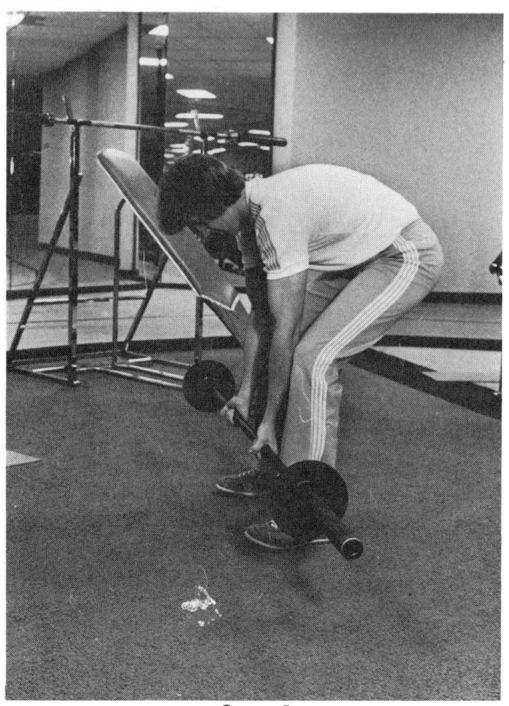

Step 1

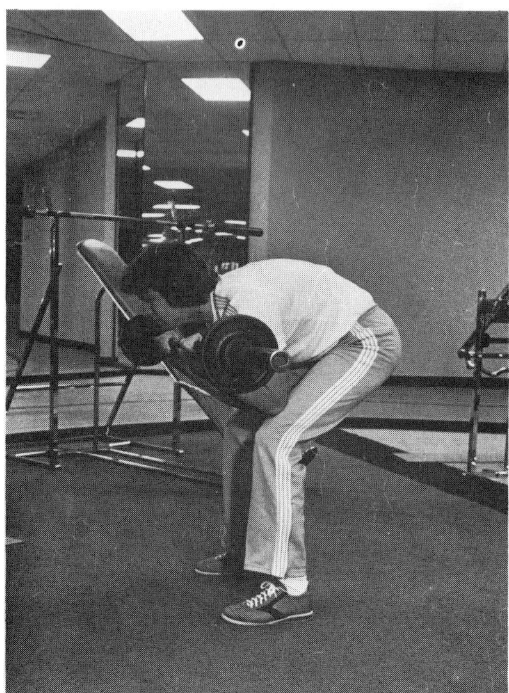

Step 2

BENTOVER BARBELL CURL

Dumbbell Curls

Curls can be done with dumbbells in all of the ways mentioned above for barbells. Consequently, there is the *standing two-arm dumbbell curl,* the *preacher stand, or Scott bench dumbbell curl,* and so on. There are also some curls that can be done only with dumbbells, and they are primarily useful for shaping, refining, and peaking. The standing barbell curl is the mass builder. The dumbbell curls are the polishers.

Incline Bench Dumbbell Curls

Lie back on an incline bench at about forty-five degrees from the floor. Grasp a dumbbell in each hand and let them dangle at your sides. Without swinging them up, raise them slowly at a slight angle to your sides so that you won't hit either your sides or the bench. At the top of the movement, your elbow will be bent at about ninety degrees. Don't allow the dumbbells to fall into your shoulders, because this would release the tension on the biceps. Let the dumbbells down slowly to the starting position and repeat.

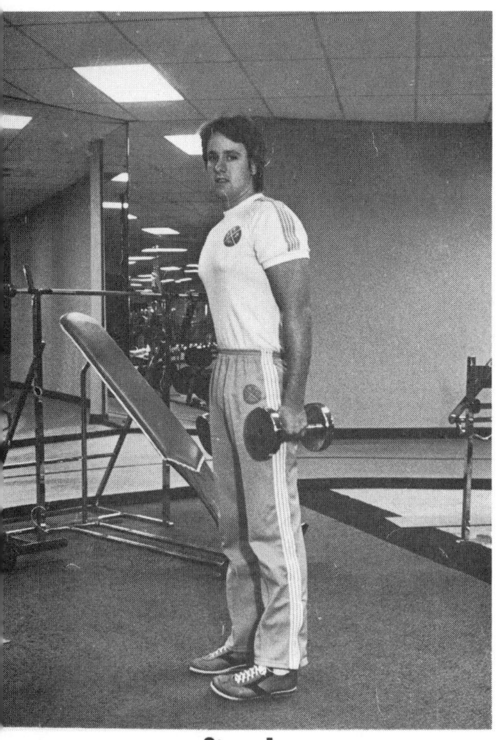

Step 1

Step 2

DUMBBELL CURL

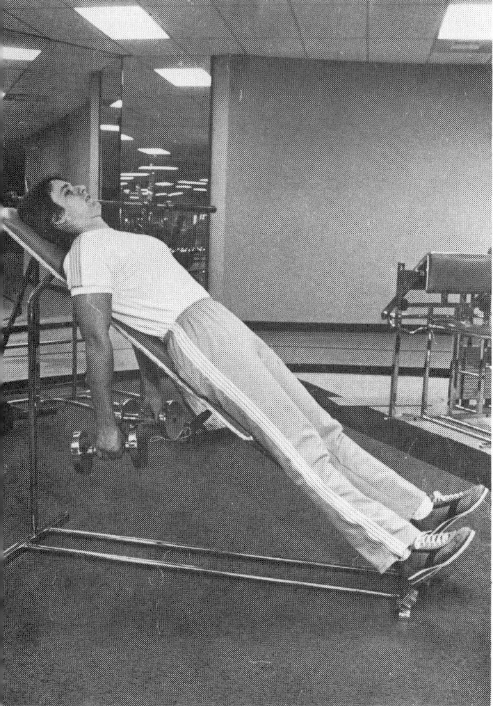

Step 1

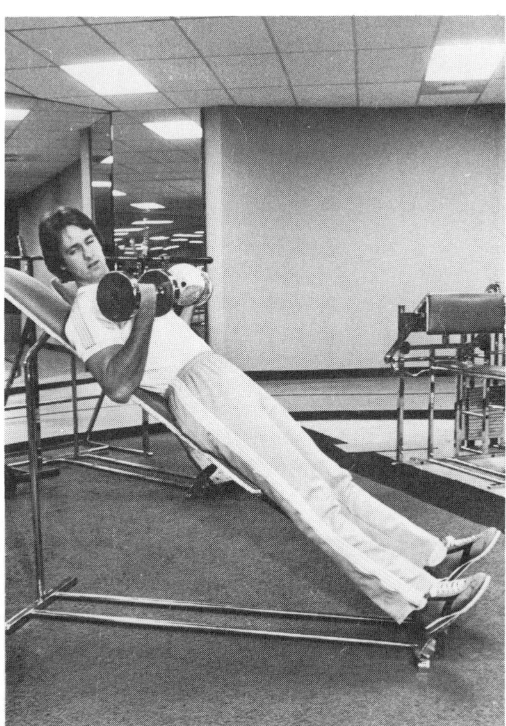

Step 2

INCLINE BENCH DUMBBELL CURL

Incline Bench Alternating Dumbbell Curls

This one is done the same way as described above, but this time bring the dumbbells up one at a time.

Standing Alternating Dumbbell Curls

For this, you stand erect and bring the dumbbells up one at a time.

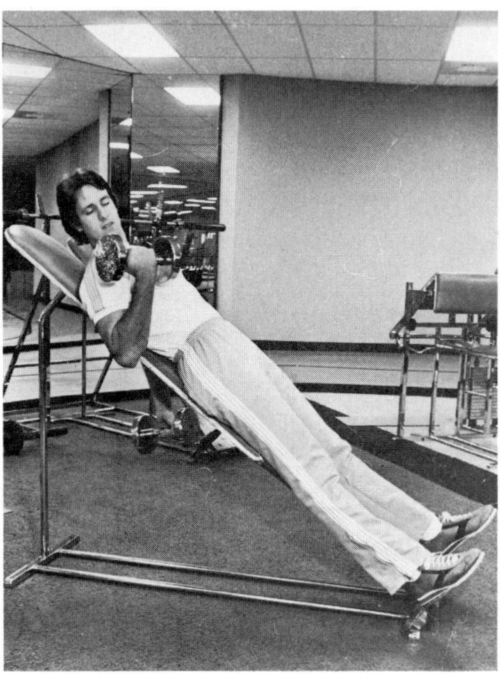

INCLINE BENCH ALTERNATING DUMBBELL CURL

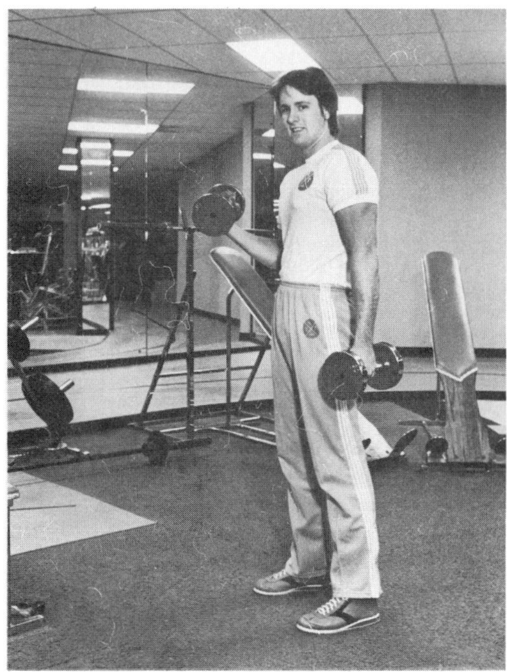

STANDING ALTERNATING DUMBBELL CURL

Bentover Concentrated Dumbbell Curls

Grasp one dumbbell in either hand, bend at the waist until the dumbbell is almost touching the floor. Bring the weight up to your shoulders, then let it back down slowly. Some bodybuilders bring the dumbbells to the chest, but this tends not to peak the biceps as fully as bringing them to the shoulders. Resist the temptation to swing the weight up. Do ten reps with each hand.

Seated Concentrated Dumbbell Curls

This is a popular exercise, and will build a high peak on the biceps. Sit on a bench, knees apart, with a dumbbell lying on the floor between your

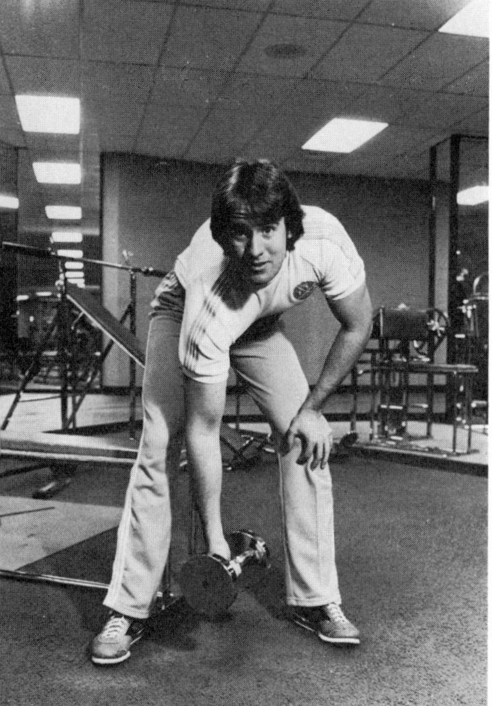

Step 1

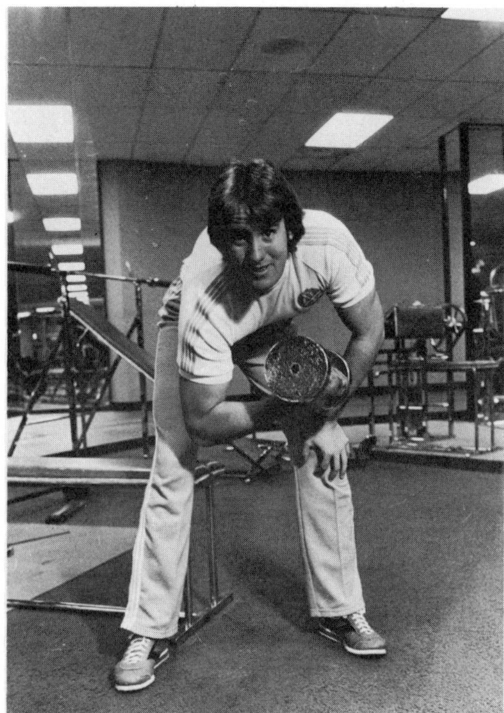

Step 2

BENTOVER CONCENTRATED DUMBBELL CURL

feet. Reach down and grasp the dumbbell with both hands, bracing your elbow against the inner thigh. Curl the weight slowly up to a point close to your chin, then let it down slowly.

Dumbbell Curls Against an Incline Bench

Grasp a dumbbell in one hand, stand behind an incline bench, and let your arm lie on the bench fully extended. Bring the dumbbell up in a curling motion until your forearm is perpendicular to the plane of the bench. Slowly lower and repeat.

Pulley Work for the Biceps

Immobilize your elbows against your knees, grasp the bar of a pulley machine, and perform a curling motion until the hands reach the chin. This exercise doesn't require much weight to be effective, and it will sometimes give you a peak contraction that you can't get from any other type of curl. The easiest way to do the movement is in a seated position in front of a

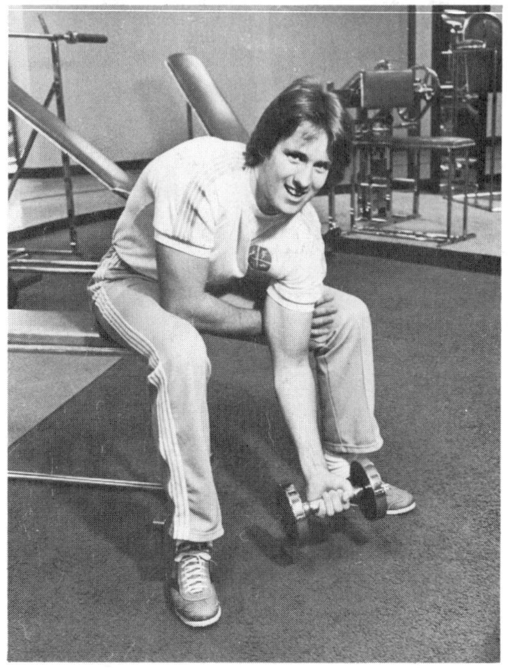

Step 1

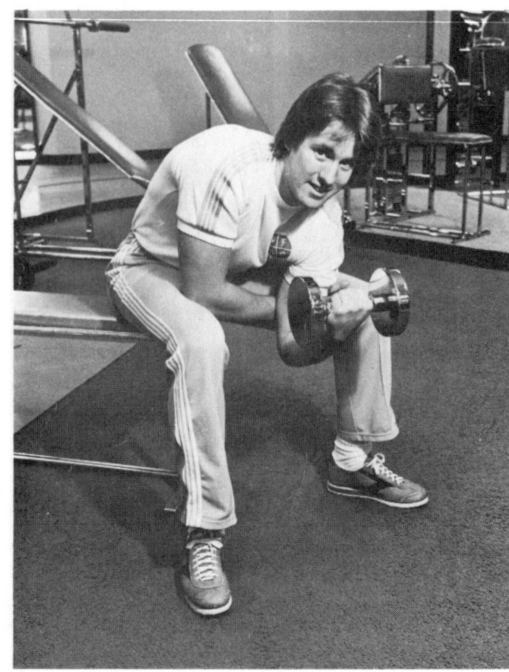

Step 2

SEATED CONCENTRATED DUMBBELL CURL

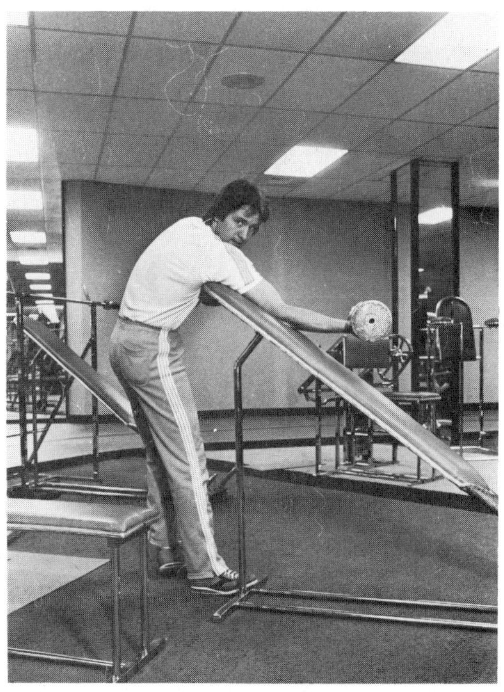

Step 1

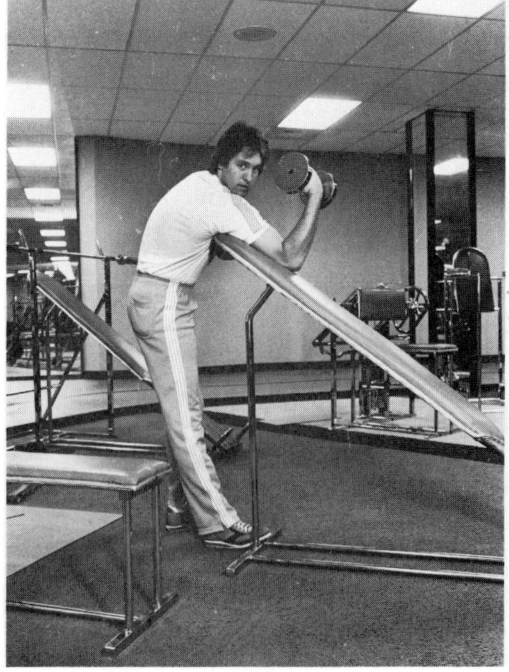

Step 2

DUMBBELL CURL AGAINST AN INCLINE BENCH

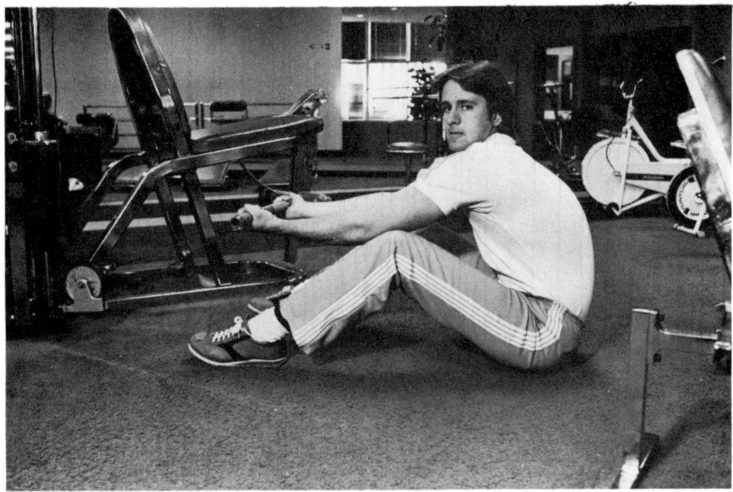

Step 1

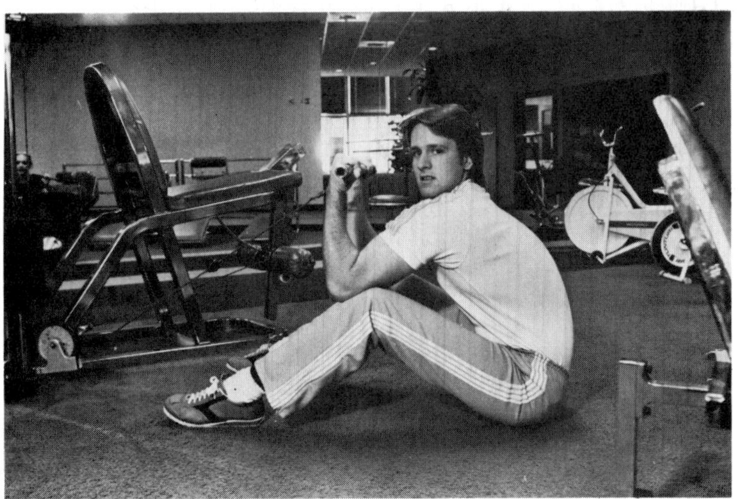

Step 2
PULLEY WORK FOR THE BICEPS

low-pulley machine. If you don't have access to a low-pulley machine, lie on your back, put your feet against the frame of a regular flat pulley machine, and try curling movements down toward your chest.

A Few Special Tips on Biceps Movements

In all the biceps exercises listed above, we've stressed that you shouldn't swing the barbell or dumbbells up, but should keep the movement strict. This is especially true if the purpose of the lift is to put the final shaping on the mass you've already built. However, if you are trying to build mass, you might find it useful to cheat a little in the regular standing barbell curl, in order to force yourself to use heavier weights. Cheating can sometimes get you through sticking points, those troublesome plateaus of strength and size that plague us all at one time or another. Further, if you swing the weight up and then take full advantage of what's called "negative" movements—letting the bar down in strict position—you will further jar the muscles into greater performance. Joe Weider of Weider International, the same Weider who pioneered the set system, also has pioneered what he calls the "Cheating Principle" as a prime way to get past sticking points into greater strength and mass.

At the other end of the spectrum, when you are refining and shaping, you might find it useful to rotate your forearms as you bring dumbbells up in a curling movement. As you may remember, this is called supination, and it involves beginning the curling motion with the hands pronated—palms facing you—and ending the motion with the palms still facing you, having gone through a 180-degree rotation. If you want to get an idea of how this works, hold your upper arm vertically against your side with the elbow bent so that the forearm is at a 90-degree angle to the upper arm. Now tighten your biceps while turning your clenched fist until the palm faces the floor. Keep your eyes on your biceps and slowly rotate the fist until the palm is facing the ceiling. See how the biceps ball up? When you do supinating curls, the biceps do the same kind of balling up, and under severe pressure.

Supinating curls, of course, can be applied to any of the dumbbell curls. At the top of the movement, try to twist your hand as far as it will go to peak the biceps fully. Try it for several weeks and you'll see and feel the difference.

When you do any curling movement, don't allow the biceps to relax at the top of the movement. If you do, you'll release the tension on the muscle, and the movement will lose its muscle-building effect. Also, it helps you concentrate mentally on contracting the biceps during the movement. Stare at the biceps, push everything else out of your mind, and concentrate on making every contraction the absolute maximum. Tense the biceps before you start the movement, and hold that tension in *addition to the tension caused by the movement itself* all the way through the movement. It gets results.

Reverse Curls

Except for the supinating curls, all of the curls described above can be done in what is called the reverse curl movement. Instead of beginning the curl with the palms facing front and ending with them facing back, do the opposite: begin with the palms facing back and end with them facing the front. This will work the biceps in a different way, and it will also work

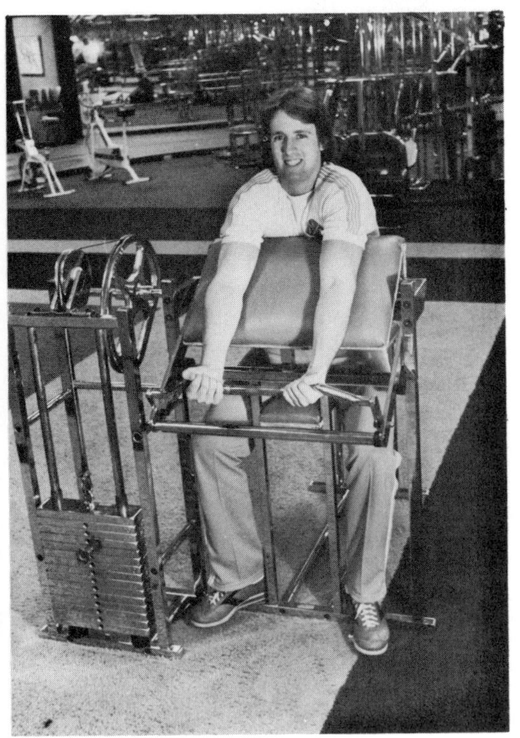

Step 1

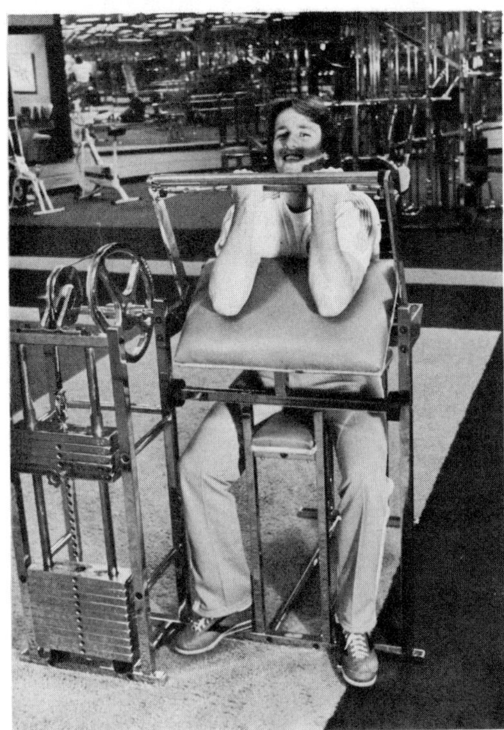

Step 2

MACHINE CURL

the top of the forearm. Be careful that you do not use too much weight in this variation, because you will not be able to handle as much as you use in the regular curls.

THE TRICEPS

Now let's move on to the other muscles of the upper arms, the triceps. This muscle group constitutes two-thirds to three-fourths of the total mass of the upper arm, so you can readily see why really big arms depend so much on triceps development.

Few people have large triceps naturally, while almost everybody has some biceps development. Perhaps that's because we pull things toward us more often than we push things away. The triceps are used in making pushing motions with the hands, and must be exercised with such motions. Nothing looks funnier than an arm with huge biceps and little triceps development, so don't neglect the triceps.

First, do the following exercises, which have already been described:

The military press (see page 158).

The bench press (see page 139).

The press behind the neck (see page 158).

Parallel-bar dips (see page 146).

The incline bench press and decline bench press (see pages 141–142).

All of the exercises listed above are compound exercises, which work more than one muscle in a muscle group at the same time. While the military press works the shoulders, it also works the triceps. While the bench press is a chest builder, it is also a triceps builder. The press behind the neck begins with a deltoid movement but ends with the triceps doing most of the work. The parallel-bar dip begins with a pectoral flex but ends with the triceps getting a good burning workout. The incline bench press, either with a barbell or with dumbbells, is a great pec shaper and is also a strength and size builder for the triceps.

There are other triceps exercises, however, that isolate the work of that muscle group. Here are the best ones.

French Curls, or Triceps Extensions

This exercise has many variations, all of which are based on a single premise: any motion that begins with the arm bent and ends with the arm straight, especially if the elbow movement is restricted, constitutes an intensive, isolated triceps movement. All of the various extensions, or French curls, are done with the elbow as nearly stationary as it is possible to keep it, and the movement is done in an arc. Ideally, the upper arm is also immobilized so that all the work is done by the triceps.

Seated Triceps Extensions with a Barbell

Sit on a bench, preferably with your back braced (try sitting with your back against a preacher stand), and start the movement with your elbows pointed at the ceilings, upper arms almost vertical, grasping a bar with both hands. The bar should be in a position behind your head at the base of your neck. Without allowing the upper arms to move from their vertical orientation, lift the weight in an arc until it almost overhead. Maintain the tension on the triceps, and slowly lower the weight to the starting position.

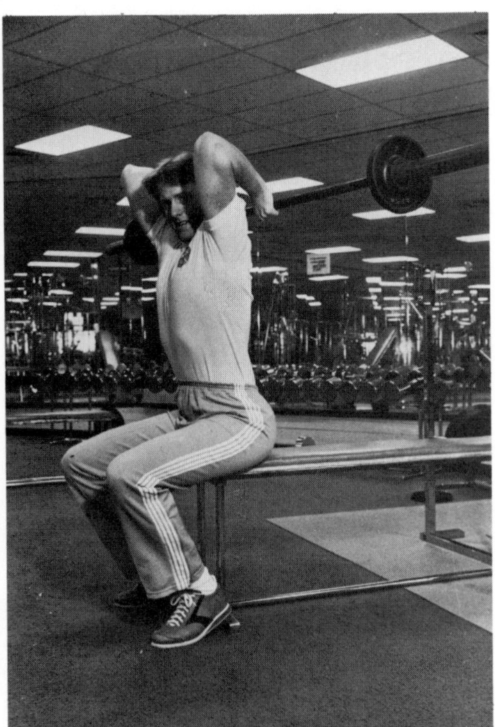

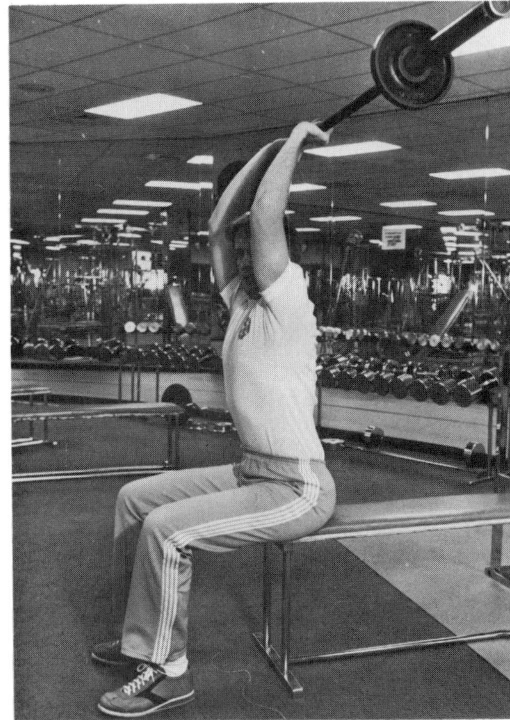

Step 1 Step 2

SEATED TRICEPS EXTENSION WITH BARBELL

Standing Triceps Extensions with a Barbell

This is done as described above, but from a standing position. It may be harder for you to maintain the immobility of the upper body and the upper arms in this position, but the movement should be the same.

Reclining Triceps Extensions with a Barbell

Lie on a bench (preferably in the same position as you would be in for the straight-arm pullover—see page 149) and hold a barbell at the top of your head so that your elbows are pointed toward the ceiling and your upper arms are vertical. Push the weight in an arc until your arms are almost fully extended over your face. Lower and repeat.

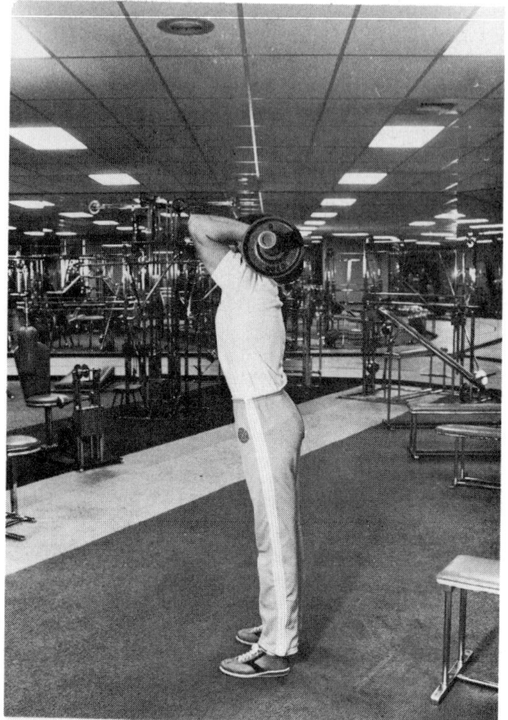

Step 1

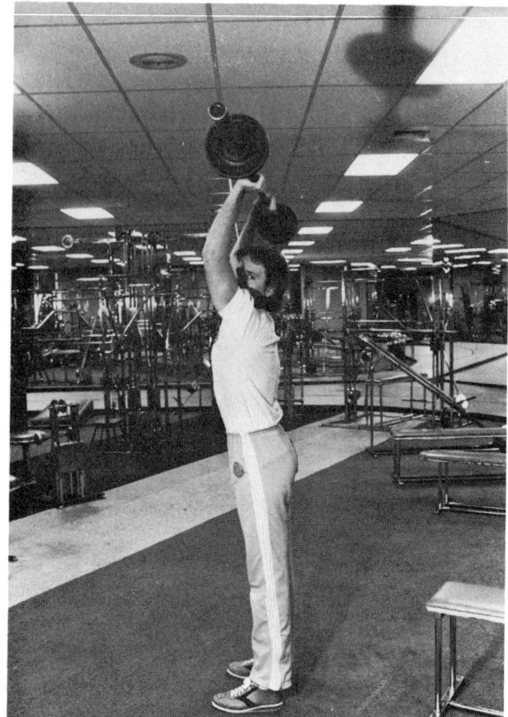

Step 2

STANDING TRICEPS EXTENSION WITH BARBELL

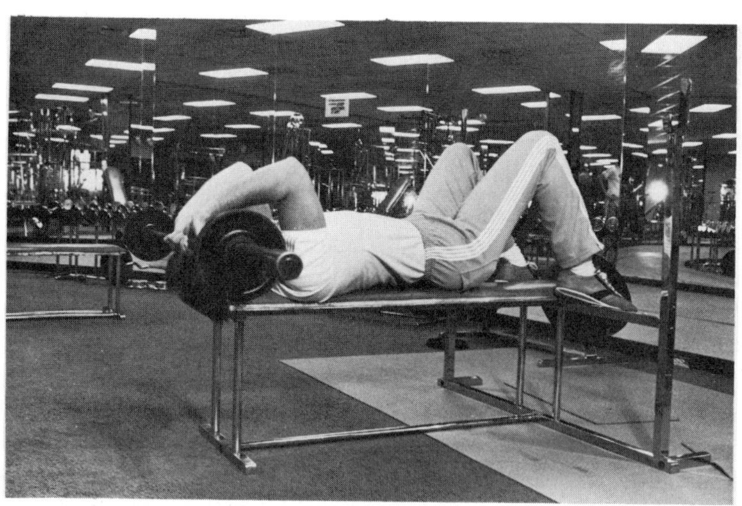

Step 1

RECLINING TRICEPS EXTENSION WITH BARBELL

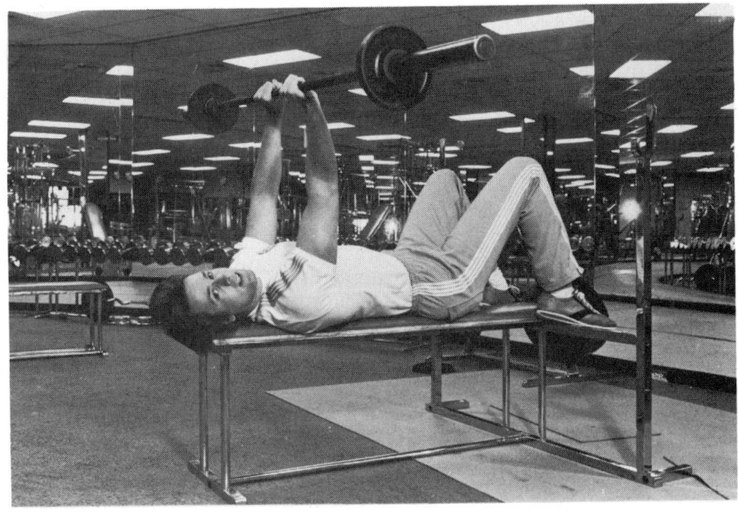

Step 2

RECLINING TRICEPS EXTENSION WITH BARBELL

Triceps Extensions with Dumbbells

All of the triceps extensions described above can be done with dumbbells, with the result that the triceps are worked in a slightly different way each time. Further, with the dumbbells it is harder to maintain upper arm and elbow immobility; thus you use the tie-in muscles in your shoulders and chest for a more complete workout of the arm and shoulder area.

You can also do any of the extensions described above in an alternating fashion with dumbbells, raising them one at a time. One additional triceps extension done with a dumbbell in a motion not described above is as follows.

Bentover One-Arm Dumbbell Triceps Extensions

Stand erect, holding a dumbbell in one hand, with your arms held loosely at your sides. Bend at the waist until your body is almost parallel to the floor. Keep the elbow of the arm holding the dumbbell against your side, and pull your upper arm up until it is parallel to the upper body. Your forearm should be vertical. Now lift the dumbbell in an arc to the back until the arm is straight. You will feel the greatest tension in the triceps at the very end of the movement. Hold for a count of one, and then slowly lower the forearm until it is vertical again. Don't move the upper arm, but keep it parallel to the upper body. Repeat with the dumbbell in the other hand.

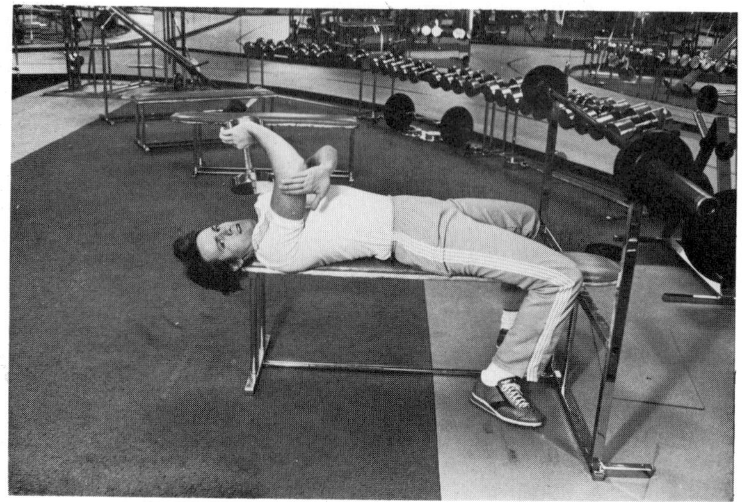

Step 1

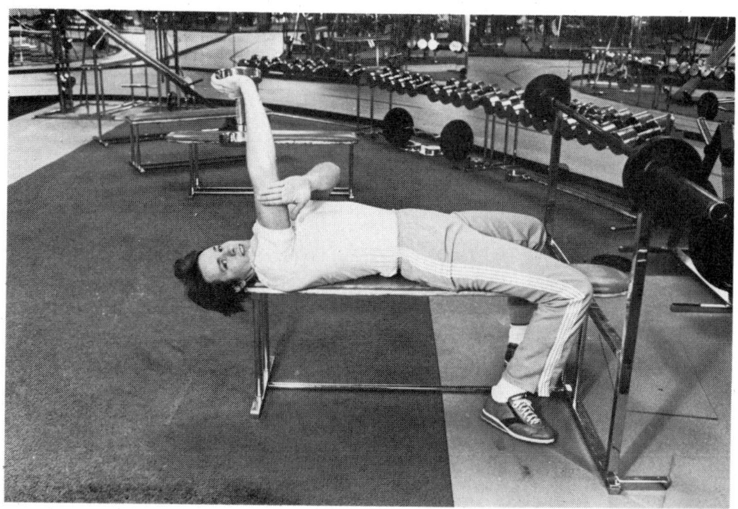

Step 2

TRICEPS EXTENSION WITH DUMBBELL (reclining)

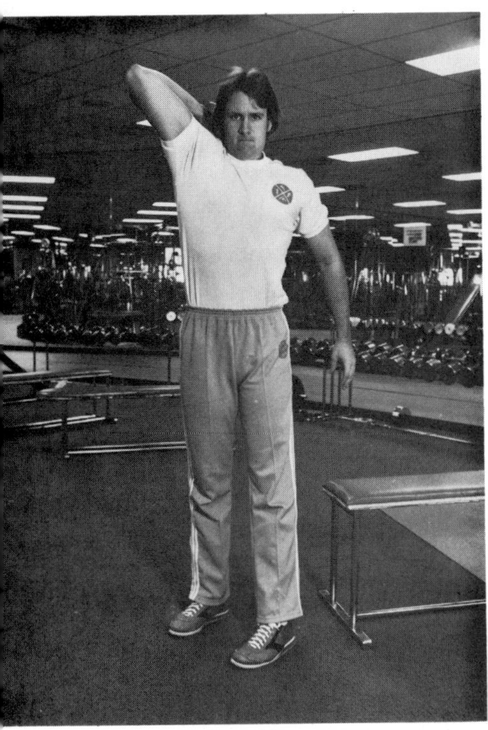

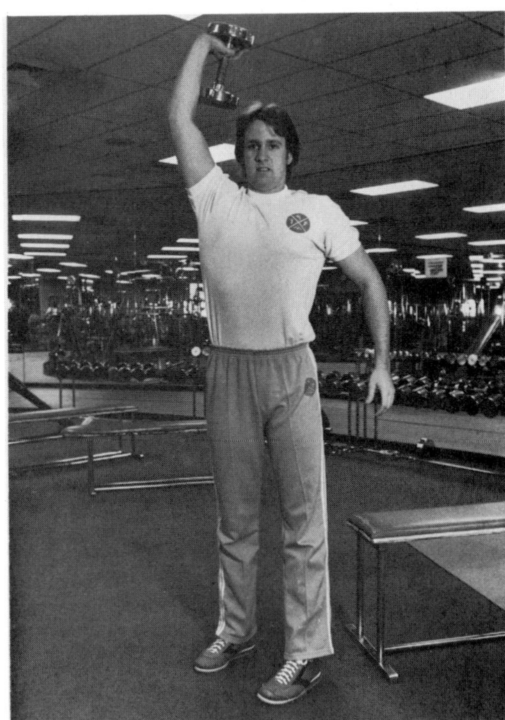

Step 1 Step 2

TRICEPS EXTENSION WITH DUMBBELL (standing)

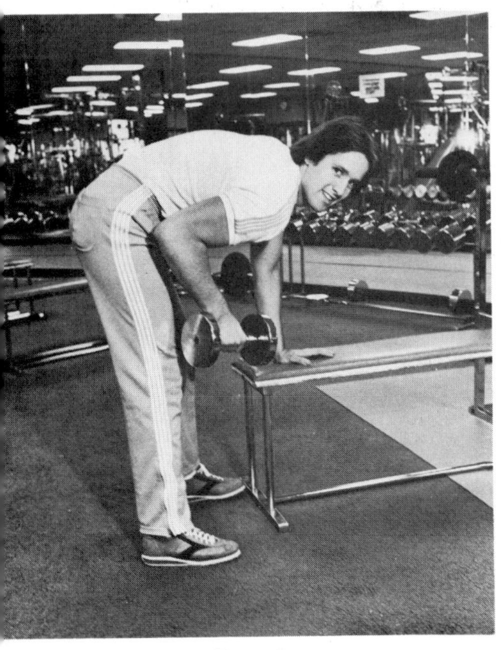

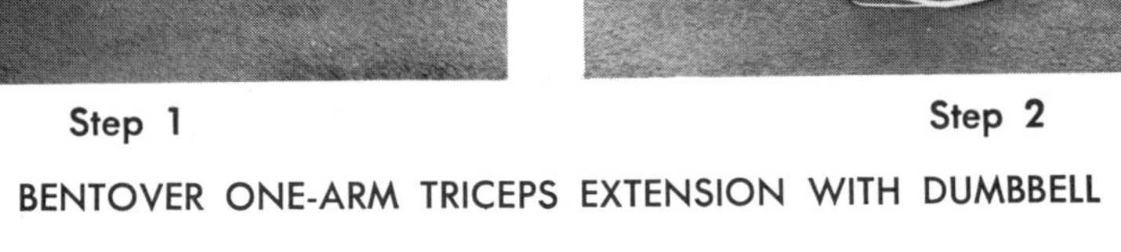

Step 1 Step 2

BENTOVER ONE-ARM TRICEPS EXTENSION WITH DUMBBELL

Triceps Extensions on Pulley Machines

Another way to isolate the work of the triceps is to use pulleys in making the extension movement. There are several ways to accomplish this, of which the most popular are as follows.

Pulley Pushdown Extensions

Stand in front of a pulley machine and grasp the bar with your hands close together, palms facing the floor. Push the bar down while keeping your upper arms and elbows immobilized. Extend the arms until they are straight, and then slowly let the bar back up.

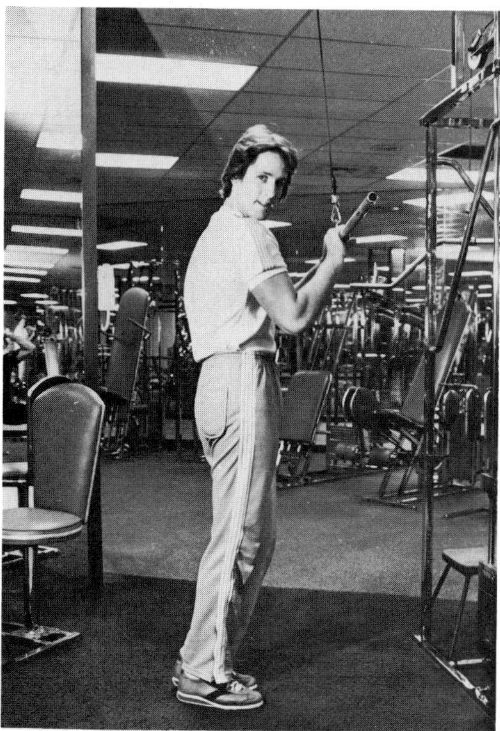

Step 1

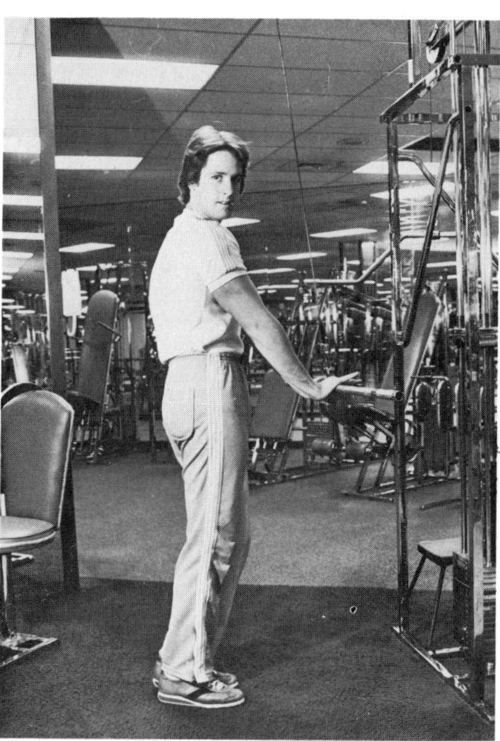

Step 2

PULLEY PUSHDOWN TRICEPS EXTENSION

Overhead Pulley Extensions

Stand with your back to the pulley machine, reach up, and grasp the bar behind your head (if the pulley bar is in a lower position when not in use, you will have to kneel with your back to the machine). Grasp the bar and pull it in an arc until your arms are straight out in front of you. Keep your elbows and upper arms immobile, and be careful not to crease the top of your head with the cable. You may be able to get a better extension if you tie a towel or fasten a strap to the pulley cable instead of a bar. This allows you to grasp the weight with the hands in a position where the palms are facing each other. Sometimes this makes for a better movement, depending on the bone structure of the individual.

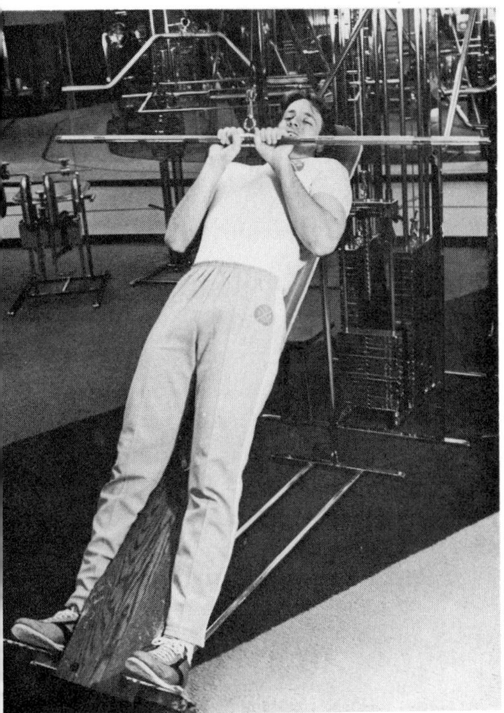

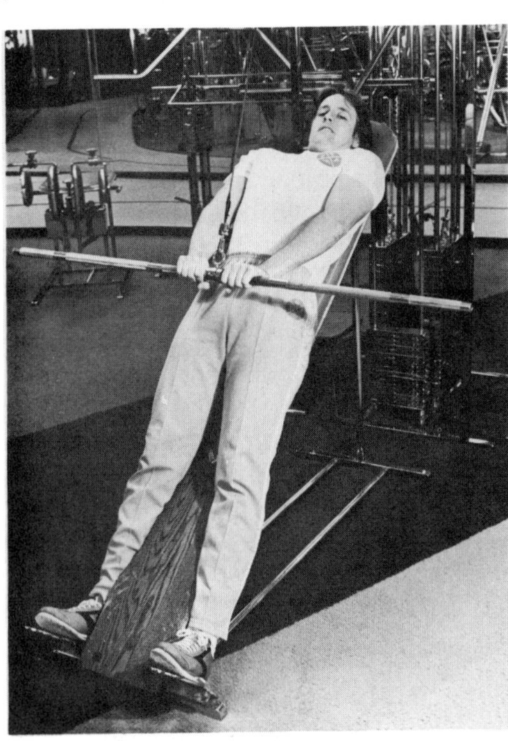

Step 1 Step 2

OVERHEAD PULLEY TRICEPS EXTENSION

THE FOREARMS

As you become able to use greater and greater poundages in the various arm movements, you may find that your triceps and biceps have outstripped your ability to hold onto the weight. This is especially true with heavy pulley work and heavy dumbbell work. It is not uncommon, especially with beginners, for the upper arm muscles to be able to lift poundages that the hands can't keep a grip on.

The way to prevent this is by working the forearms. They are similar in musculature and density to the calves, and they respond to the same kind of dogged workouts that you have to give the calves. The muscles of the forearm have two functions. Some are flexors and others are extensors. Some make the hand close into a fist and others make it open into a finger-spread. By opposing the two muscle groups, you can form a rigid, flat hand for a karate chop.

If you play the guitar or piano, you may find that you will lose your fine coordination and speed when you first start to exercise the forearm. Don't worry. Ralph has played flamenco guitar for years, as well as classical and folk guitar. Don't try to do complicated arpeggios and triplets immediately after a forearm workout, or you'll be disappointed in your performance. Simply alternate the days. Do your musical practice on off days and give those forearms a blitz on workout days. The forearms will soon adapt, and will soon reach the size that you want. Then you can put them on a maintenance routine and go back to refining your fingerwork. In the end, you'll find that you have better control with the guitar or piano than you had before you started. Here are a few ways to work the forearms.

Wrist Rolls (Palms Facing Up)

Sit on a bench and hold a barbell in your hands, palms facing up. Let your forearms rest against the tops of your thighs, with the hands in open air just past the knees. Let the wrists relax and bend downward toward the floor. Then flex the forearms, and bring the hands back up until the area between the wrist and the inside of the elbow is fully flexed. Hold for a count of two, and then slowly let the hands back down to the starting position. You won't be able to handle much weight in your hands at first, so concentrate more on the movement than on the amount of weight you are using.

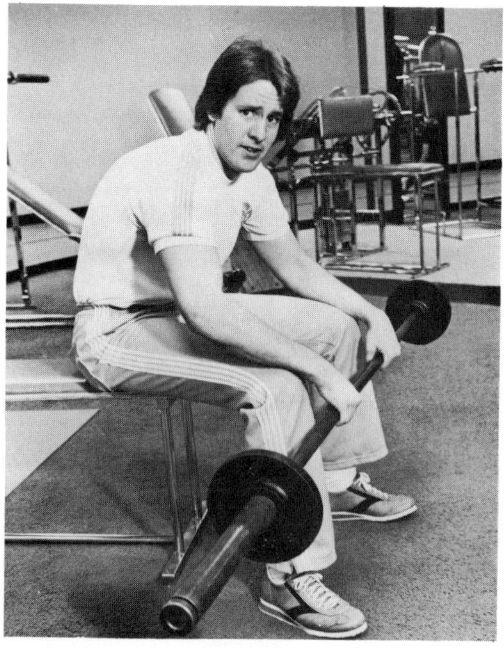

Step 1

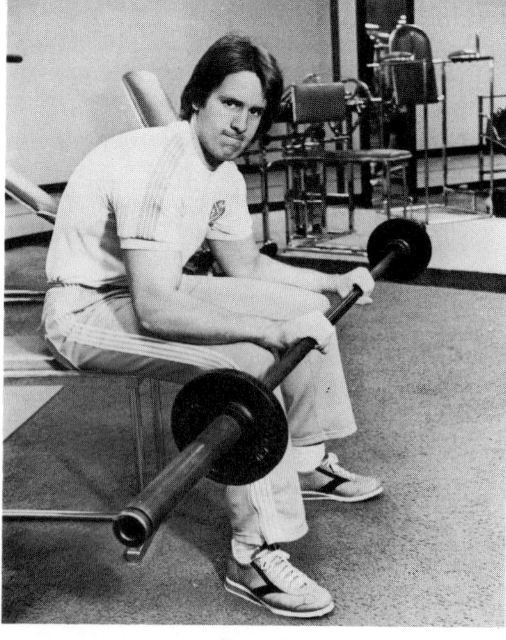

Step 2

WRIST ROLL (palms facing down)

Wrist Rolls (Palms Facing Down)

This one is done exactly like the exercise above, except that the palms are facing downward instead of upward, hence working the muscles on the other side of the forearm.

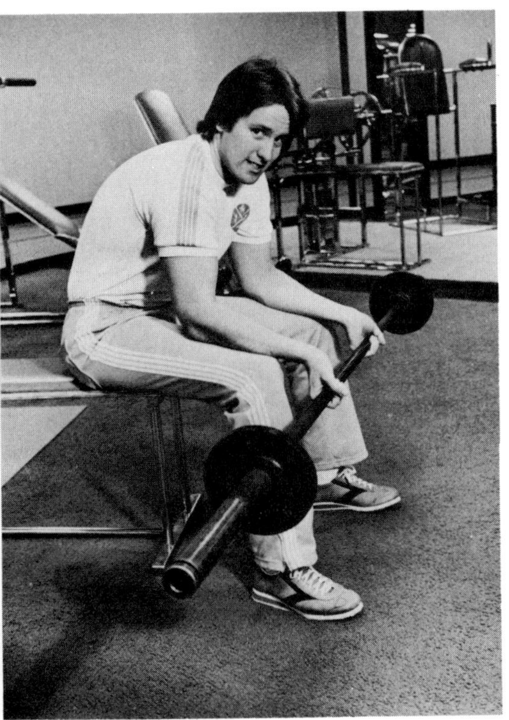

Step 1

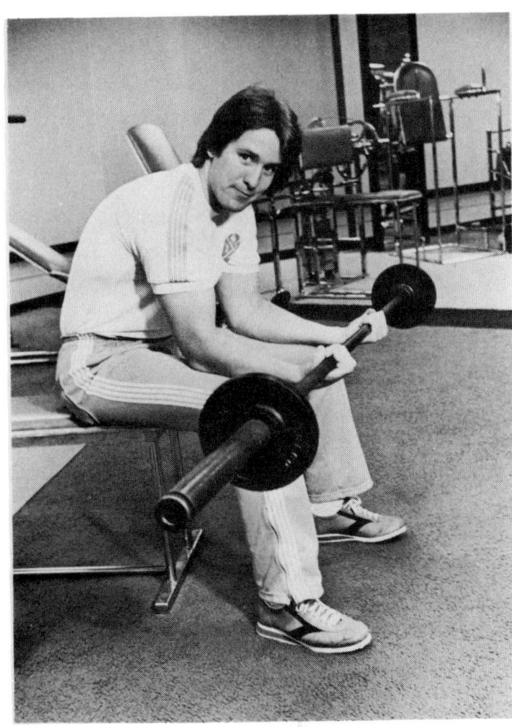

Step 2

WRIST ROLL (palms facing up)

5

HOW TO MAKE IT RUN WHEN YOU GET IT ALL ASSEMBLED

•

You've got all the parts—now all you have to do is put them together into a program that is specifically designed for the bodystyle you're after. That's what we're going to do in this chapter, and we're also going to pass along all the helpful tips on how to maximize your gains that you would get if you were enrolled in a first-class gym. First, let's talk about building for symmetry, size, and shape. Once you know how to do that, building for strength or building for cardiovascular conditioning is merely a matter of pacing yourself—adjusting the variables of workout duration and the amount of weight lifted.

You won't get the body you're after simply by showing up at the gym or dragging out of bed into the garage workout room three times a week. You won't necessarily succeed merely by going through the motions of the workouts, rushing through the sets in an effort to "get it over with" so you can get on down to the coffee shop for another Danish and sugared coffee before work. If you think it happens that way, that is probably why you are so out of shape right now.

Workouts can't be looked upon as merely means to an end. That's the basic mistake that many people make when they try to get in shape, whether they are weight training, running, playing racquetball, or just walking faster than usual. The workout has got to be something special, something you look forward to, something that not only produces the results you want but also has value in and of itself.

If you don't look at it this way, it will affect the results of the workout and you won't progress as fast as you could otherwise. There's nothing mysterious about this. It's simply that the fastest results come from *concentrated* effort. That means mental as well as physical concentration. You can't concentrate if your mind is distracted by the desire to hurry up and get it over with so you can go on to more important things.

What you are doing when you work out is this: you're creating yourself. That's right—you are creating the person you are going to be. There are few things more important than that.

Besides, once you really get into the swing of things, you'll become addicted to working out with weights, and you'll sit around and fidget until you get the chance to go back to the gym. In fact, the difficult thing for almost all beginning weight trainers is not keeping their interest up. Rather, it's resisting the temptation to work out every day.

In the four-phase program outlined in this chapter, you should work out every other day for the first three phases. You should work out two days in a row, then take a day off, for the fourth phase. Under no circumstances should you work out three or four days in a row.

Also, at the beginning you should do only one set of each exercise. You shouldn't go right into multiple sets unless you already have some experience in weight training and are already on the way toward being in shape.

You've read all the exercises and you've looked at all the photographs. You should have a pretty clear idea of how each exercise is done. Let's go over the basic principles that underlie weight training, so that you'll understand exactly what you are doing.

BUILDING FOR SYMMETRY, SIZE, AND SHAPE

When you are building for symmetry, size, and shape, you are really trying to bring your overall bodily development into a harmonious whole. Whether you have worked out before or have never lifted a barbell, you should first try to build a firm foundation of muscular mass before you start shaping any specific part of your body. To do this, you should embark on a general building and conditioning routine that works all the muscle groups, and works them as groups instead of working the individual muscles of each group in isolation. This way you'll build on something solid, and you will be able to refine and polish later. In short, you start with the chassis and work your way up.

We've talked before about sets and reps. Let's go over it again—with a few definitions:

EXERCISE — The basic unit of bodybuilding. You perform different *exercises* in order to work out different muscles. The bench press is an *exercise*.

Movement Each exercise consists of a certain movement, made with the arms, the legs, or a part of the torso. Pushing upward and away from the chest is the *movement* of the bench press.

Repetitions (reps) If you perform a certain movement, that's one *rep*. Two complete movements is two reps, and so on.

Sets If you perform the movements of an exercise ten times and then stop for a rest, you have completed one *set*.

Multiple sets If you go back to the same exercise after a short rest and perform another set, you are doing *multiple sets*.

Supersets If you perform one set of, for example, the bench press and follow it (with no rest period) with a set of incline flyes, you are *supersetting* bench presses and flyes.

Tri-sets If you do three exercises in a row with no rest, you are *tri-setting* those exercises.

Giant sets If you do, for example, a set of bench presses, followed by a set of flyes, then a set of military presses, a set of parallel-bar dips, and a final set of incline dumbbell presses—all with no rest in between sets—you are doing *giant sets*.

Forced reps If you have a spotter help you with just enough pressure to enable you to complete a rep that otherwise would be beyond your strength and/or endurance, you have done a *forced rep*.

Negative reps If you have someone help you complete the contraction portion of a movement, and then you resist the movement of the weight as it goes back to the starting position, you are doing *negative reps*.

Preexhaustion, or priority, training If you work out, say, the biceps before doing your lat work you are *preexhausting* the biceps in order to make the lats work harder. This constitutes giving *priority* to certain muscles in a sequence of exercises so that you will be better able to isolate other muscles when doing subsequent exercises.

Pushing to failure This is a popular new technique, in which you do each exercise with enough weight and for a sufficient number of reps to reach a point where the muscle affected fails to complete another movement.

Those are the nuts and bolts. Before we apply them to your routine, let's go on to the matter of workout schedules.

WORKOUT	The total collection of exercises that you perform during one training session.
STANDARD WORKOUT SEQUENCE	The *standard sequence* is to do a workout for the entire body *every other day.*
SPLIT SYSTEM	This method involves working out one part of the body (arms and upper body, for example) on one day and another part of the body on the subsequent day or another day.
DOUBLE-SPLIT SYSTEM	This system involves working out a portion of the body in the morning and another portion of the body later in the same day.

Where did this system begin? Here's a brief history. Way back in 1931, when Bob Hoffman founded *Strength and Health* magazine, he also put out some weight training courses. They were called the York Course 1, 2, 3, and 4. If you bought a York Barbell set, you got the courses. For hundreds of thousands of men in Ralph's generation, these courses constituted a beginning in weight training. Through the years, York has continued to sell barbell sets and the York courses.

During the late forties, a man named Joe Weider moved to the United States from Montreal, to found a magazine called *Your Physique.* While Hoffman's *Strength and Health* was focused primarily on weightlifting, Weider's publication was slanted toward the bodybuilding aspect of weight training. The kinds of skirmishes and feuds you might expect soon followed, and the two magazines squared off at each other. Every kid in Ralph's neighborhood waited eagerly at the newsstand each month to see what the two groups had to say about each other.

Weider wasn't so much trying to take the market away from Hoffman as he was trying to open up a new market: a market made up of all those men who wanted to have the bodybuilder's physique but were not primarily interested in competing in Olympic-style weightlifting.

What followed is history, albeit a confused one, and the skirmishes continue down to this day. Whatever else may be true, it is safe to say that weightlifting, especially Olympic lifting, is what it is today because of the efforts of Bob Hoffman and the men who followed him.

It is equally true that the development of bodybuilding in this country as a legitimate sport, the formation of the International Federation of Bodybuilders, and the current celebrity of bodybuilders is due almost entirely to the efforts of Joe Weider and his brother Ben (Ben is president of the Federation). It is impossible to describe a training routine without using the technical language codified by the Weiders. Whatever else may be said, Joe Weider's thoroughly professional *Muscle Builder* magazine was making bodybuilding respectable before *Pumping Iron* was ever conceived.

The reason for this digression is simple. When we put training programs together, we have to use the language of the field. Most of that language was codified by Joe Weider. In the same way that Isaac Asimov's Laws of Robotics have been absorbed by the literature of cybernetics, Weider's terminology has become a part of the literature of bodybuilding. Also, as in the case of Asimov's laws, the author rarely gets any credit. Thanks, Joe.

To come back to your workout program: when you perform a set of any exercise, two things are said to happen. Lactic acid is released into the muscle tissue as a built-in safeguard against injury (it keeps the muscle from contracting further), and there is a certain amount of breakdown of muscle tissue. While there is no doubt about the first item, there is much controversy about the latter. It used to be thought that muscle growth came only from the actual structural breakdown of muscle tissue. Now most researchers think that the amount of actual breakdown is small, and that muscle growth comes from the "activation" of previously dormant muscle fibers.

If you've used the right amount of weight, as you approach the eighth or ninth rep of a given exercise, you will begin to feel a burning sensation in the muscle, caused by the lactic buildup and also by the fatigue that the movement produces.

When you first start a weight training routine, you may find that you don't feel these things at all. That's because your muscles are not used to the work load you are putting on them and the fibers are not "activating" yet. Keep plugging. If you are really out of shape, you'll be sore as hell after the first workout. If you are, good. You'll know you did it right. You won't be sore again—until you change your program. So don't worry about it.

"Good" soreness comes from having really worked the muscles. It comes as a warm glow in the muscle, and you'll learn to love it. "Bad" soreness comes from pulled muscles and strained tendons. You can avoid bad soreness by going slowly at first, and building up speed and intensity as you get into the program.

The program outlined here is a 14-week program. It's designed to give you the solid foundation you'll need to do shaping and refining later on. No matter how badly you are out of shape, the program will bring you some unbelievable results. And even if you're in good shape, unless you are already an advanced weight trainer you will be amazed at the improvement you'll make. Read the description of the program below and refer to the tables on pages 195–199.

The first part of the program, phase 1, is a basic general conditioning program, designed to get you into weight training in the most constructive way. You'll do one set of each exercise, with a starting count of eight reps for arms and ten reps for legs and torso. You'll add a rep to the arms exercises and two reps to the leg and torso exercises every *third* workout day until you reach thirteen reps in the arm exercises and twenty reps in the leg exercises.

Working out every other day gives your muscles time to repair, and it gives your body time to reestablish its chemical balances. Adding reps every third workout makes the program a *progressive-resistance* program: you move to progressively higher reps with the same weight until you top out at thirteen for the arms and twenty for the legs and torso.

This is an accelerated program. Consequently, when you reach the top of the rep ladder and drop down to eight and ten reps again, you'll not only add weight but you'll add a set as well—now you'll be in phase 2. Remember: use enough weight to make those last two reps a real effort. For some people, that means adding five pounds to the arm movements. For others, it may mean adding ten pounds. Don't let yourself get caught in the old trap of poundages. While you will certainly increase your strength as you work out with weights, using too much weight will impair your ability to make gains in muscle size, especially in the beginning.

This is because muscles increase in size not so much because they are hoisting "x" amount of weight, but because "x" amount of weight is being hoisted in specific ways that cause flushing of the muscles with fresh blood and the stimulation of the brain to secrete certain growth enzymes. Ten reps with muscle failure on the last rep will result in more muscle growth than three reps with muscle failure on the third rep.

By adding a set, you will increase the intensity of your workout. You'll want to rest for about thirty seconds between reps so that the muscles will have time to recover. Otherwise you may have to reduce the poundages in order to be able to handle the additional set. Experiment and you'll quickly fasten onto how many pounds to use.

When you've made it up the rep ladder again and are ready to start phase 3, drop down, add weight, and add another set. By this time, your muscles will be "pumping up" thoroughly each time you work out. You'll find out what everybody has been talking about since *Pumping Iron* was published. The pump comes from the rush of blood and fluid into the muscle that is being worked. It's a terrific feeling, and it takes several weeks of training before your muscles begin to respond to the exercises enough to pump up. You'll know it when it happens. You'll strut around all day!

At the beginning, although your muscles won't respond so dramatically, the pumping process will be hard at work. If you've been leading a completely sedentary life and your blood isn't used to circulating very fast, you may get dizzy during the first week or so of workouts. If you have nothing structurally or organically wrong, there is probably nothing to worry about. It simply means that from a cardiovascular point of view, you're a mess. You'll get over it quickly.

By the time you get to the top of the rep ladder again, ready for phase 4, you'll be ready to split your routine. This means that instead of working out every other day, you will work out (for example) on Monday, doing the arm and upper body routine, and on Tuesday doing the leg and back routine. You'll take Wednesday off, and come back for the upper body routine on Thursday and the legs on Friday. If you are young, you shouldn't have any problem with this schedule. If you are over thirty-five, you might want to work out on Mondays and Tuesdays, skip two days, and work out again on Fridays and Saturdays. If you're over forty, as Ralph is, you may want to take more time off to let your body recover and build, working out on Mondays, Wednesdays, and Fridays but taking two days off over the weekend.

Whatever routine you settle on, try to push yourself enough so that you can at least learn what your limits are. There is such a thing as overtraining. The symptoms are nervousness, irregular pulse, tiredness, and inability to sleep. These symptoms are usually caused by the fact that you aren't giving the muscles a chance to return to normal before you launch into another workout. If you are over thirty-five and your metabolism has slowed, you may be suffering from a good case of the jitters caused by being hyperactive for the first time since adolescence.

If you do suffer from these symptoms, and you have reasons to believe that they are the result of overtraining, poor eating habits, or plain pushing yourself too far, you should see your physician and determine if anything has shown up that you should know about. Don't take any chances with yourself. Remember, the whole point of working out is to feel good, to be healthy as well as look good.

As you begin the fourth phase of the program, you will also have to fight the temptation to work out more than you should. We're really serious about this. By the time you swing into phase 4, you will be feeling better than you've felt in years, especially if high school phys ed is a dim memory. You'll get the feeling that you can walk through walls. Easy does it. The best is yet to be: the advanced workouts for which the beginning workouts were made.

In phase 4, we've added some exercises that will isolate certain muscles such as the deltoids and the biceps. Part of the reason that you will go through phase 1–3 is to get your muscles into generally good shape so that you can do isolation or concentration exercises to some advantage. If you start out with concentration movements, you will not benefit from them. Quite to the contrary, they will actually inhibit you in your efforts to lay a solid foundation.

Let's go back for a few minutes to the workout followed by our young friend Jerry at the health club. You remember him: the one who trains diligently but incorrectly.

He usually does 400 situps, 200 leg raises, 400 standing twists with a bar on the shoulders, and 200 kneeups on a leg raise machine. He will then move to the bench press and crank out anywhere from ten to fifteen sets of one to ten reps. He goes for maximum poundages every day, starting with ten reps at 135 pounds and ending with one rep at 210.

He will then slide an incline bench under the squat racks and crank out another ten to fifteen sets of incline presses. After this, he will set a slant board up against one of the other machines and crank out ten to fifteen sets of decline presses, in every case going for maximum poundages.

That's the beginning of his workout. He spends some time at the pulley pushdown bar, the lat pulleys, and at the pectoral, back, leg press, and calf raise machines. By the end of his workout, he will have ground out nearly a hundred sets, using every muscle in his body. And he does this six days a week!

Jerry is dedicated, he's serious, and he wants to be a big bodybuilder more than anything else in the world. He looks more haggard every day, and we haven't noticed any increase in size over the last three months. Everybody has tried to give him advice, but he's convinced that if four sets are good for you, ten sets must be nirvana.

Jerry is able to get away with this sort of thing because he's in his early twenties. But he's not building. He's tearing down. You want to build. You can't do it if you're in too much of a hurry. You've got the rest of your life. Train scientifically and you'll get the body you want. Train slavishly, overtrain, and you'll make no gains.

Again, we make this digression to underline the point: you're going to feel terrific by the time you get into phase 4. Don't overdo just because you are able.

At the end of phase 4, your course will probably be set for you. It's hard for us to imagine that you will quit training now that you've made such drastic improvement. The bug has usually bitten by this time, and you will have either outfitted a well-stocked home gym by now or you will have scraped up enough cash to join a health club or gym.

Also, by the time you've finished phase 4, you will have picked up enough lore to want to continue your program with a few additions and deletions. You may see that your deltoids are still lagging behind and need further concentrated effort. Look at the index of exercises, pick out a few for the deltoids, and fit them into your program. *Don't* sacrifice the basic movements, however. They're essential, and you will not have built a total foundation in only fourteen weeks. Keep up the general-conditioning, compound exercises from now on. They're your mainstay. But add isolation and concentration exercises to help balance out your physique. That's how you'll get the symmetry you want.

You'll want to change your routine from time to time after you've finished the fourteen-week program. Sometimes it helps to shock the muscles out of their rut, since the human body is so extremely adaptable—that's why we've come to the top of the evolutionary heap in one piece—that your muscles will reach sticking points. The best thing to do when they level off at some plateau is to put them through some extra work, to jar them into action.

If you're stuck on a certain poundage doing the bench press, get somebody to spot you and do some forced reps. If that doesn't work, then try negative reps. Try working the muscles to failure. This is not advisable for a beginner, because of the likelihood of injury, but when you get into advanced training, push the muscles for all they're worth. Don't overtrain like our young friend, but use extreme techniques for short periods of time to give your muscles a needed shock treatment.

If your curls are stuck, try cheating movements. Swing the bar up. Use ten more pounds than you can do in strict form (be sure to warm up first!). The same goes for the squat. If you can't make any progress, add forty pounds and do half-squats until you get used to handling a lot of weight on your shoulders.

Especially by the time you get halfway through phase 4, you could superset bench presses and flyes, military presses and deltoid raises, incline dumbbell curls and standing barbell curls or Scott bench curls. Try tri-sets or giant sets. And don't forget: when you add exercises to your program, when you work out your own phase 5, try to sequence the exercises so that you take advantage of the principle of preexhaustion. It'll make all the difference to some people.

Take a good look at yourself in the mirror before you start. Go ahead and take some photographs of yourself, both relaxed and in some of the traditional muscleman poses. It'll take nerve to do it, but you'll be thankful later on.

At the end of phase 4, take another set of photos in exactly the same poses. Then try not to jump up and down and make a fool of yourself because you look so much better.

BUILDING FOR STRENGTH

How can you alter the program and make it a strength-building program as well as a shaping and size-producing program? Easy.

In the first place, you'll make some terrific gains in strength from the program just as it stands. You'll get used to handling heavy poundages and you'll find it hard to believe that you were ever as weak as you were when you started.

Second, you will have made the necessary first step toward building strength: you will have begun a solid program to train the large muscle groups with compound exercises that will teach them to work together for maximum strength.

Third, the specialization exercises in phase 4 will begin to improve those areas that are not as well developed as the rest of your body. This is necessary for building any really lasting strength.

Now, what to do? Simply this. After you have built that solid foundation, start a routine that incorporates the exercises that support the lifts you want to make. You will have become generally strong by doing the exercises in the program. You can become "specifically strong" by specializing in those exercises that utilize the muscles that make the lifts you want to make.

Powerlifting, for example, consists of bench presses, squats, and deadweight lifts. It is a commonplace in sports medicine that the best way to improve in a certain sports movement is to do that movement. The best way to improve your bench press is to do the bench press. But you should work out all the muscles that go into the bench press as well. This means that you should pay special attention to exercises for the anterior deltoids, the pectorals, and the triceps.

And that's not all. You should remember that muscles get support from nearby muscles, so you shouldn't neglect the lateral deltoids, the latissimus dorsi, and the trapezius, not to mention the forearms (you've got to hold the damn bar, remember?) and the biceps.

Once you've built some muscle mass, you can lower the number of reps per set and go for maximum poundages once a week. Instead of doing ten to twenty reps of the bench press with the same weight, do four to ten. Start at four to ten reps, add weight and drop reps each time you do a set, and work to the point where you have to get help for one forced rep at the end.

Alternate your power workouts (fewer sets, fewer reps) with your regular workouts (more sets, more reps, more exercises). If you're really going to get into the strength groove, it's a must to get acquainted with the powerlifting guys wherever they congregate. Also, you'll find instructive articles in *Strength and Health* and *Iron Man* magazines as well as in *Muscle Builder*. Seek out the local powerlifting team. They're usually based in the YMCA or in the one heavy-metal gym that almost every city has. Watch them work out. Ask for advice. See how they do it.

Olympic lifting is the same story. Not as many people are caught up in Olympic lifting as in powerlifting, but they are around. You'll usually find them in the same place as the powerlifters. After all, their goals are the same. Only the lifts differ.

Again, the way to train for strength instead of shape and size is to go after heavy poundages, with fewer sets and fewer reps, not only in the Olympic lifts and the powerlifts but in those exercises that work the muscles that support these lifts. Don't diet so strenuously, and eat enough protein to take care of the huge demands you are going to make on your system. Weight moves weight, and although you can't flex fat, fat will increase the cross section of a muscle and some strength can be derived from that alone. Look at the heavyweight champion lifters on the Sunday afternoon sports shows sometime. The lightweight and middleweight guys will be trim, but the heavyweights will almost all be packing a lot of fat.

This book, however, isn't about becoming a champion powerlifter or Olympic lifter. It's designed to help you shape your body to the shape you want, quickly and effectively. How big you get and how strong you get is strictly up to you. Once you get to the place you want to go, you can cut back on the number of reps, sets, and exercises you do and go on a maintenance routine. Your workouts will never last more than an hour, and there will be little reason for you to work out more than three times a week.

Think about it for a moment: three hours a week, and you can look terrific, feel terrific, and be terrific. It's a small price to pay for what you get.

If you want some inspiration, you might take a look at the record book for the 1979 weightlifting championships. They're nothing less than incredible. Here are the weight-class winners.

1979 Junior National Weightlifting Championships (Olympic style)
(Chicago, Illinois, March 10 and 11, 1979)

Weight class (pounds)	*Contestant*	*Snatch*	*Clean & jerk*	*Total poundage*
		(in pounds)		
132	Joe Delago	192.75	270.0	462.75
148	Henri Peters	242.5	314.0	556.5
165	Tim Neller	275.5	341.5	617.0
181	John Julius	297.5	374.75	672.25
198	James Curry	303.0	391.25	694.25
220	Ken Clark	325.0	429.75	754.75
242	Mitch Mignano	314.0	424.25	738.25
Superheavy	John Schiechl	231.25	270.0	501.25

And that's the Junior Nationals. Now look at the Senior Nationals:

Weight class (pounds)	*Contestant*	*Snatch*	*Clean & jerk*	*Total poundage*
		(in pounds)		
114	Jon Chappell	176.3	214.9	391.2
123	Pat Omori	192.9	253.5	446.4
132	Phil Sanderson	248.0	308.6	556.6
148	Dave Jones	264.5	330.6	595.1
165	Dave Reigle	270.0	363.7	633.7
181	Tom Hirtz	325.1	374.7	699.8
198	Jim Curry, Jr.	314.1	402.3	716.4
220	Kurt Setterberg	347.2	424.3	771.5
242	Mark Cameron	363.7	485.0	848.7
Superheavy	Tom Stock	363.7	468.4	832.1

Take another look at the last two weight classes. The winner of the 242-pound class beat the total of the winner of the superheavyweight class. It ain't how much you weigh, it's how much you can lift when it comes to brute muscle strength!

And then there's powerlifting. Look at these statistics from the National Powerlifting Championships:

Weight Class (pounds)	*Contestant*	*Squat*	*Bench Press*	*Dead-lift*	*Total poundage*
			(in pounds)		
114	Chuck Dunbar	485.00	303.00	363.75	1151.75
123	Robert Lech	462.75	270.00	512.50	1245.25
132	George Hummel	451.75	325.00	540.00	1316.75
148	Jim Rush	551.00	319.50	595.00	1465.50
165	Mike Bridges	705.25	446.25	655.75	1807.25
181	Walter Thomas	694.25	440.75	683.25	1818.25
198	Roger Estep	727.50	490.50	672.25	1890.25
220	Larry Pacifico	766.00	529.00	722.00	2017.00
242	John Kuc	766.00	507.00	810.00	2083.00
275	Larry Kidney	832.00	562.00	749.50	2143.50
Superheavy	Paul Wrenn	953.25	435.25	760.50	2149.00

The next time anybody tells you that weight-trained muscles aren't really strong, show him the figures.

If you want to go the strength route, there are the mileposts. You begin to get an idea of just how powerful the human body is when you study the performance of the Olympic lifters and powerlifters. All the lifts are done with careful, precise form, and the men who make these lifts are the strongest men in the world.

Why do they lift heavy weights over their heads? Why do people race cars, shoot bows and arrows, play football, skydive, or climb mountains? Why not?

BUILDING FOR CARDIOVASCULAR CONDITIONING

Back in chapter 1, we talked about how weight training can be used for cardiovascular conditioning. Now that you know all the exercises, how to put them together, and how to do a complete workout, you can see how easy it is to alter your routine the little bit that is necessary to make it a cardiovascular conditioning routine.

All you have to do is measure your limits in terms of strength and stamina, choose poundages lighter than you would use for building size or building strength, and work out in such a way that the entire workout is one giant set. Don't rest at all between sets. Make sure that you are handling an amount of weight that will allow you to move from exercise to exercise without stopping (and without losing stamina).

Increase the number or reps for each exercise. Start with ten reps for the arms and twenty reps for leg and torso work. Instead of doing multiple sets, try doing one set for each exercise, but with double the number of reps you presently do. Do the movements quickly instead of slowly (but don't jerk the weights). Cut down the total time of the workout from one hour to forty-five minutes, and make up the time with the speed of the workout instead of by eliminating exercises.

Try to stay a little out of breath during the entire workout.. If you've done jogging, you'll know approximately what your oxygen debt will be. Don't make the debt so high that you can't repay it except by stopping the workout. It'll take you a while to sort out your limits, but you'll get the hang of it quickly enough.

The top bodybuilders use routines like this to build cardiovascular conditioning along with size and shape. By increasing the speed and the intensity with which they work out, they burn fat off their bodies and thus achieve the "cuts" between the muscles that are absolutely necessary to win contests. The secret is this: do the greatest amount of work you can do in the shortest amount of time you can do it. This will give you the maximum combination of strength, stamina, and size. It amounts to solid, hard training, and the results are well worth it if you're willing to put out the effort.

This doesn't mean hurrying through your exercises in a halfhearted way. Instead, it means that you get in there and really go at it. You make every minute count. Every exercise is done with maximum effort, whether you are "cheating" or doing it in strict form. There are no long rests between sets, no talking about your workout with other people as you try to disguise the fact that you're out of breath. No extra trips to the water fountain or to the kitchen as you try to recover from the last exercise. No stretching the workout to two hours when half that time was spent not working out.

That's the kind of dedication you need to really succeed at this game. Approach it that way and you'll get the admiration you want and deserve. You'll become a special person, and you'll soon wonder how you were ever satisfied with the sedentary life you once lived. You'll also become a little less patient with people who try to make you go off your program, who make you try to sympathize with them for never quite having the time to work out.

The time will come, and you might as well be prepared for it. Your overweight friend will be well into his third tray of junk food and his fourth beer, will heave his bulk up and look at you out of the corner of his eye, hiding the flab under his dark business suit. He'll mutter something about how you ought to act your age, how he used to to do all that stuff but he's too busy for it now. "That's kid stuff," he'll say.

And he'll be absolutely right, this man who is stumbling toward old age although he's the same age as you are.

He's right. Kid stuff. Ain't it great to be a kid again?

Here's the program. Good luck and good workout!

Exercises for Phases 1 Through 3

Exercise	*Number of sets*	*Starting number of reps*
Squats	1–3	10
Dead weight lift	1–3	10
Calf raises	1 (each position)	10
Straight-arm pullover	1–3	10
Bench press	1–3	8
Military press	1–3	8
Seated twists	1	100
Military curl with barbell	1–3	8
Shoulder shrug	1–3	10
Situps	1	20

When you finish phase 1 and again when you finish phase 2, drop back to the starting number of reps, add weight, and add another set for everything but the situps, twists, and calf raises.

Exercises for Phase 4 Split Routine

Exercise	*Number of sets*	*Starting number of reps*
Routine A: Legs and Lower Back		
Squats	4	10
Stiff-legged dead weight lift	4	10
Leg press	4	10
Leg curl	4	10
Leg extension	4	10
Seated twists	1	100
Calf raises	2 (each position)	10 (each position)
Bentover rowing (elbows at the sides)	4	10
Situps	1	40

Routine B: Arms and Upper Body

Bench press	4	8
Flyes	4	10
Military press	4	8
Seated lateral raises	4	10
Incline dumbbell curls	4	8
Parallel-bar dips	4	10
Scott bench or military curls	4	8
Bentover twists	1	30
Shoulder shrugs	4	10
Front abdominal crunches	4	15

Sets and Reps Schedule for Phase 1

Day	*Sets*	*Reps*
Sunday	1	8/10
Monday	0	off
Tuesday	1	8/10
Wednesday	0	off
Thursday	1	9/12
Friday	0	off
Saturday	1	9/12
Sunday	0	off
Monday	1	10/14
Tuesday	0	off
Wednesday	1	10/14
Thursday	0	off
Friday	1	11/16
Saturday	0	off
Sunday	1	11/16
Monday	0	off
Tuesday	1	12/18
Wednesday	0	off
Thursday	1	12/18
Friday	0	off
Saturday	1	13/20
Sunday	0	off
Monday	1	13/20
Tuesday	0	off

Sets and Reps Schedule for Phase 2

Day	*Sets*	*Reps*
Wednesday	2	8/10
Thursday	0	off

Friday	2	8/10
Saturday	0	off
Sunday	2	9/12
Monday	0	off
Tuesday	2	9/12
Wednesday	0	off
Thursday	2	10/14
Friday	0	off
Saturday	2	10/14
Sunday	0	off
Monday	2	11/16
Tuesday	0	off
Wednesday	2	11/16
Thursday	0	off
Friday	2	12/18
Saturday	0	off
Sunday	2	12/18
Monday	0	off
Tuesday	2	13/20
Wednesday	0	off
Thursday	2	13/20
Friday	0	off

Sets and Reps Schedule for Phase 3

Day	*Sets*	*Reps*
Saturday	3	8/10
Sunday	0	off
Monday	3	8/10
Tuesday	0	off
Wednesday	3	9/12
Thursday	0	off
Friday	3	9/12
Saturday	0	off
Sunday	3	10/14
Monday	0	off
Tuesday	3	10/14
Wednesday	0	off
Thursday	3	11/16
Friday	0	off
Saturday	3	11/16
Sunday	0	off
Monday	3	12/18
Tuesday	0	off
Wednesday	3	12/18

Thursday	0	off
Friday	3	13/20
Saturday	0	off
Sunday	3	13/20
Monday	0	off

Sets and Reps Schedule for Phase 4

Days	*Routine*	*Sets*	*Reps*
Tuesday	A	4	10
Wednesday	B	4	8/10
Thursday	0	0	off
Friday	A	4	10
Saturday	B	4	8/10
Sunday	0	0	off
Monday	A	4	12
Tuesday	B	4	9/12
Wednesday	0	0	off
Thursday	A	4	12
Friday	B	4	9/12
Saturday	0	0	off
Sunday	A	4	14
Monday	B	4	10/14
Tuesday	0	0	off
Wednesday	A	4	14
Thursday	B	4	10/14
Friday	0	0	off
Saturday	A	4	16
Sunday	B	4	11/16
Monday	0	0	off
Tuesday	A	4	16
Wednesday	B	4	11/16
Thursday	0	0	off
Friday	A	4	18
Saturday	B	4	12/18
Sunday	0	0	off

That's the weight training–bodyshaping program. Follow it carefully and take the days off as indicated. You should weigh in and take your measurements on the first day of phase 1 and also on the first days of phases 2, 3, and 4. Then take them one more time on the last day of phase 4 and compare them with what you were at the start. If you started fat and out of shape, you'll be slimmer and harder. If you started skinny, you'll show some solid muscle.

Here's a chart to put your vital statistics on. Girth measurements should be taken both relaxed and flexed. You might also find it interesting to take measurements before and after workouts to see how much you are pumping up.

	Start phase 1	*Start phase 2*	*Start phase 3*	*Start phase 4*	*End phase 4*
Weight	( )	( )	( )	( )	( )
Height	( )	( )	( )	( )	( )
Calves	R( )L( )	R( )L( )	R( )L( )	R( )L( )	R( )L( )
Thighs	R( )L( )	R( )L( )	R( )L( )	R( )L( )	R( )L( )
Hips	( )	( )	( )	( )	( )
Waist	( )	( )	( )	( )	( )
Chest	( )	( )	( )	( )	( )
Shoulders	( )	( )	( )	( )	( )
Neck	( )	( )	( )	( )	( )
Upper arms	R( )L( )	R( )L( )	R( )L( )	R( )L( )	R( )L( )
Forearms	R( )L( )	R( )L( )	R( )L( )	R( )L( )	R( )L( )

6

KEEPING IT RUNNING AT HOME, AT WORK, AND ON THE ROAD

•

As you become more and more immersed in the fascinating world of keeping in shape, you'll find that you resent the time you have to take away from your workouts. You'll look forward to them and you'll arrange your time around them so that you can spend as much time as possible exercising.

When this happens, you've got the fever, and the only hope for you is to reconcile yourself to the fact that it really is better to be healthy than sick, to look good rather than bad, to be slim, trim, lean, and mean rather than fat, sloppy, puffy, and fading fast.

Working out will change your life for the better, no doubt about it. It'll rearrange your priorities in such a way that you'll be around a lot longer than you might have thought. If you belong to a gym or health club, you'll find a world of ordinary guys who like to feel good and who are dedicated to pumping that iron.

If you have a home gym, you'll probably have to learn how to explain it all to visitors. Don't worry about the weights lying all over the living room. They're very hi tech anyway, and if you have the money to buy a chromed set, you can think of them as sculpture.

You'll especially resent interruptions in your newly established routines, and you'll find yourself eventually involved in the old juggling act between home, office, trips out of town, and trying to keep the shape you put so much effort into developing. That's what this chapter is for. To give you a few tips on survival *as* the fittest.

EXERCISES TO DO WITH YOUR FAVORITE PARTNER

If you have a home gym, introduce her to the iron. Show her the before-and-after photos of Valerie and she'll see the point. Even if she's exactly the way you want her to look right now, you'll find that a good workout, especially if you do it together, will bring out a glow from both of you. No, it's not a flaky idea. Double workouts are the most erotic things going, and the sooner you find it out the more fun both of you will have.

Of course, you can act as a spotter for her in some of the weight training exercises. And you can have a lot of fun teaching her how to get the most out of an intensive workout. Show her some of the leg raises for any cellulite she may have begun to collect around her hips. Careful, though. Include her in your workout world not as an implicit criticism. Do it because it's fun, it's healthy, and it's an absolutely *fine* way really to get to know each other.

While you're knocking around the weight room, here are some exercises you can do together, just to get the feel of things. We call them the "witchy workout," because all you need is a broomstick and room to stretch out. They'll cast a spell on you (and her).

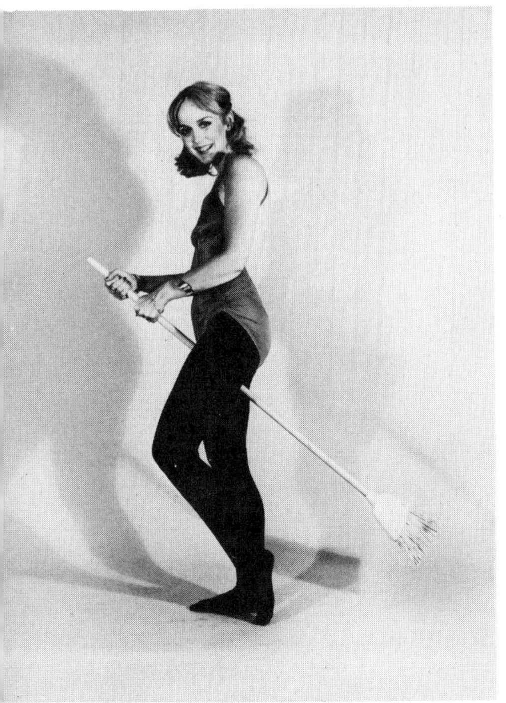

Step 1

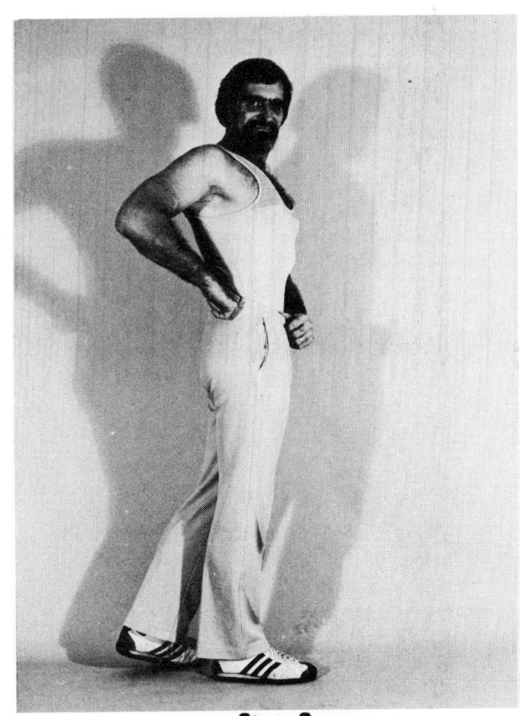

Step 2

BASIC EQUIPMENT FOR THE WITCHY WORKOUT

BROOMSTICK PULLDOWNS

Raise the broomstick overhead and stand about two feet apart, facing each other, clasping the broomstick in your hands (the hands should be about shoulder width apart, palms facing downward). Now take turns trying to keep each other from bringing the broomstick down. The one pulling will work the lats, the pecs, and the serratus muscles. The one resisting will get a good shoulder workout. Do ten reps.

BROOMSTICK SHRUGS

Let her lie on the floor on her back, holding a broomstick above her face at arms' length. Reach down and grasp the broomstick the way you would for a regular shoulder shrug. You'll lift her upper body off the floor as you do the shrug. Change places and let her try. Ten reps.

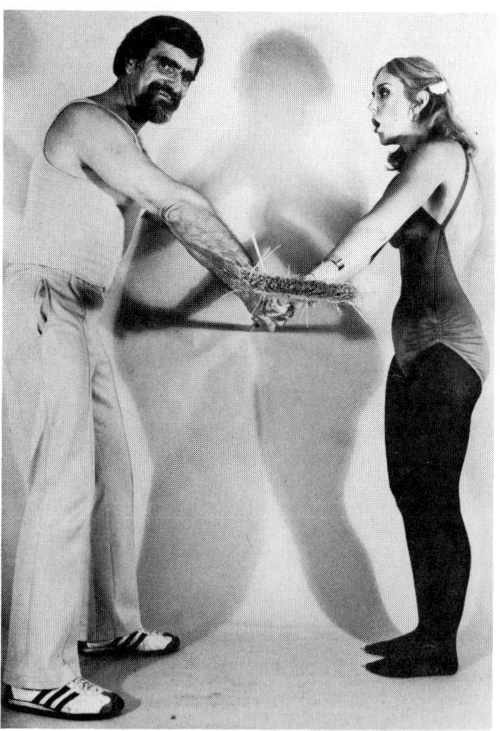

BROOMSTICK PULLDOWN

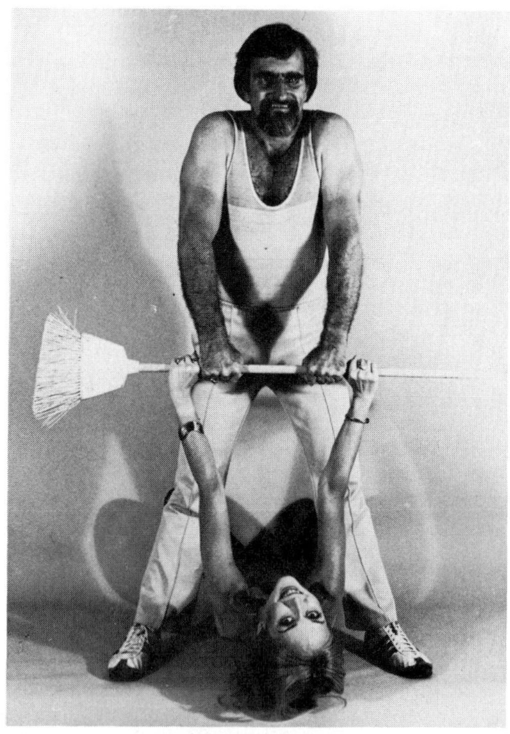

BROOMSTICK SHRUG

BROOMSTICK CURLS

Hold a broomstick the way you would for a regular military curl. Have her stand facing you, with her hands grasping the broomstick palms downwards, as in a military press. Have her push down on the broomstick as you try to curl it. Now let her try. Do ten reps.

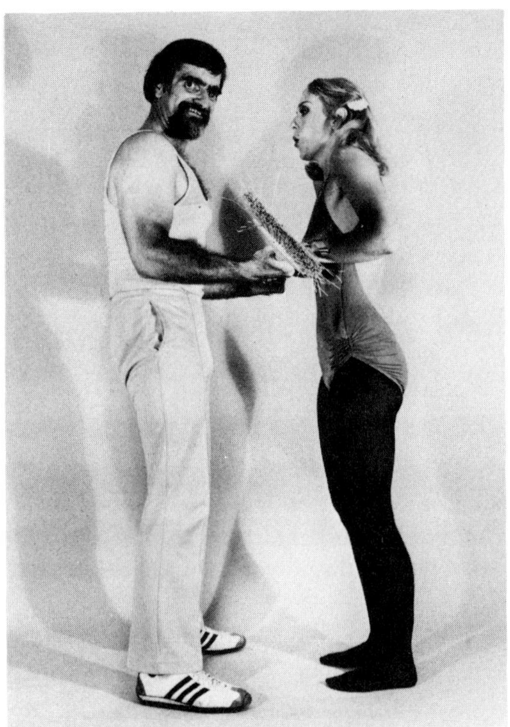

BROOMSTICK CURL

BROOMSTICK SQUATS

Stand facing each other, with your feet flat on the floor, each holding onto the broomstick. Lean back so that your arms are almost straight. Since you'll be the heavier one, let her lean back farther to keep the two of you balanced. Now do a squat, keeping the arms straight as you go down. Go all the way down and then rise slowly. After twenty reps, you'll have no choice but to fall into each other's arms.

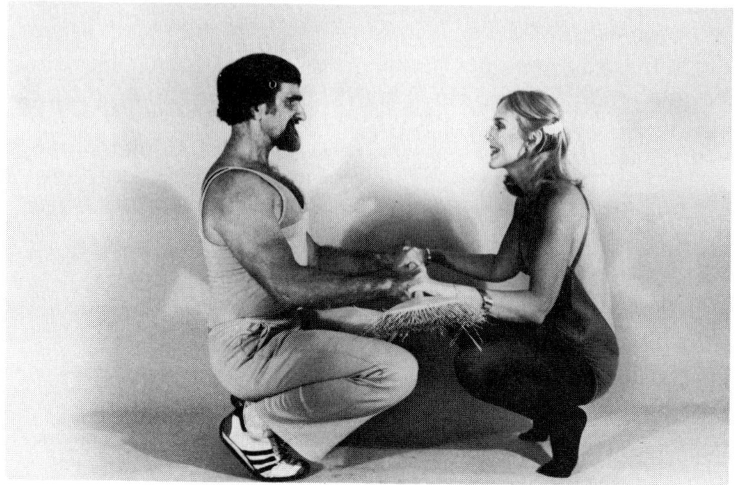

BROOMSTICK SQUAT

BROOMSTICK ROWS

Sit on the floor facing each other, legs spread in "V's," with her legs lying across yours. Reach toward each other and grasp a broomstick with your hands palms down, about shoulder width apart. There are three ways to do this exercise: one for the lower back, one for the upper back, and one for the lats.

For the upper back, sit close enough together so that each of you alternating can do the rows with your arms perpendicular to the floor. Use your bodies to give resistance.

For the lower back, keep your arms straight and bend from the waist. Be careful, because you can really exert some pressure on those lower vertebrae.

For the lats, do the motion the same way that you would do low-pulley rows. Keep the arms close to your sides and try to bring the broomstick to a point right under the pecs. If you can't reach the broomstick, get closer together. Do ten reps.

BROOMSTICK TWISTS

Here's a good one that will give you enough pep to finish the workout. Stand facing each other, holding the broomstick at arms' length between you, arms perpendicular to the floor. Hold the broomstick steady while she does the old-fashioned twist dance-step as she hangs onto the broomstick to keep her upper body from moving. Do about twenty reps and then trade. Put on an old Chubby Checker record.

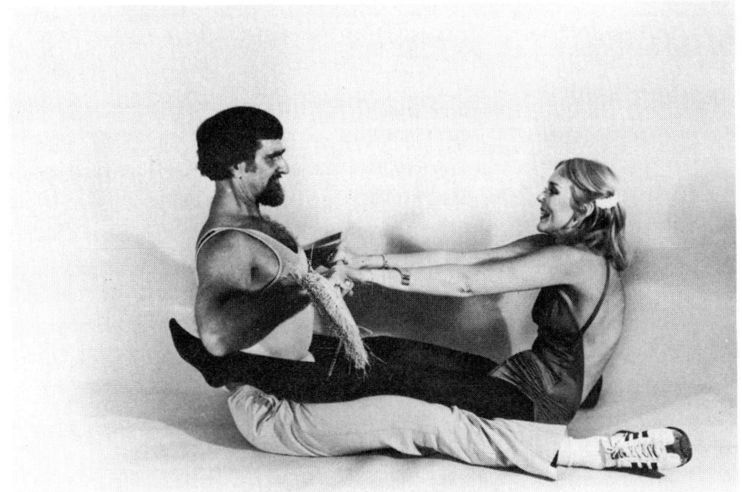

BROOMSTICK ROW

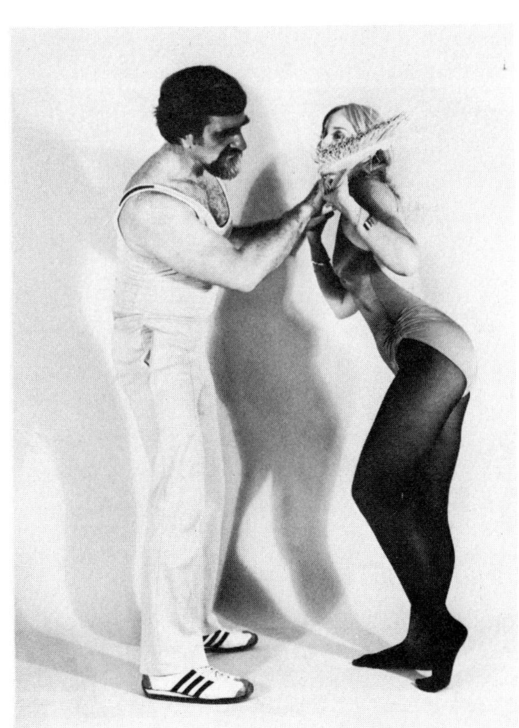

BROOMSTICK TWIST

BROOMSTICK BENCH PRESSES

If you don't have a bench, you can do this one on the floor, the couch, the bed, or anyplace where a person can lie on his or her back comfortably. The one on the bench holds the broomstick as a barbell would be held for the regular bench press, and the partner sits, lies, or leans on the broomstick enough to make it hard to do the movement. Use your imagination. Got it? Now do the exercise. Use your imagination again. Do ten reps.

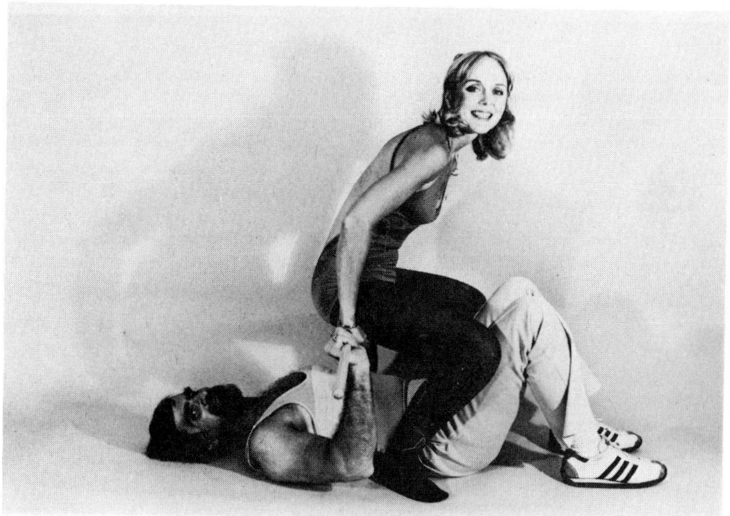

BROOMSTICK BENCH PRESS

BROOMSTICK PRESSES BEHIND THE NECK

Stand like spoons, with her nestled close to your back. Hold the broomstick behind your head, the way you would for a behind-the-neck press. Have her grasp the broomstick and try to keep you from lifting it. She'll probably succeed. Now let her try. Let her succeed again. Ten reps should do the trick.

BROOMSTICK LEG EXTENSIONS

You'll need to sit in a chair for this one. Have her kneel in front of you (this may take some coaxing), holding a broomstick against the front of your ankles. Try to do a leg extension as she tries to keep your feet down. Now you try it, so that you can keep your perspective.

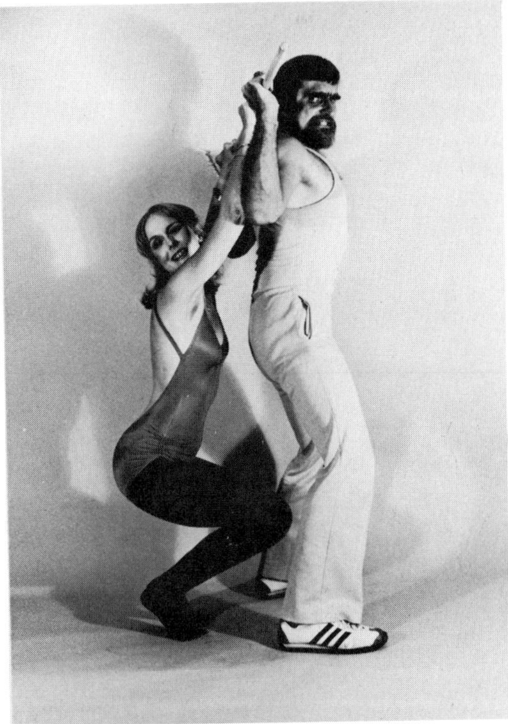

BROOMSTICK PRESSED BEHIND THE NECK

BROOMSTICK CALF RAISES

Another one in a chair. Place the broomstick across your knees. Have her lean over toward you, grasping the broomstick with her hands, arms almost straight. Now do calf raises. Do a lot of them. Then let her do a few while you rest.

That's it from head to toe. Don't forget to take your measurements before and after the workout, so that you can see if you've made any improvement. Don't be disappointed if your gains are only temporary.

Take her measurements.

And try not to overtrain.

OFFICE EXERCISES

So you haven't been working out since you got that new job or that long-sought-after promotion? Sure, you *mean* to work out, but the hours seem to get longer, the job more demanding, and the stack of work in your briefcase

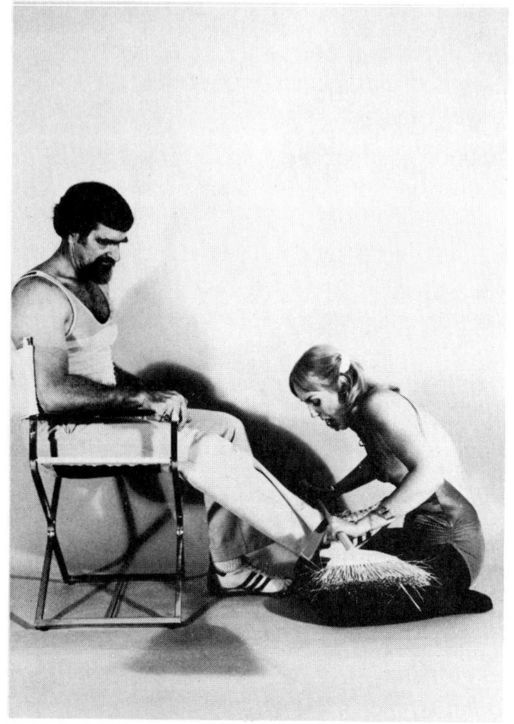

BROOMSTICK LEG EXTENSION

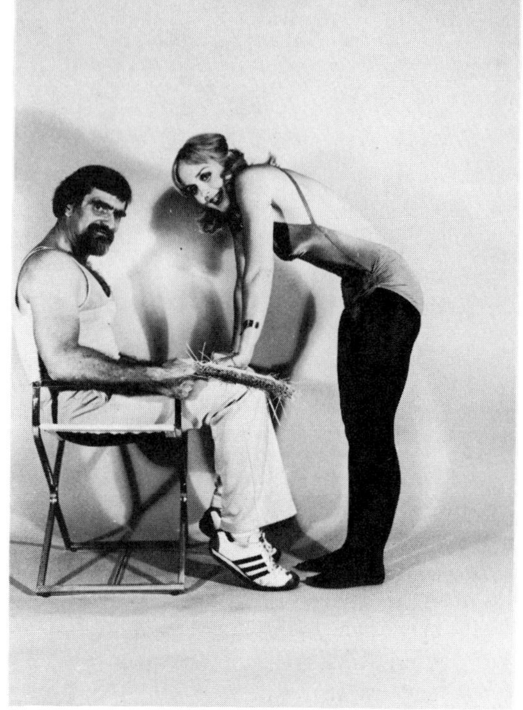

BROOMSTICK CALF RAISE

bigger every day. Health clubs don't open until 9:00, and you have to get up at 6:30 as it is to fight the traffic and get to your desk by 8:30. You stay late nearly every day, and by the time you've finished fighting rush-hour traffic the club is closed. Saturdays and Sundays—well, you *deserve* at least one day off, and by the time you've done a few errands, some odd jobs around the house, the week's laundry and grocery shopping, plus a little serious tube-watching, disco-ing, and visiting, the weekend's over.

Who really has time to exercise? you wonder. No one—at least no one who's admitting it! Fifty-four percent of the people surveyed in the recent Perrier fitness poll said that lack of time was the chief reason they didn't get enough exercise. At least you're not alone in your plight.

But don't despair. Everyone has periods in his or her life when work is so demanding, intense, or physically exhausting that there's hardly a spare moment in the day. Don't worry: use some of that office time as exercise time.

Yes, you heard us right. You can make use of those short "dead spaces" before and after work, during lunch, at morning and afternoon coffee breaks, and at other odd moments during the day to help yourself at least maintain a fitness level until things slow down a bit. If you add up the average office worker's "free" hours during the day, you'll find quite a lot of usable time—fifteen to twenty minutes before work, fifteen more minutes during the morning coffee break, twenty to thirty minutes (minimum) during lunch, fifteen minutes in the afternoon break, and another ten to fifteen minutes after work. That's anywhere from an hour to an hour and a half, depending on your particular schedule and its flexibility. If you're in sales or PR or another slot that requires many outside appointments, your time may be even more usable. A half-hour gap between appointments might not even get you into the gym and in your workout gear, but it's certainly ample time for a good arm or upper back routine.

So take a "health break"! The advantages are too numerous to name. You'll feel better the rest of the day—more alert, more energetic. Your performance on the job will improve. You'll actually be capable of thinking more clearly because of the increased oxygen supply to your brain. You'll be less sluggish and less susceptible to "four o'clock slump." You'll look better and more rested to your coworkers and clients. Best of all, you'll no longer be plagued by guilt feelings when you see those Executive Bells lying in your coat closet at home. Instead, the weights will be at the office stored in your credenza, and you'll be on a program that allows you to fit your workouts to your working day and vice-versa.

Now let's get started with those health breaks. They started in Japan, as you know, in an effort to make office workers more energetic, alert, and relaxed during the workday. Many American firms are now incorporating fitness breaks into their day. If your firm is one of those new, health-conscious ones, terrific. If not, you'll have to do some scheduling on your own.

First, think in terms of small chunks of usable time. It may help to keep a diary or notebook of a week's worth of typical workdays and then analyze your findings at the end of the week. Let's say you arrive at work ten to fifteen minutes early each day. Probably you like to leave home a little early to avoid the traffic jams or the long lines waiting for the commuter train or the bus. If your office opens at 9:30 and you're there at 9:00 sharp, you've got a good fifteen minutes before the others arrive in which to do stretches and toners.

There are other usable segments of time, too. Take the morning break—typically at about 10:00. Whether it's formalized or just an informal custom, many offices take time out for "coffee and . . ." at about that hour. What do you do with that time—head for the coffee shop downstairs and settle back with a Danish? That means 300-plus calories, too much sugar, and a poor use of those fifteen minutes besides! Take another health break, and you've now logged a full half-hour of exercise.

Lunchtime! To many of us, that means time to head for the nearest deli, pastry shop, fast-food emporium, or local watering hole and nosh our way through several glasses of the local brew, a sandwich high in fats and refined carbohydrates, and a big slice of pie or cheesecake. Or we go the high road, and polish off an expense account lunch of a small filet mignon, baked potato with sour cream and bacon bits, salad with croutons and blue-cheese dressing, all the rolls and butter in the tempting little basket, and perhaps a scoop of chocolate ice cream to top things off. Then we wonder why we feel so lifeless and seem to get nothing done all afternoon.

Of course, some business lunches are unavoidable. But how many days do you head for the junk food place or the Grease 'n' Oil when you could use the hour for other things? If you brown-bagged it, for example, you could take a full half-hour for your lunchtime exercise break and still have time to enjoy a thermos jar packed with cottage cheese or tuna, vegetable sticks, fresh fruit, and low-fat farmer cheese (or mozzarella) and *still* have time for a ten-minute stroll to the corner newsstand before the company fat cats came back from their three-martini lunches. If brown-bagging it is just too complicated, at least train the building's coffee shop to save a big salad or plain hamburger for you. Or carry a thermos of your favorite protein drink ready to shake and pour.

By now, you should have logged an honest hour of exercise. Add another five to ten minutes of quick stretches and bends when the four o'clock slump is ready to hit and another ten while you wait for the traffic to clear before you start home. No time to exercise, you say? You've packed a full hour and twenty minutes into your office day without interfering with scheduled office work. You feel terrific and you've staved off the Big Mac/fast food/martini/pastry cart circuits—the biggest traps for bored and tired office workers. Don't you feel great?

What about equipment? Here you'll have to learn to be inventive and resourceful. But you might start with one of the on-door exercisers (Weider Enterprises made the originals, but the copies are about as good). Add a set of eight-pound Executive Bells (Sears or any good department or sporting goods store has them) and a set of ankle weights or iron boots. Invest $29.95 and get one of the 110-pound "Lift for Life" sets—it has a collapsible folding bar that you can travel with, as we do. The weights range from five to twenty-five pounds and can be stacked in your credenza or filing cabinet.

Also, learn to use ordinary office furniture as "props" for your program. Hook your feet under the credenza or desk to do situps. Do dips between two strong-backed chairs. One of the greatest things about weight training is that it requires so little space (Valerie did all the training described in *Body-sculpture* in a two-bedroom Chicago high-rise; she now follows the program in a small townhouse). If you have a small amount of clear space in your office, or can make one by shifting around some chairs, you can do side leans, squats, pullovers, flyes, situps, leg raises, and a variety of other exercises.

What's a good office routine? Take a look back at the section on individual exercises. Then read the program starting on page 211. It outlines a good general conditioning routine for your largest chunk of time (usually before work or at lunchtime), plus some specific exercises that can be done for relaxing, stretching, and toning anytime, anywhere—sitting, standing, even walking.

One note before you get started: try to reserve your biggest block of time for that general conditioning routine. It consists of nine exercises that mostly need to be done in multiple sets (at least two sets per exercise) with moderately high repetitions for maximum effectiveness. Not that the ten- or fifteen-minute exercise period isn't effective, and not that you can't benefit yourself in terms of general toning, relaxation, and stretching if you flex a muscle ten times on the way to the water cooler. Generally speaking, any exercise is better than no exercise, and flexing a muscle ten times on your way from desk chair to water cooler, while it won't build muscle or increase cardiovascular fitness appreciably, *will* help you at least maintain some muscle tone until you can go through a more sustained workout. If five minutes a day is all you can spare, then do five minutes a day. But try to devote at least a portion of lunchtime or before-work time to this routine:

General Conditioning Routine for the Office (Before Work, After Work, on the Lunch Break)

Stretching and limbering exercises—three minutes.
"Good morning" exercise—two sets, ten reps.
Squats—two sets, ten reps.
Twists—do for five minutes by clock or timer.
Pullovers—two sets, ten reps.
Situp crunches—one set, thirty reps.
Leg raises—one set, thirty reps.
Curls—two sets, ten reps.
Bench press (on floor)—two sets, ten reps.

Exercises for Shorter Breaks

Select ten minutes' worth of the following:

Category 1: Sitting-down exercises (to be done while sitting at a desk, taking a break from typing or writing, waiting for a meeting or appointment, talking on the telephone, dictating, reading mail or reports, etc.).

A. For the upper arms: sit upright in the desk chair, press your palms down tightly on the sides of the chair seat, and using only your arms, lift your body off the surface of the seat; hold for a count of ten, relax for a second or two. Repeat ten to twelve times. Tensing the upper thighs at the same time makes this exercise a leg toner as well.

B. For firming the pectoral muscles: hold your arms at shoulder height and grab your wrist firmly (as if you were pushing up your sleeves); do the movement until you feel the pull in your pectoral muscles; hold for a count of three and repeat ten to twelve times.

Alternate pectoral exercise: make a "steeple" with your fingertips by pressing them hard together as you pull your shoulders forward and together; again, hold for a count of three and repeat ten to twelve times.

C. For the ankles (do standing or sitting down): sit with your knees crossed one over the other; point the foot of thc top leg toward the floor, then raise the foot, arching it as much as possible; circle the ankle to the left, then to the right, repeating ten to twelve times with each foot. Standing position: back up against the wall and raise one leg, supporting your knee with both hands; make foot circles as described above.

D. For the neck: sit erect in the desk chair, hands folded behind your head; without moving your body, push your head down until your chin rests on your chest; resist the motion by pushing the head against the arms. Repeat ten to twelve times.

E. Another neck exercise: hold your right hand under your chin, supporting the chin with your left hand, fingers curled; push the chin up while pushing your head down, thus providing resistance to the movement; lower the chin and relax. Repeat eight to ten times.

F. For overall posture and as a tension-reliever: place your fingers at the base of your neck and point your chin toward the ceiling; try to make the elbows touch behind your neck. Repeat the motion slowly five times.

G. For the gluteus maximus (buttocks): either seated or standing, tighten the gluteus maximus muscles and hold to a count of five; release the tension and repeat ten times, working up to twenty-five. Note: you should also feel some tension and stress in the upper thighs if you do this one correctly.

H. A stomach tightener: while sitting at the desk, exhale so that your stomach appears distended; then suck in, tightly contracting the stomach muscles, and hold to a count of five. Repeat five times, working up to twenty-five.

I. Calf flexes: sit at the desk, both toes pointed; lift the heel of your right foot off the floor, flexing the calf muscle as you do so, and hold to a count of five; relax and repeat the motion with the left foot. Alternate legs, doing ten to twelve repetitions for each leg.

J. For the arms and neck: rest your head on the desk and place your hands on the edge of the desk; push down hard on the desk with your fingers and also your forehead until you feel tension in your arms and neck; hold for a count of five and repeat ten to twelve times.

K. Another stomach tightener: while sitting at the desk, lean forward and place your hands firmly under your thighs; then press down with your hands and at the same time push up with your toes until you feel the strain in your abdomen and waist; hold to a count of five and repeat ten to twelve times.

L. Head rolls: drop your head to one side and let the weight of the drooping head bring it forward in a completely relaxed position; continue the roll to the other side and bring the head back up. Repeat three to five times.

M. Shoulder roll: sit up straight in the desk chair and slowly roll both shoulders forward, up, and back. Let your elbows move forward on the upswing, then pull back as your chest juts out. Arms and shoulders should move together in a smooth, continuous circle. Repeat three to five times, then reverse directions and repeat.

N. Leg stretches: while sitting at the desk, stretch your legs high under it, toes touching the underside of the desk; press feet upward as if to touch the underside of the table; hold to a count of six, relax, and repeat ten to twelve times.

Category 2: Standing-up exercises (to be done while standing in line, waiting for a meeting or appointment, even for a bus or taxi; waiting for the Xerox machine or in line at the company snack bar).

A. For the upper thighs: stand erect with a book, telephone directory, or other heavy object—perhaps a large briefcase or bag—between your feet; push your heels together against the object (as if you were trying to bring them together) until you feel the tension in your thigh muscles; hold to a count of five, then relax. Repeat fifteen to twenty times.

B. Leg and derrière firmer: stand in the doorway with your left knee against the door frame; place your hands on the frame at chest level and push with your hands and knees until you feel the tension in your buttocks; hold to a count of five and repeat with the right knee. Alternate legs, ten to twelve repetitions each.

C. For the lower back: stand erect, feet about a shoulder's width apart; bend over slowly, letting your arms dangle in front of you. Think of the exercise as a relaxer and simply let your upper body fall limp as if you were a rag doll. Gradually sink a little lower until you feel the pull in the backs of the upper thighs.

   Do this one for fifteen seconds, then return to an upright position. To do as a leg stretch, add the following movement: as you bend lower, try to touch your face first to the left knee, then to the right one. Feel the pull in your thighs and hamstrings as you try to reach your knee. Keep doing this stretch—at first only a partial movement—until it becomes easier. Start with one slow repetition, work up to five.

D. For the lower back: stand with your back to the wall, feet nine to twelve inches in front of you; contract the stomach muscles so that your back flattens against the wall; tuck your chin in and try to flatten your neck against the wall also; hold for three to four seconds, then relax. Repeat ten to twelve times. This is also a super exercise for good posture.

E. A standing stomach-flattener: bend over, knees in a slight crouch, back parallel to the floor with the hands above the knees on the lower thighs; exhale, letting the stomach muscles relax totally; now, without inhaling, contract the stomach muscles, pulling everything up and under the rib cage; hold to a count of five, relax, and repeat fifteen times.

F. A deep-breathing exercise: stand straight with your arms held to the sides; then slowly raise your arms, lift your chin up, and inhale slowly; hold for a few seconds, then exhale as slowly as possible, letting your hands come together comfortably in front and allowing your head to drop slowly. Repeat several times during the day as needed.

G. For the upper shoulders and upper back: stand erect with arms extended about shoulder level, straight in front of you; make a loosely clenched fist to make the motion easier; then pull your arms back as far as they can go, trying to make your shoulder blades touch. Do twelve to fifteen fast repetitions.

H. For the upper arms: lean on the back of a chair, supporting yourself with your arms, in a "slumping" position; now raise yourself up until your arms are fully extended and you feel the tension in both arms and shoulders; hold for a count of three, then relax. Repeat three times and work up to eight or ten repetitions.

Category 3: Walking exercises (to be done on the way to other parts of the office complex, the Xerox machine, the coffee shop, the conference room, the rest room—anywhere where you are in motion, including on the street).

A. Stair climbing: one of the most effective ways to shape and tone hips, thighs, and calves. If there are stairs in your office building, use them in preference to an elevator or escalator. If your office is on a high floor, try walking up one flight, then two, then three, gradually increasing until you are walking up (and down) first halfway, then all the way.

B. Calf and ankle shaper for stairs: tiptoe upstairs without touching your heels to the steps; at the top, relax; then, holding onto the bannister for balance, tiptoe downstairs. If no one is watching and the stairs are not too steep, tiptoe *backward* for best results!

C. For the gluteus maximus again: as you take each step, either in climbing stairs or in normal walking, make a conscious effort to tighten the "glut" muscles until you feel the tension in the lower buttocks and upper thighs as you walk. Hold the tension to the count of three for each leg.

D. For general conditioning: make your walking work for you by moving at a faster pace than normal—really *walk,* don't saunter—and also by carrying a load: a dictionary, a telephone book, the state insurance code, the real estate listings for your city, a Dictaphone, or a tape recorder. Make a conscious effort to walk the length of the office suite several times a day—also to the coffee shop, conference room, supply room, Xerox room, or whatever else is within easy range of your office. Do this whenever you feel tired or drowsy instead of reaching for the pastry wagon or heading to the coffee machine for a cup with double cream and sugar.

E. For the arms: swing your arms vigorously as you walk, alternating arms. In more secluded parts of the building, or in the park at lunchtime, make windmills by swinging the arms in a circle, first to the front, then to the sides as you walk.

F. More general conditioning: add weight! Winter coats count, as do briefcases, totes, shopping bags, sacks of groceries. If you shop at lunchtime, don't have your purchases sent home—carry them back to the office and then home. And don't succumb to the temptation of taking a bus or cab in good weather. Remember that simple walking can burn from 150 to 300 calories an hour, depending on your pace.

Feel better? After a week or so of these routines, you should begin to feel better—more alert, more rested and energetic, trimmer, less inclined to fall victim to the four o'clock slump. Try to couple your office routines with some supplementary routines on weekends. An hour on either Saturday or Sunday in the gym or with the weights at home plus a brisk walk/jog/run or an hour of your favorite sport the next day should add up to an impressive fitness program even for a busy man like you. As your strength and stamina increase, you may find that you prefer to do stretches and limbering before work or on lunch hour and save the main workout for after work, at home or in the gym. Whichever way you schedule, the important thing is to keep at it. Don't let a missed workout end your program. Just pick up the next day and go on from there. No backsliding!

In addition to the programs we've described above, there are other alternatives. Many gyms—more and more in the major cities, in fact—are opening at 6:00 or 7:00 A.M. to accommodate the before-work crowd. For over a year, we started our workouts at 6:30 A.M. in order to make a mandatory 7:30 breakfast meeting before the workday began at 8:30. Do some investigation—your company may be located near a health club, family fitness center, branch of the Y, or gym so that you can run in before work or at lunch, have a short workout of thirty to forty-five minutes, shower, and be at the office fresh and rarin' to go when everyone else is still on the commuter train, sitting in traffic, or just paying the lunchtime check.

Better yet, many companies are now catching on to the secret that the Japanese have known for decades—that refreshed office workers are more accurate, harder workers, and more productive—and are incorporating the "health break" idea into the official corporate day. Many companies are now building their own gyms or weight rooms and are encouraging employees to go at certain intervals during the day. Some of the more enlightened even conduct classes or have instructors on duty at specified hours during the day. They're finding it's a terrific way to keep their employees happier, more relaxed, and in better shape.

A few minuses: equipment in these corporate workout studios tends to be geared to the "average" (read nonathletic) man or woman, so look for lots of chrome machines and few free weights. Also, there's apt to be less of a variety of equipment than in the local health club, Y, or spa. If classes are offered, you can likewise expect them to be geared to the "average" office worker—lots of floor exercises, stretching, and limbering rather than a full weight training course. If you're an advanced devotee of the weights, the workouts may prove a bit elementary for you.

Still, a company that follows this policy is to be commended. If you're in a policymaking position or can influence the top men and women in your outfit to support, finance, or build a company gym, by all means do it. As an alternative, consider a group enrollment or special discount rate at a nearby health club; there may even be one in your building that would welcome a group enrollment from your office. Any way you cut it, the health-break idea is a marvelous, very efficient—and very politic—way to raise morale, productivity, and the general level of fitness awareness of the company. It's good for the employees' collective health and psyches, good for corporate image and PR, and most of all, good for *you*. Try it—you'll like it!

ON-THE-ROAD MAINTENANCE

So you've got the office routine all organized. The Executive Bells are in the credenza and the bar hidden away behind an impressive breakfront. You've organized your lunch hours and before-work moments to add up to an impressive hour of exercise a day. Plus the half-hour run or swim after work, and the five-mile runs on weekends—not to mention those long Saturday and Sunday mornings when you and your lady head out to the local spa or gym.

You're getting in shape—in fact, you're already looking pretty good—when suddenly things go straight to hell in the office. The corporate game players are at it again, and it's fox-in-the-henhouse time every morning as things get juggled, priorities rearranged, and positions moved like pawns on a chessboard. Suddenly you come in one day after you've spent the previous day on a client call to find your desk in the parking lot, so to speak. Vice-president Klutzmann has reassigned you to sales, and by next week you're living out of your briefcase, an overnight bag, and the back seat of your car. One-day trips to the next city, overnight stays in Austin or Des Moines or Milwaukee, two-day stints with the big accounts on the Coast, week-long conferences, and national sales meetings. And first thing you know, your workout schedule—and physique—are a thing of the past.

We all know the cycle: up too early, bad airlines food, too much coffee—and maybe just one Bloody Mary to calm the jitters—followed by a mad dash from the airport, a wild taxi ride, a rush out to meetings or sales calls, a Big Mac for lunch, then an afternoon on the run until dinnertime: time to collapse in the motel's watering hole with the *beeg* margarita and then go on, an hour later, to a steak with all the trimmings (after all, it's *their* money), another libation or two or three, and finally to bed. Next morning same scenario, different city. You drag home two days later—tired, puffy, and about three pounds heavier—and work like a dog to get back in shape again. And then a week later you wake up in Dubuque or Tulsa or Dallas and the whole downward spiral starts again.

It's a rough life for anyone, especially for the fitness buff, who thrives on schedule, regularity, and a workout routine he can count on. But you really don't have to succumb to the martini-and-marbled-steak syndrome. Here are a few tips to get you started on that traveling fitness program:

1. First of all, try to regularize your travel schedule to whatever extent you can. It's not so much the travel as the sheer unpredictability that plays havoc with even the most dedicated exerciser. If you can set up a schedule that allows you to travel on "off" days in your workout program (see the previous chapter) and still maintain your three or or four days a week with the weights, that's not so bad—not nearly as nerve-wracking as the schedule that literally prevents you from planning a day or two in advance.

   You might try breaking up your out-of-town work into several short trips instead of one mammoth one. Three short two-day jaunts can allow time in between to make up for the missed workout. But a two-week layoff often constitutes serious backsliding. Keep the travel short for best results—at least you can work out on the days you're home.

2. Stick to your diet on the road. Again, that's often close to impossible, but with a bit of planning ahead, it *can* be done. Many airlines allow you to order low-calorie or salt-free meals *if* you notify them in advance. If worst comes to worst, skip the airline meal entirely and sip coffee (black), tea or mineral water in flight. Most airlines also offer diet soda and fruit juice as an alternative to the booze and and soft drink wagon.

   Try to plan adequate breaks for mealtimes instead of dashing into the nearest fast-food haven or Ptomaine Tavern. For emergencies, keep some dried fruit, unsalted nuts, granola bars, raisins, or protein tablets in the car for a quick source of energy. Make a habit of eating a larger breakfast or lunch and less dinner while you're traveling. Nothing is worse at the end of a harried but inactive day than to pack away three martinis and a huge steak with baked potato and sour cream, salad with heavy dressing and croutons, and dessert. You can easily consume 3,000-plus calories in one such meal!

   As an alternative, look for a simple broiled or grilled chicken or fish entree—minus sauce, cream, or butter. Lemon and herbs are tastier and better for you. Skip the potato or eat only the skin and leave the insides. Forget the butter and sour cream and have a small salad with plain oil-and-vinegar dressing. Substitute espresso for the dessert. If you finesse the martinis and go for the current "in" drink of chilled Perrier with a sliver of lime, you've knocked a substantial number of calories off your night's intake. You'll sleep better and wake up refreshed instead of stuffed and bloated.

   Hard to do? Sure it is, but the alternative is harder. The extra pounds that you put on during your two-day binge can take you a week or more to lose again through hard dieting and extra workouts. Keep the caloric intake down—more important, eat the right things and stray from your normal diet as little as possible—and you'll find that your waist stays proportionately trim.

3. If you can arrange it and have some choice in the matter, try to travel to a city with a health club. Check out your local spa or gym in advance (preferably before you join and sign your name on the dotted line to the contract with X Acceptance Corporation). Tell them you'll be on the road a lot when you join, and ask if they have affiliates in other cities. Many of the leading health clubs are part of large chains or have affiliates in large and medium-sized cities. For example, the Presidents/First Lady Club in Houston is part of the same chain as the Chicago Health Clubs and has over 1,200 affiliates in cities large and small all over the United States. All you have to do to get a workout in a strange city is to look up the right affiliate in advance, make sure it's open (best to call for hours when you arrive), and head over when you have a short break in your day. The quality of

the equipment and the type of machines and free weights will be familiar to you, since, chances are, it's what you use at home every time you work out.

4. An alternative to the above: try to get your company to put you up in a hotel or motel with a small health club or gym. That's often hard to locate in a small town, but lodgings in the major cities often offer health clubs, steam baths, saunas, indoor pools, and other health-related extras as part of their "package." In Chicago, for example, the Continental Plaza and the Marriott, to name only two, have weight rooms for guests. So does the Lake Geneva Playboy Club and many other resorts under the sign of the big bunny. The hotel or motel club is *not* a heavy-duty lifting room—it isn't intended as such—but it *will* give you a place to relax, work out, and stay in shape until you get back home. If you know the city well, request a hotel-with-health-club in advance. If not, and the company is paying for your accommodations, do a little detective work in advance and try to spot the places with workout facilities. Another bonus: the clubs often open early for just such dedicated souls as you!

5. No gym or hotel club? Try the local Y. Many towns, large and small, have excellent facilities at both downtown and suburban Y's, and you can usually arrange for a short-term visitor's pass for a couple of days. At worst, you'll have to go as the "guest" of a friend or acquaintance in the city. Check into it. Often the clubs, especially in off-seasons and slow hours, will be happy to see another face at the door. The equipment varies from city to city, as do hours and regulations governing who uses what when. But check out what's available by phone. Large downtown Y's will often have superb weight training equipment, and some of the smaller suburban clubs are surprisingly well equipped.

6. If you're a runner, walker, or jogger, make use of the local high school or college track or running course in summer, or try to get into the gym in winter. Again, you'll have to check out what arrangements (if any) can be made for visitors. But you may end up getting the use of the equipment free, or with a token payment of a few bucks. Same goes for the community fitness centers, suburban health clubs, and family-style Y's. It's certainly worth the 20¢ phone call to inquire!

7. If you're really stuck in Nowhere, USA, and there is no Y, health club, gym, or local school facility for miles around, make use of what you have. Most motels will have at least a small pool. Swim a decent number of laps in early morning, midafternoon, or before dinner—anytime when the kiddies and rubber sea monsters aren't in evidence. Run around the motel grounds or parking lot before your day starts or later in the evening. Explore the local scenery with a before-dinner

walk, run, or jog. Again, you don't have to duplicate the exact workout schedule that you do at home. Just do a few miles or enough laps in the pool to keep yourself from backsliding all the way to your prefitness days. An added plus: the exercise relieves tension, keeps you out of the local watering holes, reduces appetite, and makes you sleep like a two-year-old, regardless of how hectic your day might have been.

8. If all else fails, try traveling with some light equipment of your own. The Weider exerciser, an ingenious little contraption you can hang on any hotel or motel doorknob or fasten to a bureau drawer, is a very packable device. It fits nicely into a corner of your suitcase or duffel. Same for a jump rope—you can stuff it into a shoe if you're short of space. Add jogging shoes, tennis socks, swim trunks or jogging pants, a lightweight tee shirt or tank top, and a pair of Executive Bells, and you've got the makings of a decent little motel-sized gym. You might also try to find one of the lightweight collapsible bars that you can carry disassembled in a long garment bag or duffel (we carry ours with us when we travel—but an umbrella will also do for seated twists in a pinch!). Take a pedometer, and you can jog in place in the room while you watch the morning news if the weather's bad. Remember that a fifteen-minute workout is good, twenty minutes are excellent, and a half-hour is next to godliness when you're on the road! *Don't* try to duplicate your entire routine from home—you'll end up feeling guilty, frustrated, or both. Look on all this as a "maintenance routine" only, and you'll feel virtuous about the whole thing. The object is to do *something* toward fitness that day, not to rival The Hulk.

   OK, let's say you're really in Nowhere and there's nary a gym in sight. Or worse still, you're in the big city with a million gyms—all of which open at 9:00. Your first meeting, naturally, is at 8:30; it's now 6:00 A.M., pouring rain (or snowing); the pool is closed for the winter, and all your neighbors are peacefully sleeping it off—no fair running up and down the halls at this hour! What to do? Well, try the following quick wake-up routine for starters. Do it while you watch the "Today" show, and then have a leisurely, low-calorie breakfast in the coffee shop.

Good-morning exercise (use a collapsible bar or umbrella; if neither is available, hold an Executive Bell or the local phone book behind your head). Do twenty to twenty-five reps.

Situps (hook your feet under the bed or bureau) or *crunches* (cross your feet in the lotus position and you won't need the bureau). Do twenty to thirty reps.

Leg raises, regular or alternating (use a pillow or extra blanket as an exercise mat). Do thirty reps. As an alternative, use the Weider exerciser on your doorknob for the alternating raises.

Seated twists (use a collapsible bar or umbrella; otherwise, clasp your hands behind you for the standing twist; hold your arms out to the sides for seated ones). Do for three to five minutes by the clock.

One-legged calf raises (stand on one foot, the other leg resting on the opposite knee; this allows you to use the entire weight of your body as your "weight" for the exercise). Do fifty reps for each leg.

Squats (use the collapsible bar or Executive Bells; work for high repetitions done very fast). Do twenty-five to thirty reps without pausing—more if time and your condition permit.

Dips (use a sturdy chair with *very strong* arms). Do twenty to thirty reps.

Lunges (use a collapsible bar or Executive Bells). Do twenty to thirty reps.

Stretches (select seven to ten of your favorites from the sections on yoga, dance, and karate stretches and use them as a wind-down). Do a minimum of five reps for each stretch.

Jogging (jog in place or around the room for ten to twelve minutes, depending on the time available; use a pedometer if you're curious about distances). If the space is large enough, or if the hallways are available, try jumping rope instead.

What about exercising while you're actually in the process of traveling—exercising en route? We don't really recommend jogging up and down the aisles of a 747 or trying to do calf raises or crunches while you're speeding down the freeway. But you *can* give yourself a treat with a short exercise break when you make a pit stop, if you're driving or busing it. (Some dedicated joggers, wer'e told, run around the service station for a few laps while the oil is being checked!) You can certainly stop long enough to do five minutes or so of the stretching and limbering exercises given in chapter 3. Even a minute or two of simple stretches will make you feel more alert, less tense, and less prone to freeway fatigue or drowsiness.

If you're a car, train, or plane passenger, the process is even simpler. Many of the office exercises in this section are equally good for travel—especially the sitting-down exercises. Shoulder shrugs, neck rolls, and a variety of simple stretches are good relievers of tension and fatigue when you travel. If you stop en route, some standing twists, shrugs, the good-morning exercise, and a few side leans will give you an "energy break." If you need something more strenuous, try jumping or running in place for a minute or two.

Air travel brings with it a whole host of special problems. To begin with, there's the airline food—usually high-calorie and smothered in sauces and breading. We've said it before, but it's worth repeating: *abstain!* Order a low-cal snack or opt for juice, diet soda, mineral water or coffee/ tea/ milk (skim). One reason for passing up the booze cart, besides the calories, is that alcohol dehydrates you. Air travel is drying enough anyway and the combination of the two can make you arrive at your destination feeling fatigued and disoriented. You're already a victim of jet lag before your feet touch the ground!

To combat the syndrome, drink plenty of fluids, skip the alcohol, pass up the munchies, and keep yourself active on a long flight. Try a few in-flight exercises. True, your range of movement is limited, especially if you're going tourist class. But try to keep your circulation revved up, especially if it's a long flight (three hours or more). Otherwise fluid begins to collect in your lower body and your circulation seems to grind to a halt. For longish flights, try these three simple exercises, plus shoulder shrugs and neck rolls to relieve upper body fatigue:

1. If you're sitting with your seat belt fastened, spread your feet apart and put all your weight on them (imagining that you're standing up while doing this exercise will make it easier). You should feel some sensation—a mild burning—in your thighs and buttocks as you tense, hold the pressure for a count of three, then relax. Do sets of twenty to thirty reps at intervals during the course of the flight.
2. Place your hands on top your thighs and try to place all your weight on your left foot. Bend your upper body slightly to the left. Keep your shoulders down, rib cage up. Relax. Now shake or shrug your shoulders and repeat on the right side. Do sets of twenty to thirty reps for each side at intervals during the trip.
3. Fluid retention in your lower legs and ankles? Even people who normally have no fluid retention problems at all often leave a long flight with slightly swollen ankles. To combat this tendency, do ankle rotations. Make circles with your toes while seated, one leg crossed over the other. Do the motion both clockwise and counterclockwise. If you've space in front of you or beside you, try to elevate your feet for at least part of the trip.

Besides these three basics, there's also an isometric exercise for the abdomen you might want to try. As you sit in your seat, try to pull your rib cage up and your stomach in as far as it will go. Hold for a count of five, relax, and repeat. It's a good though simple waist exercise and reminds you to pull in your stomach. Besides, it's a good reminder to say no to the pastry and martini carts, pass on the "light meals," and stick with "coffee or tea for a lighter me."

By the way, you'll probably not find yourself alone doing in-flight exercises. A year or so ago, Lufthansa pioneered the idea of shaping up in the air with recorded exercises on the music channels of its 747's and DC-10's. The airline has a pamphlet of exercise and diet tips called "Fitness in the Chair," and SAS has its own seven-minute film of mini-workout tips. Some of the airline magazines and pamphlets put in the pockets of the seat in front of you will also have workout and stretching tips to keep you from turning to stone on a coast-to-coast flight.

One final tip. Let's say you're returning home from a four-day convention or sales trip. You get back home on a 5:30 P.M. flight, spend an hour fighting the traffic from the airport to your residence. Allow an hour or so for unpacking and general reentry. Don't push yourself. You need time to "come down"—to unwind and reenter your normal routine and atmosphere. Don't rush right out to the gym or jogging track unless you really feel that a light workout would relax you. Give yourself anywhere from a few hours to a full twenty-four before you hit the workouts full steam again. Even then, go slow. Make the first workout a lighter one. You can cut back by a few reps, or drop back on the weight by a few pounds. Rest a minute extra between sets. Even if you've really made an effort to stay in shape, you may still find that your layoff makes you a little slower than usual. Don't push it. Warm up adequately, go through a thorough but light version of your usual routine, and you'll find yourself back in terrific shape in a workout or two. There! Didn't all that on-the-road fitness effort help in the end?

7

EPILOGUE: STAYING IN CONCOURS CONDITION

•

So you've finally got the bod in the shape you want? Congratulations! It's been an uphill battle, but you've made it. Your 99-day program is over and you're noticeably leaner, more muscular, trimmer, and less flabby than you were at the beginning. Your heart no longer beats like a trip-hammer when you walk up a flight of stairs—these days, in fact, you're more apt to *run* up them, two at a time. You can run that three-mile track without ever really getting out of breath. You look forward to your every-other-day workout at home or in the gym. Weekends, you no longer hang out in front of the TV with beer or soda in hand; now you're more apt to think of "recreation" as a few sets of tennis, ten laps in the pool, a brisk bike ride, or a long walk.

Along with all this, you're probably noticing some changes in yourself, too. People are beginning to look at you differently. Other men, even good friends, are just a little envious of your broader shoulders, trimmer waist, more muscular arms. Women are beginning to sit up and take notice again. Bosses and prospective bosses are impressed. Your subordinates at work are more deferential. Clients give you better treatment. You find it easier to get those accounts or to make new sales. Family and close friends are just plain amazed.

What you're finding is an old truth: clothes may not make the man, but a new body certainly does help. The better-looking, more muscular, trimmer man exudes self-confidence and positive vibes. He's a winner, destined for good things on the job and in his social life. Unfair though it may be, we still equate good looks, muscularity, neatness, and trimness with success. Fat, excessive skinniness, or a sloppy appearance spell "failure." The man who is a consistent winner today is the one who looks fit and healthy, well dressed and trim. You've already gone a long way toward making yourself over into the "winner" image: you've got the new bodystyle. Now let's talk about the upholstery. First, there's grooming:

1. Get a good haircut. Invest a few extra bucks, if you must, in a good tapered, blunt cut, slightly layered if you have very thick hair. The best one is medium length and can be either blown-dried or finger-dried. Although many *outré* hairdressers say that the fluffy, blow-dry look is on its way out and the latest thing is slicked-back hair, try for a length versatile enough to go either way. If you decide to opt for a hair oil or cream, pass up the old-time greasy kid stuff and insist on the new, lighter-textured creams that hold the hair in place without making you look like a refuge from the set of *Grease*.

2. Care for your hair with a slightly alkaline shampoo (ask your barber for advice or experiment on your own). Remember that the job of any shampoo is simply to cleanse the hair as thoroughly as possible. Conditioners basically are simple—they make the hair *feel* smoother and silkier to the touch and prevent snarling or tangling. Select a low-pH conditioner (one that's slightly acid in nature) that is not too creamy—otherwise you'll end up with the greasies again.

   The hot combs and compact blow-dryers (minus the asbestos) are still the best grooming aids for men. Invest in a good one—perhaps a small compact model that you can travel with. That, plus a good shampoo and conditioner, is all you need to keep your hair in top shape. If you want a bit more body to your hair, you might try a natural henna rinse; the new "neutral" or "natural" hennas give body without changing the hair color. You'll get a nice shine and healthy luster to your hair without a "colored" appearance.

3. Pay attention to your nails. Make sure your diet is high enough in protein and calcium to give you the basis for strong nails. Every five to eight days, soften your cuticles by a hot shower or a soak in hot, sudsy water. Scrub the nails with a nailbrush, push the cuticles back, trim off hangnails. Buff the nails lightly for a smoother look and shape the ends with an emery board or diamond file. File lightly and firmly, at a slight angle to the nails, so that you get a rounded, curved effect. Always file the nails dry; wet nails that are filed often split and crack.

4. Start paying attention to your skin. Remember you have the advantage over your lady—you shave every day and thus scrape off the dead cells that the skin normally sloughs off by itself at a much slower rate ("exfoliation" is the fancy term for it). As a result, your skin remains young-looking longer than hers!

   The best thing you can do for your skin, besides shaving every day, is to wash it with a superfatted soap (one with extra fats or oils added). Try Neutrogena or a hypoallergenic soap if you are subject to skin rashes or allergies. If you have dry patches, use an unscented cream like Nivea or one of the good new Clinique for Men products as a moisturizer. There are some excellent new lines of men's skin products coming out every month. They are *not* male "cosmetics," but simple, basic skin products: a skin scrub (usually a fine-grained scrubbing paste), a cream for dry areas, and a good soap. Most will also include a bronzer to help you along if the last three weekends have been rainy. They're also instant camouflage for dark circles and are good pick-ups if you have to face an early morning TV or photo session—they do wonders for that pasty, gray look in mid-January.

Now that you're all nicely cleaned and polished, let's talk about that new upholstery. No, you don't have to turn peacock or look like a walking ad for *Gentleman's Quarterly*. But chances are that you now find yourself more interested in what you put on your back. You *can* wear some of the sharp new styles much more easily if you're neither too fat nor too thin. Things that looked grotesque on you before you started your training program now look fantastic. Here are some quick-and-easy guidelines to help you dress to hide any lingering trouble spots:

1. If you still have some thickness in the waist area, don't wear a tight belt pulled over (or just below) a protruding stomach. Posture and exercise are the keys to "holding it in," and not an extra-tight belt. Avoid super-narrow belts, huge ornamental buckles, big hat brims, wide ties, big collars with spreading points, and toe ornaments on shoes. Plain neutral or dark medium-wide belts and plain gold or silver buckles are best for you. Good dark or neutral leather belts are always in fashion and now that the webbing belts are so popular, try one in a neutral or khaki tone for casual wear. Forget the red and green stripes, even if it *is* Gucci—it only makes your waist seem thicker.

2. If you're still a bit heavy, don't wear windowpane checks, big plaids, art deco or art moderne patterns, or electric day-glo colors. Keep yourself in one color, or shades of the same color range, and you'll appear pounds lighter than you are. Save the contrasting outfits and super-hot colors for your stringbean friends. Ditto for ties—don't wear them too long, too short, or too wide. Fortunately, the super-wide ones are out anyway, as are big florals, psychedelic prints, and hunting scenes (unless they're by Ralph Lauren). The most slimming tie is a medium-length, medium-to-narrow-width tie in a solid, small foulard, Ivy League, or "rep" pattern, or diagonal stripe. The new silk and wool knits are excellent, too, unless they're a fuzzy knit.

3. Stay away from turtlenecks unless they are thin, flat-ribbed, and a lightweight knit; if they are too form-fitting, they can accentuate a double chin or bulging waistline. Keep them *outside* your pants unless you're really slim. Use open-necked shirts to give you the illusion of more neck, less chin.

4. Stay with single-breasted suits with fairly narrow lapels, slightly fitted jackets, and pinstripes or solid, dark colors for the best and slimmest look. Large windowpane checks or plaids, *outré* colors (salmon, rust, moss green), and ice-cream pastels will all add pounds. So will a really tight-fitting continental cut. You can take a slightly fitted jacket, but stay away from those nipped waists and flared vents unless you are skin-and-bones thin.

5. Use color in your outfit in small ways: a dark red or burgundy pocket handkerchief, a small pattern in your tie, a darker-color initial on your shirt, perhaps one good piece of jewelry. Remember, the more you can keep your outfit in one color, or tones of one color range (e.g., beige suit, pale brown shirt, rust foulard tie, beige and brown pocket handkerchief), the neater and trimmer you'll look.

6. Don't wear very heavy, fuzzy tweeds or other thick fabrics if you're still on the heavy side. The best fabrics for you are smooth and lightweight: gabardine, thin wool flannel, light knits, a fine-wale corduroy.

7. Don't try a style that is too avant-garde, or conversely, get stuck with what *Columbus Forum* once dubbed "the total Cleveland look" of pastel leisure suits. A classic, conservative cut is best for you. Narrowish lapels and broader shoulders make the most of that new physique. Pants should be well-fitting and clean-lined, with straight legs (a very slight flare at most—no elephants or baggies, please).

8. If you have "love handles" on the side, stick with loose-fitting tops (polo shirts or loose sweater tops that go comfortably over pants). Keep your coat and/or vest on, unbuttoned or partially buttoned if it's still tight. Stay away from the tight belts and pick loosely fitting blazer-style jackets. Some of the "unconstructed" jackets and shirt-jackets are super. Skip the body shirts and tight-fitting silks until you have a waist like John Travolta's.

9. To make shoulders look broader, try fitted polo shirts, lightly padded shoulders, tank tops, or tee shirts if you're well on your way to achieving that coveted bodybuilder's look. If you've got it—or are getting it—flaunt it!

10. If you still look a little too much like your skinny kid brother, fake the size and bulk with contrasting colors, texture (corduroy, shearling, suede, leather, heavy knits, and tweeds), lighter colors, layers of clothing (a fisherman's knit sweater over a pullover topped with a heavy jacket). Skip the tight polos, Lacoste shirts, tanks, and tee shirts until you've built up some muscle in those skinny arms.

Now, let's say that you've just emerged from a lifetime as the neighborhood fat or skinny or shapeless boy. All of a sudden, you're sleek, svelte, and moderately good-looking. For the first time in your life, you're able to buy "normal" clothes. If you're starting from scratch, or close to it, try these basics to get you through the first months with the "new you":

Three or four cotton or cotton-blend shirts(pale solids, including blue and white; pinstripes, chalk stripes, tiny checks).

One navy blue or gray flannel three-piece suit (can be pinstriped or solid).

Three or four ties (solids, foulards, reps, diagonal stripes in silk or silk blends).

A navy blue blazer.

Three pairs of sport slacks: gray flannel, camel flannel, tan corduroy.

Two pairs of jeans for casual wear.

Two or three polo shirts for casual wear.

Plain slip-on loafers, dress shoes, and boots for rain or winter.

A trenchcoat, overcoat, or lined raincoat in beige, dark blue, or navy.

ACCESSORIES:

A watch in plain gold or silver (or stainless steel) with a plain metal or leather band.

Cuff links.

Two or three good leather belts with plain gold or silver buckles. A good leather wallet, an attaché case or briefcase, and an appointment book.

A simple dark umbrella.

A gold or silver pen.

No matter how impeccable your clothing, hair, nails, and skin, you'll also want to pay attention to other details. Make sure, in addition to your daily shower and shampoo and shave, that you de-lint or de-fuzz your clothes and air them thoroughly before they're hung up again, polish shoes (and if necessary, your other leather accessories), and keep your dry cleaning up to date. If your bodystyle changes have outstripped your clothing, go ahead and spend the money on alterations to make sure your clothes fit the body you *now* have. Have that vest tapered, take in the waistline on your favorite slacks, make sure your new blazer conforms perfectly to the extra two inches you've added to your shoulders. It costs, of course, but it's well worth the extra money. And don't forget, while you're at it, to have shoes resoled or reheeled, briefcase and watch straps repaired, and all leather goods thoroughly cleaned. All little touches, but important to the spiffy image you're building for yourself.

So much for the right upholstery. Now let's make sure you're getting the right fuels for high performance. First, remember some facts you learned early on in the section on diet. The big problem for most people is not *taking* it off but *keeping* it off. Nearly any diet that lowers caloric intake will take off ten to fifteen pounds if you stick to it for a minimum of two weeks. There's nothing hard or mysterious about it. But then what happens?

The May 30, 1979, *New York* magazine gives us an alarming statistic: we as a nation spend over $10 billion a year trying to lose weight, but 95 percent of those who do lose gain it all back—usually with interest. And that's within a six-month to one-year period! (Obesity in this respect is a little like cancer: the longer you can go without a recurrence, the more likely you are to be permanently "cured.") The tragedy is that most people seem physically or psychologically unable to maintain their new svelte selves. If you can keep it off for six months, the body gets "reprogrammed" for the new lighter weight and things get easier all around—if, and only if, you're willing to pay the price of eternal vigilance. So here are some tips and ideas to keep you putting the right stuff into that newly streamlined body of yours:

1. Learn to think of yourself not as "naturally thin" but as "artificially thin." Don't think of yourself as "fat"—that's destructive behavior—but don't be misled by appearances either. Just because you *look* thin now doesn't mean you'll always *be* thin. The same foods and bad eating habits that led to the overweight in the first place can lead you right back along the same path. Try to overcome the cycle by staying on a balanced but fairly strict diet.
2. Keep a strict watch on your weight by weighing yourself every morning. Then the instant the unwanted pounds come back, you can take them off. Remember that "new" fat (which is largely water) is often easier to lose than "old" fat, which is often real, honest-to-goodness solid *fat*. The easiest way to take off weight is to lose it at once. Learn to compensate for a binge or a celebration—a party, holiday, or vacation—as soon as it's over. It's almost impossible to gain more than two or three pounds of real fat in a short period of time. If you show a five-pound gain on the scales over a weekend, rest assured that at least half is fluid plus the weight of the food itself. But take it off anyway; take it *all* off, and right away. Go back on your original strict diet for five days, a week, or whatever it takes to lose the excess baggage. Then resume your maintenance routine.
3. Set limits for yourself. Give yourself a range of three-to five pounds, but no more, beyond which you simply won't go. Let's say your bottom weight is 165. That's the weight at which you feel most comfortable, look best, fit into your clothes nicely, and have plenty of energy. Below that weight you look haggard and feel weak; above that, you're pudgy and bloated. Your aim, then, should be to stay as close to that weight as possible. If you're sick with flu, you can drop a pound or two but no more. If you go on vacation and overeat some delicious Polynesian (Greek, Italian, Mexican, French) food, you may go three pounds over. But no more! Set a top range for yourself and stick to it. Make sure the range is realistic and then allow yourself to deviate as little as possible. It's better for your skin, your

muscle tone, your health, and your overall condition if your weight changes as little as is humanly possible. Plus: establishing such strict limits gives you a feeling of being constantly in control, and control spells power. We like to feel powerful in this way because it means that we, not the food or the party or the vacation or our friends, but *we* are in control. Remember that just because the food is there doesn't mean you have to eat it. In fact, knowing that you can occasionally allow yourself a small wedge of pastry, a taste of sauce, a hot slice of bread, a quarter of a pizza, means you're less likely to feel the mad impulse to stuff yourself with junk food. You have the choice and so you choose not to eat just at that time—especially if it's inferior food anyway. Barbara Edelstein tells women, "If you're going to cheat, make sure it's gourmet." The same goes for men—and 90 percent of the time, you'll be safe.

4. Occasionally you'll backslide and need more than a simple cutback in calories to start losing those pounds once again. What you really need is Men's Week at the Golden Door or the Ashram, right? But who has the bucks or the time for these fancy resorts? Not you—but you might just try recreating one of their weekends with your lady at home or making use of the local spa, gym, or resort. Try this for a schedule. Start the day early with a brisk walk, jog, or run, followed by a weigh-in, sauna, and shower. Next is breakfast (low-cal, of course), followed by your stretching and limbering exercises and a good workout with the weights. Have a midmorning break for a shower or steam bath and some fresh juice or mineral water. For relaxation before lunch, swim or do water exercises and try a massage (she does you; you do her). Whip up a low-calorie lunch (a big do-it-yourself salad bar is ideal), and then take another walk, jog, or run. Another juice break, more stretching exercises, another shower, and you're ready for vegetable-juice "cocktails" and a low-calorie dinner. Spend the evening quietly listening to records or tapes and sipping Perrier-on-the-rocks in frosted glasses. Try this routine for two days and see if you're not pounds lighter and much more refreshed and relaxed than after the usual weekend nibbling, noshing, sipping, and sitting.

5. As for the maintenance diet: there's no simple magic formula, as you might guess. Your body's chemistry is unique and complex, and therefore much of the program will have to come from trial and error. But here are some general marks of a good diet to help you maintain what you have and continue to make gains and refinements in the future:

   A. The diet provides an adequate number of calories to keep your body in top running condition—that is, it allows for adequate energy for work, recreation, workouts, and emergencies.

B. It allows adequate water, carbohydrates, fat, protein, minerals, and vitamins for your bodily processes to continue in top form.

C. It provides a minimum of six glasses of fluid a day (there's no maximum: adults can tolerate up to eighty glasses a day if they have normal kidneys).

D. It provides adequate carbohydrates, particularly of the long-chain variety: whole grains, potatoes, pastas, vegetables, and fruits. Skip the refined carbohydrates, but include at least some of the foods listed above in your daily diet, even if you're working for high definition.

E. It contains adequate fat to provide resting muscle energy and energy for late spurts in endurance sports or exercises after the muscles are already depleted of glycogen. Stick with low-fat products such as mozzarella, hoop, and farmer cheeses; low-fat yogurt; skim milk; safflower and wheat-germ oil; lean beef; fish and fowl; avocados, and nuts.

F. It contains adequate protein to rebuild body tissues and provide the eight essential amino acids. It's important to take in enough protein, but don't fall for the myth that you "can't eat too much protein." Excess protein, like excess anything, is stored as fat. You'll need one gram of protein daily for each two pounds of body weight if you are on a moderate program like the one described in this book; one per pound if you're on a superheavy regimen. Then, and *only* then, should you be eating eight eggs and two pounds of hamburger for breakfast. Six small balanced meals are better for the moderate exerciser.

G. It contains adequate minerals (the basic chemicals found in the soil, important to proper heartbeat, muscle contraction, water levels in the body, and conduction of nerve impulses). The major minerals you need are sodium, potassium, magnesium, and calcium. In addition, you need trace amounts of such minerals as chromium, copper, iodine, iron, nickel, tin, and zinc. Ordinarily a balanced diet supplies these, but check your multivitamin pill for added minerals if you're on a restricted diet for any length of time.

H. It provides adequate amounts of vitamins A, B-complex, C, D, E, and K. Again, a balanced diet supplies most of these, but deficiencies can be covered with good multivitamins. The B group is the source of deficiency for most dieters, but some plain toasted wheat germ, plain bran flakes, and brewer's yeast will prevent B deficiencies without adding more than 100 calories total to your daily intake.

I. It is low in cholesterol, salt, refined sugar and flour, junk and processed foods, and anything containing saturated fats. These are the real killers in terms of cardiovascular disease and obesity—they add pounds and inches without adding much of nutritional value.

One final note on all this. There's a myth abroad in the land that it is inordinately expensive to eat well, get adequate diet supplements, and stay in top shape. Not so. Most of our food dollars go for processed, frozen, canned (translate: sweetened or syrup-packed or oversalted) "junk" and "convenience" foods. Gloria Swanson and William Duffy, authors of *Sugar Blues,* said in a 1976 interview in Chicago that their average weekly food bill for all their specially prepared organic and natural fare was several dollars less than that of the average New York family on welfare! True, protein costs, and so does fresh produce, and so do supplements. But take away the potato chips and nachos and dips and cookies and ice cream and Twinkies, and the figures suddenly become impressively less. Vitamins last forever; so does a large can of brewer's yeast or protein powder and a jar of plain wheat germ. And who ever *finishes* a box of plain bran flakes?

The point of all this is simply that you *can* maintain your high-performance condition with a minimum of running costs. A full 110-pound set of weights can cost as little as $29.95. An average health club or gym membership can run as low as $21 a month. At those prices, who can afford *not* to be healthy?

And now, good-bye and good luck with your new bodystyle! We've enjoyed helping you shape it, trim it, sculpt and slim and build it. We've told you what to eat, what supplements to take, how to get your lady to join you, how to build a program, and how to create a maintenance routine. We hope you're "hooked" by now and will keep on the new program for years to come. After all, you can't trade yourself in for a new model next year. But then, with the terrific shape you're in, who would want to?